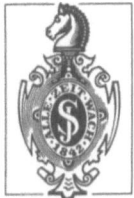

International Boehringer Mannheim Symposia

Cardiac Glycosides

Edited by

G. Bodem and H. J. Dengler

With 125 Figures and 70 Tables

Springer-Verlag Berlin Heidelberg GmbH 1978

International Symposium, Bonn, Germany, January 27–29, 1977

Priv.-Doz. Dr. med. Günter Bodem
Prof. Dr. med. Hans J. Dengler
Medizinische Universitäts-Klinik, D-5300 Bonn-Venusberg

ISBN 978-3-540-08692-5   ISBN 978-3-642-66904-0 (eBook)
DOI 10.1007/978-3-642-66904-0

Library of Congress Cataloging in Publication Data. Main entry under title: Cardiac glycosides. (International Boehringer Mannheim symposia) "International symposium, Bonn, Germany, January 27-29, 1977." Includes bibliographical references and index. 1. Cardiac glycosides-Congresses. I. Bodem, G., 1939-II. Dengler, Hans J. III. Series. RM349.C37   615'.711   78-2501.

Table of Contents

1   Evaluation of Different Methods for Determining Serum Concentrations
of Cardiac Glycosides

(V.P. Butler, Jr.) 1

2   A New Simple Assay for Determining Digoxin Serum Levels

(K. Stellner) 22

3   Chloroform-Extractable and Polar Metabolites Examined With Different
Assays

(U. Gundert-Remy, K. Koch, and V. Hrstka) 28

4   Studies of the Metabolism of Digoxin and Digitoxin Using Double
Isotope Dilution Derivative Methods

(D.S. Lukas) 36

5   Occurence and Chemical Nature of Polar Water-Soluble Digoxin
Metabolites

(H.F. Benthe) 52

6   Pharmacokinetics and Metabolism of Digitoxin in the Human

(H.F. Vöhringer and N. Rietbrock) 64

7   Dihydrodigitoxin, a Metabolite of Digitoxin in Humans

(G. Bodem and E.v. Unruh) 74

8   Enterohepatic Circulation of Digitoxin Metabolites in the Dog
(G. Ch. Oliver, L.A. Santini, G. Griffin, and R. Ruffy)   85

9   β-Methyl-Digoxin, a New Lipophilic Digoxin Derivative
(W. Schaumann)   93

10   Tissue Distribution of Cardiac Glycosides
(J. Kuhlmann, N. Rietbrock, and B. Schnieders) 109

11   Plasma-Tissue Distribution of Different Cardiac Glycosides
(D. Larbig and R. Haasis) 126

12   Significance of Plasma Concentration of Digoxin in Relation
to the Myocardial Concentration of the Drug
(J. Coltart) 135

13   Influence of Thyroid Function on the Pharmacokinetics of Cardiac
Glycosides
(H.J. Gilfrich and T. Meinertz) 159

14   Effect of Jejunoileal Bypass on the Bioavailability of Digoxin in Man
(F.I. Marcus, D. Perrier, and M. Mayersohn) 167

15   Bioavailability of Digoxin in Renal Insufficiency and Heart Failure
(E.E. Ohnhaus) 181

16   Bioavailability Studies: Their Influence on the Clinical Use of Digitalis
(T.R.D. Shaw) 187

17   Comparative Pharmacokinetics of Various Digoxin Preparations in Man
(P.F. Binnion) 199

18   Digoxin Pharmacokinetics and Their Relation to Clinical Dosage Parameters

(H.J. Dengler, G. Bodem, and H.J. Gilfrich) 211

19   Clinical Interpretation of Serum Concentrations of Cardiac Glycosides

(T.W. Smith, L.H. Green, and G.D. Curfman) 226

20   Assessment of Digoxin Action by a Pharmacodynamic Biochemical Method

(D.G. Grahame-Smith and J.K. Aronson) 242

21   Relationships Between Doses, Plasma Levels and Cardiac Effects Under Digitalis Treatment

(G.G. Belz and R. Erbel) 254

22.1 Therapeutic Implications of Digoxin Kinetics in Impaired Renal Function

(W.J. Jusko) 265

22.2 Peak Plasma Digoxin Concentration and Cardiotoxicity

(B.F. Johnson, D.J. Chapple, R. Hughes, J. LaBrooy, and I. Smith) . 273

22.3 Biliary Excretion of β-Acetyl-Digoxin in Man

(U. Klotz) 284

23   Digitoxin Pharmacokinetics in Patients With Renal Disease

(L. Storstein) 292

24   Increased Digitalis Tolerance in Uremic Patients

(P. Kramer, E. Stroh, D. Matthei, F. Teiwes, and F. Scheler) 304

25   Digitoxin and Digoxin in Patients With Chronic Renal Failure and on Hemodialysis

(B. Grabensee, U. Peters, T. Risler, and F. Grosse-Brockhoff) 317

26 International Patterns of Clinical Use and Toxicity of Digitalis Glycosides: Report From the Boston Collaborative Drug Surveillance Program

(D.J. Greenblatt). 326

27 Pharmacokinetic and Clinical Effects During the Predistribution Phase of Digoxin Treatment

(P. Reissell, V. Manninen, and O. Lokki). 335

28 Digitalis Intoxication: Clinical and Experimental Work

(P.F. Binnion). 346

29 Digitalis Intoxication: Specificity of Clinical and Electrocardiographic Signs

(W. Doering and E. König) 358

30 Treatment of Digitalis Intoxication

(H. Jahrmärker) 367

31 Biologic Effects of Specific Antibodies in Reversing the Pharmacologic and Toxic Effects of Digoxin

(V.P. Butler, Jr., T.W. Smith, D.H. Schmidt, and E. Haber) 374

32 Reversal of Digitoxin Toxicity and Modification of Pharmacokinetics by Specific Antibodies

(H.R. Ochs and T.W. Smith) 384

33 β-Methyl-Digoxin Disposition During Spironolactone Treatment

(U. Abshagen). 392

34 Digitoxin Disposition Under Rifampicin Treatment

(U. Peters, T.U. Hausamen, and F. Grosse-Brockhoff). 401

35 Is There a Need for New Cardiac Glycosides? For More Blood Level
    Determinations?
    (G. Kaufmann) 410

    Subject Index 423

List of Contributors

U. Abshagen
Medizinische Klinik und Poliklinik, Klinikum Steglitz, Hindenburgdamm 30,
D-1000 Berlin 45

G.G. Belz
Flößergasse 6, D-5400 Koblenz-Kesselheim

H.F. Benthe
Pharmakologisches Institut, Universitäts-Krankenhaus, Martinistraße 52,
D-2000 Hamburg 20

P.F. Binnion
201 S. 18th Street, Philadelphia, PA 19103/USA

G. Bodem
Medizinische Universitäts-Klinik, D-5300 Bonn-Venusberg

V.P. Butler
Department of Medicine, Columbia University of Physicians & Surgeons,
630 West 168th Street, New York, NY 10032/USA

J. Coltart
St. Thomas' Hospital, London, S.E. 1., England

H.J. Dengler
Medizinische Universitäts-Klinik D-5300 Bonn-Venusberg

W. Doering
II. Medizinische Abteilung, Städtisches Krankenhaus, München-Schwabing,
Kölner Platz 1, D-8000 München 40

H.J. Gilfrich
II. Medizinische Klinik und Poliklinik der Universität Langenbeckstraße 1,
D-6500 Mainz

B. Grabensee
I. Medizinische Klinik A der Universität, Moorenstraße 5,
D-4000 Düsseldorf 1

G. Grahame-Smith
MRC Unit University Department of Clinical Pharmacology,
Radcliffe Infirmary, Oxford OX2 6HE, England

D.J. Greenblatt
Clinical Pharmacology Unit, Massachusetts General Hospital,
Boston, MA 02114/USA

U. Gundert-Remy
Medizinische Universitäts-Klinik, Abteilung für Klinische Pharmakologie,
Bergheimerstraße 58, D-6900 Heidelberg

H. Jahrmärker
Medizinische Klinik Innenstadt, Universität München,
Ziemssenstraße 1, D-8000 München 2

B.F. Johnson
Burroughs Wellcome Co., 3030 Cornwallis Road, Research Triangle Park, N.C.
27709, London, England

W.J. Jusko
Clinical Pharmacokinetics Laboratory, Millard Fillmore Hospital,
3 Gates Circle, Buffalo, NY 14209/USA

G. Kaufmann
Ärztehaus Sonnenberg, Freiestraße 211, CH-8032 Zürich

U. Klotz
Dr. Margarete Fischer-Bosch-Institut für Klinische Pharmakologie, Robert-Bosch-
Krankenhaus, D-7000 Stuttgart

P. Kramer
Medizinische Klinik und Poliklinik Humboldtallee 1, D-3400 Göttingen

H.J. Kuhlmann
Institut für Klinische Pharmakologie, Klinikum Steglitz Hindenburgdamm 30,
D-1000 Berlin 45

D. Larbig
Innere Medizin III, Medizinische Universitäts-Klinik, Otfried-Müller-Straße,
D-7400 Tübingen

D.S. Lukas
New York Hospital, Cancer Center 1275 York Avenue, NY 10021/USA

F.I. Marcus
Department of Internal Medicine, College of Medicine University of Arizona,
Tuscon, AZ 85724/USA

H.R. Ochs
Medizinische Universitäts-Klinik, D-5300 Bonn-Venusberg

E.E. Ohnhaus
Inselhospital Bern, Medizinische Klinik Freiburgstraße, CH-3010 Bern

G.Ch. Oliver
Cardiology Division, Jewish Hospital 216 South Kingshighway, St. Louis.
MS 63110/USA

U. Peters
I. Medizinische Klinik A der Universität, Moorenstraße 5, D-4000 Düsseldorf

P. Reissell
Kivelä Hospital, Helsinki-26, First Department of Medicine, University of
Helsinki, Helsinki-29 and Technical University, Espoo, Finland

W. Schaumann
Boehringer Mannheim, Medizinische Forschung
Sandhoferstraße 116, D-6800 Mannheim 31

T.R.D. Shaw
Department of Cardiology, Western General Hospital, Edinburgh, EH4 2XU,
Scotland

T.W. Smith
721 Huntingdon Avenue, Boston, MA 02115/USA

K. Stellner
Boehringer Mannheim, Biochemica Werk Tutzing, D-8132 Tutzing

L. Storstein
Medical Department B, University Clinic, Rikshospitalet, Oslo, Norway

H.F. Vöhringer
Institut für Klinische Pharmakologie im Klinikum Steglitz der Freien Universität
Berlin, Hindenburgdamm 30, D-1000 Berlin 45

Introduction

In spite of old vintage and 200 years of clinical use, digitalis remains an interesting therapeutic agent, to clinicians as well as to the pharmacologist, the biochemist, and colleagues in other diciplines of theoretic medicine.

When a drug, however, has so many attractive facets, it seems proper and advisable for the success of a scientific meeting to focus on a number of well-defined aspects.

This symposium was devoted to pharmacokinetics, drug metabolism, analytic procedures, blood level determinations, and their interpretation both for therapeutic and toxic situations. Considerable progress has been made during the last years in this area of digitalis research. The time was suitable for a critical reappraisal of facts and theories and for future planning. Our main intention was to relate analytic data and biochemical findings to clinical problems and questions. Despite the undoubtedly basic character of clinical pharmacology, it is nevertheless an applied science which should help to develop the rational basis of therapeutics.

We are particularly grateful to the active participants who bore the burden of preparing presentations and — even worse — manuscripts. At the same time we are well-aware that many other active research groups would have been able to contribute in this way, but our program was limited because of the short time available. Their knowledge is included in the discussion parts of the meeting, so we hope a well-balanced description of the present state of affairs emerged in this volume.

Finally, we would like to express our gratitude to Boehringer Mannheim and their representatives who sponsored this meeting and were of great help as regards the organization.

The editors also acknowledge the secretarial work and assistance as a translator of Mrs. Ines Nandi.

G. Bodem and H.J. Dengler
Medizinische Universitäts-Klinik
Bonn-Venusberg

1 Evaluation of Different Methods for Determining Serum Concentrations of Cardiac Glycosides[1]

V. P. BUTLER, JR.[2]

Two centuries have passed since Withering first reported that digitalis "has a power over the motion of the heart, to a degree yet unobserved in any other medicine" (Withering, 1937). Although digitalis glycosides are now widely used in the therapy of congestive heart failure, the dosage of digitalis preparations must, as in Withering's day, be carefully adjusted to the needs of each individual patient in order that an optimal therapeutic effect may be achieved without the development of toxic side-effects because, as Withering noted, excessive digitalis "occasions sickness, vomiting. purging, giddiness, confused vision, objects appearing green or yellow . . . slow pulse . . . cold sweats, convulsions, syncope, death" (Withering, 1937). Developments in the first 6 decades of this century which have enhanced the physician's ability to adjust digitalis dosages to the specific needs of individual patients have included: the isolation of highly purified cardenolides, the recognition of the effects of digitalis on the electrocardiogram, a better definition of the effects of cardiac glycosides on myocardial contractility, conduction, and automaticity, and an appreciation of the role of electrolyte disturbances in facilitating the development of digitalis toxicity (Butler, 1972).

In the 1950s and 1960s, the use of radioactively labeled digitalis preparations made possible, for the first time, the direct measurement of cardiac glycosides and their metabolites in the blood, urine, and tissues of man and of experimental animals, thereby providing great insight into the pharmacokinetics of digitalis preparations (Okita et al., 1953; Doherty et al., 1961; Marcus et al., 1964; Marks et al., 1964; Doherty and Perkins, 1966; Doherty et al., 1967; Doherty, 1968; Ewy et al., 1969). Studies with tritiated digoxin, in particular, provided evidence that this drug is metabolized at a relatively slow rate and that its disappearance from the body is dependent, in large part, on its renal excretion (Doherty, 1968). These studies also provided evidence that there is a relationship between the serum level of this glycoside and its concentration in the myocardium and other tissues. (Doherty and Perkins, 1966; Doherty et al., 1967). Doherty et al. found myocardium-to-serum concentration ratios from 17:1 to 35:1 (mean 29:1) in man (Doherty, 1968) and pointed out that the relative constancy of these ratios in the

---

1 This work has been supported by research grants from the United States Public Health Service (HL 10608) and from the New York Heart Association.
2 Recipient of an Irma T. Hirschl Career Scientist Award.

face of large differences in total body digoxin stores "indicates that the serum-digoxin level is related to the cardiac-muscle digoxin level and that a serum digoxin determination . . . should be of definite value in clinical assessment of digoxin cardiac content" (Doherty et al., 1967). Under ordinary conditions, less than 1% of the total body digoxin is present in the vascular compartment (Doherty, 1968), and serum concentrations of digoxin and other cardiac glycosides are so low that it was not possible, until recently, to measure these concentrations. In the past decade, however, several new techniques (Table 1.1.) have been developed for the determination of serum or plasma concentrations of cardiac glycosides. As Doherty had predicted (Doherty et al., 1967; Doherty, 1968), these methods all have proved to be cf great value to the physician in determining the dosage of digitalis to be administered to patients requiring this drug (Butler, 1972; Smith and Haber, 1970; Butler, 1970; Smith, 1972; Bodem and Gilfrich, 1973; Duhme et al., 1974; Butler and Lindenbaum, 1975; Smith, 1975; Grosse-Brockhoff and Hausamen, 1975; Huffman et al., 1976). It is the purpose of this review to compare these methods for determining serum digitalis concentrations with special reference to their specificity, rapidity, and suitability for routine clinical use.

Immunoassay

Cardiac glycosides are relatively small molecules with molecular weights in the 500-1000 range and are too small to be immunogenic by themselves. To obtain antibodies to cardiac glycosides, it is necessary to conjugate these pharmacologic agents as haptens to antigenic protein carriers (Butler and Beiser, 1973; Beiser et al., 1976). For this purpose, periodate-oxidized glycosides have been coupled to albumin carriers by the method of Erlanger and Beiser to form synthetic glycoside-

Table 1.1. Digitalis Assay Methods

Biochemical methods
    Immunoassay
        Radioimmunoassay
        Enzyme immunoassay
    Competitive protein binding assay
        Enzymatic isotope displacement assay
    Inhibition of red Cell ^{86}Rb Uptake
    Inhibition of $(Na^+ + K^+)$-ATPase

Chromatographic Methods
    Double isotope dilution derivative assay
    Gas chromatography
    (High pressure liquid chromatography)

---

protein conjugates as shown in step 1 of Figure 1.1. (Butler and Chen, 1967); alternatively, the 3-0-succinyl derivative of digitoxigenin, the digitoxose-lacking cardioactive aglycone derived from digitoxin, has been conjugated to albumin carriers by the carbodiimide and mixed anhydride methods (Oliver et al., 1968). Rabbits immunized with these conjugates form antibodies to the albumin carriers, but more importantly, they also form antibodies capable of binding digoxin in the first instance (Fig. 1.1, step 2) and of binding digitoxin in the latter case. Antidigoxin antibodies from selected antisera possess a high affinity and great specificity for digoxin. For example, certain digoxin-specific antibodies have been shown to bind digoxin at least 20 times more effectively than they bind digitoxin or dihydrodigoxin, a digoxin metabolite (Butler and Chen, 1967; Smith et al., 1970; Butler et al., 1974), although digoxin differs structurally only slightly from these two closely related compounds (Fig. 1.2.).

The radioimmunoassay procedure is based on methods developed by Berson and Yalow for the assay of insulin and other peptide hormones (Yalow and Berson,

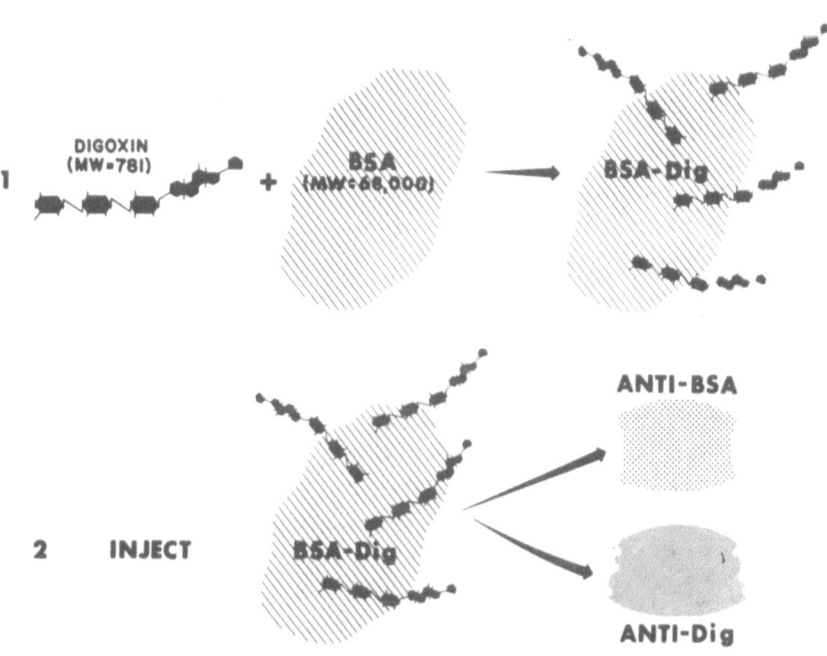

Fig. 1.1. Production of antibodies to digoxin. (Withering, 1937). Digoxin (Dig) is chemically conjugated as a hapten to a protein carrier such as bovine serum albumin (BSA) by the periodate oxidation method. (Butler, 1972). Rabbits immunized with BSA digoxin conjugates form antibodies that bind, but do not precipitate with, digoxin. The bivalent antidigoxin molecule shown here is capable of binding one digoxin molecule at each of its two binding sites. Animals form antibodies to the protein carrier, BSA, but such antibodies have no effect on most immunoassay systems. (Reproduced with permission from the New England Journal of Medicine (Butler, 1970)

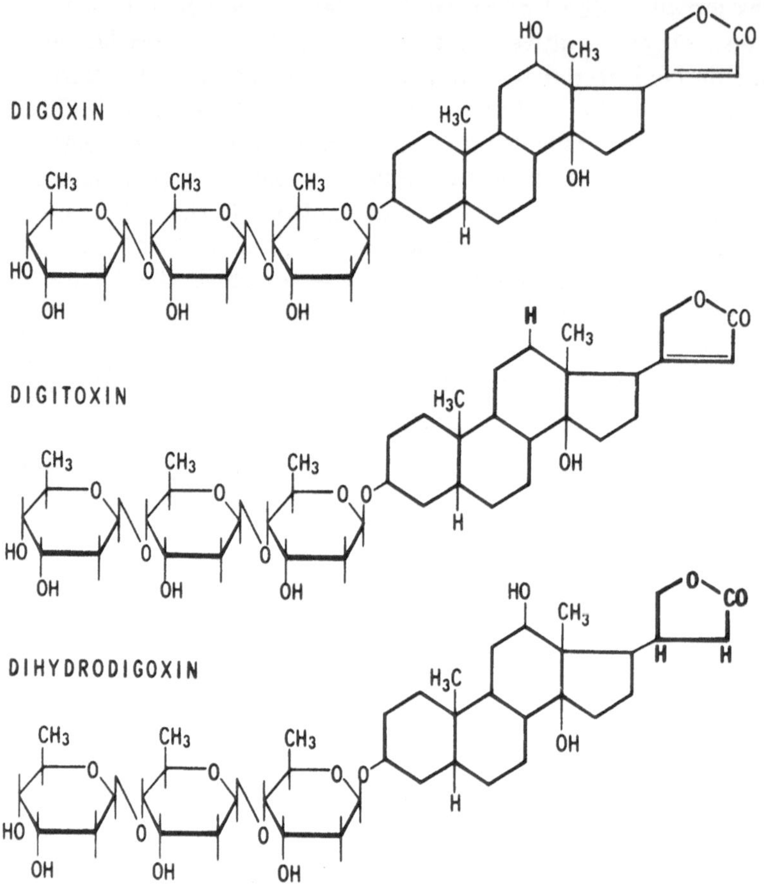

Fig. 1.2. Structural formulas of digoxin, digitoxin, and dihydrodigoxin. All three glycosides consist of aglycones (steroidal portion and lactone ring) shown at right and glycosidic portions (consisting of three digitoxose sugar molecules) shown at left. Digitoxin differs from digoxin only in that it lacks the hydroxyl group at the C-12 position in the aglycone portion of the molecule. Dihydrodigoxin differs from digoxin only in that its lactone ring is saturated (Reproduced with permission from the Annals of the New York Academy of Sciences (Butler et al., 1974)

1964; Berson and Yalow, 1967). The underlying principle is that nonradioactive glycoside (in known standard solutions or in patients sera) will compete with radioactively labeled glycoside for combining sites on antidigitalis antibody. If one mixes varying quantities of unlabeled digitalis with a standard amount of radiolabeled glycoside, the amount of radioactivity bound by a standard amount of antibody will decrease as increasing amounts of unlabeled glycoside are added. A standard curve can then be constructed (Fig. 1.3) from which the concentration of digitalis in a given patient's serum can be determined on the basis of the decrease it causes in the binding of radioactive glycoside by specific antibody (Oliver et al., 1968; Smith et al., 1969).

4

A large number of radioimmunoassay procedures has now been described, differing principally in the method by which antibody-bound labeled glycoside is physicochemically separated from unbound ("free") labeled glycoside. In the dextran-coated charcoal method (Herbert et al., 1965), sera to be tested and standard glycoside reference solutions are added to test tubes. Tritiated glycoside (Smith et al., 1969) or a radioiodinated digitalis derivative (Oliver et al., 1968) is then added. After mixing, a small volume of dilute antiserum is added, followed, after a brief incubation period, by the addition of a suspension of dextran-coated charcoal. Essentially all nonantibody-bound radioactivity is rapidly adsorbed by the charcoal. The charcoal and nonantibody-bound labeled glycoside are removed from suspension by centrifugation, and the supernatant solution, containing the antibody-bound radiolabeled digitalis, is removed and assayed for radioactivity (Smith et al., 1969; Smith, 1970). More recently described methods have employed antibodies coupled to a solid matrix or support; in these solid-phase methods, the unbound radiolabeled digitalis remains in solution and is measured as an indicator of the extent of antibody-binding in each tube (Line et al., 1973). Radioimmunoassay methods have been described to date for several cardiac glycosides and related compounds, including digoxin (Smith et al., 1969), digitoxin (Oliver et al., 1968; Smith, 1970), ouabain (Selden and Smith, 1972), gitoxin (Lesne, 1972), gitaloxin (Lesne, 1972), proscillaridin (Belz et al., 1973), acetyl strophanthidin (Selden et al., 1973), and β-methyl-digoxin (Härtel et al., 1973; Haasis et al., 1975).

Because the immunoassay procedures reported to date have employed antisera with specificity for the aglycone portion (Fig. 1.2) of the digitalis molecule (Butler and Chen, 1967; Oliver et al., 1968; Smith et al., 1970), metabolic breakdown products of cardiac glycosides containing the intact aglycone (e.g., digoxigenin and its mono- and bisdigitoxosides (Doherty, 1968) will react significantly in these procedures. Metabolites in which the aglycone has been altered may also react but to a lesser extent. Because these closely related compounds react in digitalis immunoassay procedures (Smith et al., 1970), the term "immunoreactive" might be more accurate in describing results. The fact that immunoassay methods will detect metabolites of cardiac glycosides constitutes a theoretic disadvantage, but in practice, serum immunoreactive digoxin and digitoxin concentrations have correlated well with values obtained by other methods and with the clinical state of the patients studied. In the case of digoxin, this correlation may reflect the findings that very little of this glycoside is metabolized in man (Doherty, 1968) and that most of its known metabolites (digoxigenin and its mono- and bisdigitoxosides) are both cardioactive and immunoreactive (Butler, 1972). In the case of digitoxin, metabolic degradation is more extensive (Doherty, 1968), and the contribution of inactive metabolites to the serum concentration of immunoreactive digitoxin is not yet clear (Oliver et al., 1968). Although this has not been a major limitation in a practical sense, the precise role of metabolites in radioimmunoassay procedures has not yet been clearly delineated.

Although the antibodies in most antidigitalis sera are directed largely toward the aglycone portion of the digitalis molecule, all antisera to cardiac glycosides that have been characterized cross-react to some extent with other glycosides and aglycones (Butler and Chen, 1967; Oliver et al., 1968; Smith et al., 1970). This cross-reactivity may create a problem if it is not known with certainty which glycoside a patient is receiving. For example, because serum digitoxin concentrations are generally ten times as great as serum digoxin concentrations, serum from a digitoxin-treated patient will give a substantial but potentially dangerous and misleading value if subjected to a digoxin assay procedure. Results in digitalis radioimmunoassays are meaningful only if it is known with certainty that the patient is receiving the corresponding glycoside and not a related preparation (Butler, 1972).

A weak cross-reactivity of antidigoxin antibodies with certain steroid hormones has been directly demonstrated (Butler and Chen, 1967), but there is no evidence that any steroid hormone of man will interfere, at clinically encountered concentrations, with the binding of radioactive digoxin (Smith et. al., 1969) or digitoxin (Oliver et al., 1968; Smith, 1970) by their corresponding antibodies in the assay systems currently in clinical use, and serum from subjects who have not received digitalis therapy has had no effect on these assay systems. It is well-known by immunologists that different antisera (even those obtained from a single animal on different occasions) may vary greatly in their specificity (Smith et al., 1970). Before a given antidigitalis antiserum is introduced into routine use, it is essential that it be demonstrated that its binding of radiolabeled digitalis is not inhibited by high concentrations of steroid hormones or by serum from individuals not receiving digitalis therapy (Butler, 1972; Oliver et al., 1968; Smith et al., 1969; Smith, 1970).

Antidigoxin sera vary not only in their specificity for digoxin but also in their affinity for the glycoside (Smith et al., 1970). It is now well-recognized that, in some instances, the dissociation rate of digoxin-antibody complexes is sufficiently great to cause a temporally related variability in results as dissociated digoxin is progressively adsorbed to charcoal as a function of variations in the duration of the charcoal incubation step in the dextran-coated charcoal immunoassay procedure (Meade and Kleist, 1972; Smith and Haber, 1973; Smith and Skubitz, 1975). Thus, it is important to assess the effect of slight variations in the duration of the charcoal incubation step on the binding of glycoside by antibody before a given antiserum is selected for use in a dextran-coated charcoal immunoassay procedure.

The presence of a radioisotope in a patient's serum is a potential source of error in the radioimmunoassay method, particularly since many of the patients in whom serum digitalis determinations are requested have complicated medical problems requiring the diagnostic administration of radioisotopes, but the digitalis concentration can be accurately determined if appropriate control tubes are included in the assay procedure (Butler, 1971). The possibility of reporting a spuriously low serum digitalis concentration is of course great when the presence of the isotope in the patient's serum is not suspected by the laboratory. Dual-channel liquid scintillation spectrometers can be adjusted to detect γ-emitting isotopes in specimens being assayed, but if a radioiodinated digitalis derivative is used in the assay procedure, a blank serum tube containing only serum should also

6

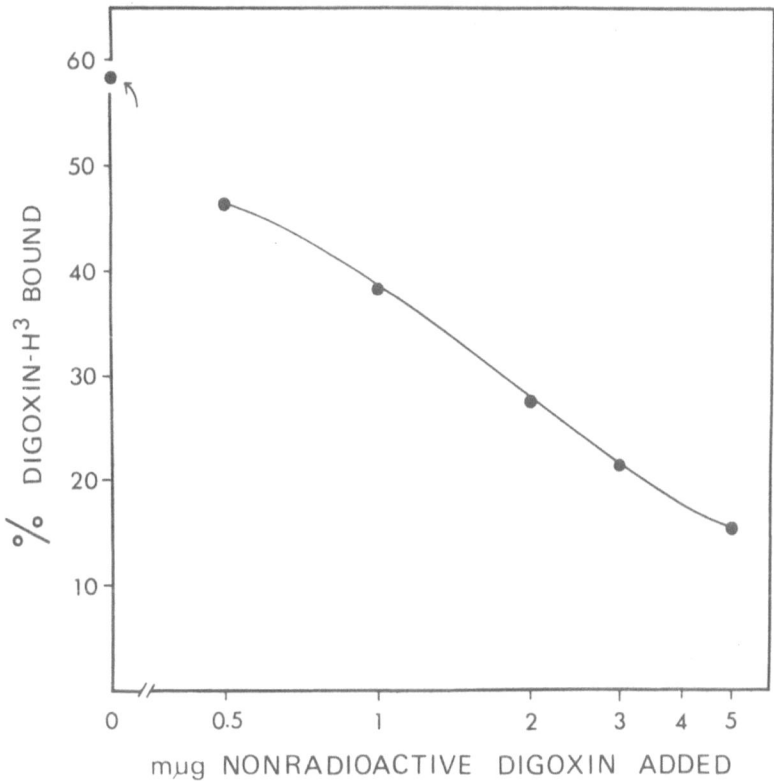

Fig. 1.3. Representative standard curve for digoxin radioimmunoassay. In the presence of increasing concentrations of nonradioactive digoxin (in known reference standard solutions), the percentage of digoxin-[3]H (3 ng) bound by a constant amount of antidigoxin antibody (50 μl of a 1:2500 dilution) decreases from 59% in the absence of unlabeled digoxin to 16% in the presence of 5 ng (mμg) of unlabeled digoxin. Under identical conditions, if a patient's serum reduces the binding of digoxin-^{3}H to 29%, this serum contains 2 ng digoxin per ml. (Reproduced with permission from the New England Journal of Medicine (Butler, 1970)

be counted to minimize the possibility of error from this source (Butler, 1971; 1972).

Another potential source of error in the radioimmunoassay method is the fact that certain sera (especially when obtained from uremic subjects) produce chemiluminescence for variable periods of time after addition to liquid scintillant. Such chemiluminescence subsides with time but for a few hours may falsely raise the counts observed in the scintillation spectrometer. If one does not have the time to ascertain that successive counting determinations are relatively constant, the inclusion of a control tube (without added ^{3}H-glycoside) in the assay procedure should suffice to detect the production of such chemiluminescence by test serum (Butler, 1971).

The use of radioactively labeled digitalis preparations in radioimmunoassay procedures constitutes an inconvenience, particularly in clinical chemistry laboratories. One approach to this problem has been the development of an enzyme immunoassay procedure for the measurement of serum digoxin concentrations. This method takes advantage of the fact that antibodies to digoxin inhibit the enzymic activity of a digoxin-glucose-6-phosphate-dehydrogenase conjugate; the concentrations of digoxin in test serum specimens can be determined by the extent to which these specimens reverse this inhibitory effect of antidigoxin antibodies (Rosenthal et al., 1976).

If antisera of proper specificity and high affinity are selected and if potential sources of error are kept in mind, digitalis immunoassay procedures represent the simplest and most convenient methods for the measurement of large numbers of serum or plasma digoxin concentrations. Small volumes of serum (0.1 ml or less) can be analyzed without any requirement for prior extraction. A large number of specimens can be analyzed within a few hours, and the procedure can readily be adapted to new semiautomated or totally automated immunoassay systems. Tritiated glycosides and radioiodinated digitalis derivatives of high specific activity are commercially available. Antisera may be readily prepared and characterized or, alternatively, they may be purchased commercially. If stored properly, antibodies are stable for many years, and 1 ml of a satisfactory antiserum may be employed in more than 100 000 determinations.

Competitive Protein Binding (Enzymic Isotope Displacement) Assay

The cell membrances of all mammalian cells thus far tested contain a digitalis-sensitive sodium-and potassium-dependent ATPase (Skou, 1965) capable of binding cardiac glycosides (Schwartz et al., 1968). Brooker and Jelliffe have prepared tissue homogenates rich in this ATPase from guinea pig brain and have shown that these homogenates are capable of binding radioactive ouabain (Brooker and Jelliffe, 1972). Nonradioactive digoxin, ouabain, and other cardiac glycosides will compete with tritiated ouabain for binding sites, and, as in the radioimmunoassay procedure, if varying quantities of unlabeled digitalis are mixed with a standard amount of ouabain-^{3}H, the amount of ^{3}H bound by a standard amount of $(Na^+ + K^+)$-ATPase will decrease as increasing amounts of unlabeled glycoside are added. A standard curve very similar to that used in the radioimmunoassay procedure (Fig. 1.3) can be constructed from which the concentration of glycoside in a test serum can be determined on the basis of the decrease it causes in the binding of ouabain-^{3}H by the enzyme preparation. (Brooker and Jelliffe, 1972).

In this method, 5 ml of serum are extracted with 30 ml of chloroform and the extract evaporated to dryness. The dried extract is redissolved in a mixture of toluene and Tris buffer, following which the toluene is discarded. Ouabain-^{3}H in buffer is then added, followed by a small volume of guinea pig brain homogenate. After 30-60 min of incubation, the suspension is centrifuged and the supernatant solution containing the nonenzyme-bound ouabain-^{3}H is poured into a counting vial containing liquid scintillation mixture and assayed for radio-activity in a scintillation spectrometer (Brooker and Jelliffe, 1972). This method has been used for the measurement of digoxin, digitoxin, and ouabain (Brooker and Jelliffe, 1972; Belz and Pflederer, 1975; Marcus et al., 1975).

Since cardioactive metabolites of cardiac glycosides also interact with $(Na^+ + K^+)$-ATPase, this assay method detects these metabolites, while noncardioactive metabolites are considerably less effective in displacing ouabain-[3] H (Belz and Pflederer, 1975; Marcus et al., 1975). The fact that this assay method, like immunoassay procedures, will detect cardioactive metabolites constitutes a theoretic disadvantage, but for reasons similar to those discussed above in the immunoassay section, this fact has not been a major disadvantage to date in a practical sense.

There are three significant practical limitations to this method: 1. A 5 ml specimen of the patient's serum is required. 2. A chloroform extraction of serum is necessary, following which the authors report 77% recovery of digoxin. Not only is this extraction somewhat inconvenient, but this step carries with it the hazard of variability in per cent recovery of digitalis inherent in all serum extraction procedures. This hazard has not been a problem to the originators of the method and no correction is made for losses in the extraction procedure. Conceivably this hazard could create problems if the method were employed on a large scale in a routine clinical chemistry laboratory. 3. New batches of ATPase, which may vary in their binding characteristics, must be prepared from time to time and characterized for use in the assay procedure. In all other respects this method appears to be as convenient as the radioimmunoassay procedure, and as with the radioimmunoassay, large numbers of specimens can be processed within a few hours. In one respect, the radioreceptor assay is more convenient that the radioimmunoassay procedures employing tritiated glycosides. Since an extract (rather than whole serum) is subjected to assay, the presence of radioisotopes in test serum, the production of chemiluminescence, and quenching (with the resultant necessity to determine counting efficiency and insert corrections) have not been problems with the radioreceptor assay.

Inhibition of Red Cell [86] Rb Uptake

It is well-known that extremely low concentrations of cardiac glycosides will inhibit the uptake of certain monovalent cations, notably potassium and rubidium by human red blood cells (RBC) in vitro (Skou, 1965; Shatzmann, 1953). Lowenstein and Corrill took advantage of this fact and developed an assay method in which the ability of cardiac glycosides to inhibit [86] Rb uptake was used as the basis for their quantification in plasma. In this method, glycoside is extracted from plasma with dichloromethane; after evaporation to dryness, the residue is dissolved in saline and washed RBC are added. After a period of equilibration, [86] RbCl is added; after an hour or more of incubation, the RBC are washed and their uptake of [86] Rb is determined. Glycoside concentration is determined by comparing [86] Rb uptake in extracts from patient's plasma with a standard curve obtained by plotting RBC [86] Rb uptake against concentration of the same glycoside in known reference standard plasma specimens simultaneously subjected to the same extraction and assay procedure (Lowenstein, 1965; Lowenstein and Corrill, 1966). This method has been applied to the study of plasma from patients receiving digoxin, digitoxin, and proscillaridin (Lowenstein, 1965; Lowenstein and Corrill, 1966; Bertler and Redfors, 1970; Belz et al., 1974a, b). As with the competitive protein binding assay method, cardioactive metabolites interact with $(Na^+ + K^+)$-ATPase and inhibit ^{86}Rb uptake (Kaufman and Belpaire, 1973).

Inhibition of cation transport, as employed in this method, represents a biologic rather than a chemical assay of digitalis. As such, it is susceptible to interference from other physiologic and pharmacologic substances that may affect cation transport. When first described, this method detected significant quantities of digitalis-like activity (the ability to inhibit RBC ^{86}Rb uptake) in plasma from patients not receiving cardiac glycosides, and plasma concentration ranges of digoxin were higher than those determined by other methods (Lowenstein, 1965). These observations suggested that substances other than digitalis were being detected by this method. The introduction of improvements into the extraction and assay procedures has resulted in greater specificity and the determination of serum digoxin concentrations in better accord with those obtained by other, more specific methods (Lowenstein and Corrill, 1966; Bertler and Redfors, 1970).

The extraction procedure and the RBC washings make the method less convenient than the radioimmunoassay and radioreceptor assay. A moderate number of specimens can be conveniently assayed in a 7-h period (Bertler and Redfors, 1970). The ^{86}Rb has a relatively short half-life (18.7 days) and must be purchased at regular intervals. Human RBC must also be obtained (usually in 500-ml units) at regular intervals (Lowenstein, 1965). It should be emphasized that these are minor limitations and that this method has been employed by many laboratories to obtain much useful information concerning the clinical pharmocology of digoxin and digitoxin.

Inhibition of $(Na^+ + K^+)$-ATPase

Cardiac glycosides have been shown by Skou to be capable of inhibiting the sodium- and potassium-dependent "transport" adenosinetriphosphatase [$(Na^+ + K^+)$-ATPase)] system of mammalian cell membranes (Skou, 1965). After extracting digitoxin or digoxin from human plasma, it is possible to determine the glycoside content of this extract by comparing its ability to inhibit $(Na^+ + K^+)$-ATPase with the ability of known reference glycoside standards to inhibit the same enzyme preparation. After extraction of plasma with dichloromethane and evaporation of the solvent, the dried plasma extract is taken up in a buffered reaction mixture containing Na-K-ATPase from hog brain homogenates and containing appropriate concentrations of Mg^{2+}, Na^+, and K^+ required for ATPase activity. After 15 min of princubation, ATP is added and a 15-min incubation carried out. The reaction is stopped by the addition of cold trichloroacetic acid and ATPase activity assayed by the release of inorganic phosphate. Glycoside concentration is determined by comparing $(Na^+ + K^+)$-ATPase inhibition in extracts from patient's plasma with a standard inhibition curve simultaneously obtained with varying concentrations of glycoside standards on the same $(Na^+ + K^+)$-ATPase preparation (Bentley et al., 1970; Medzihradsky et al., 1971; Burnett and Conklin, 1971).

The $(Na^+ + K^+)$-ATPase system employed in this assay procedure is labile and theoretically susceptible to many environmental influences. To date, no inhibition of this ATPase system has been caused by extracts of plasma from patients not receiving digitalis. The effect of digitalis metabolites on this assay system is not known. As with the competitive protein binding and ^{86}Rb uptake inhibition methods, one might anticipate a contribution of cardioactive metabolites to plasma digitoxin values obtained by this technique.

The extraction procedure and the necessity for a large number of control tubes, particularly those for "nontransport" ATPase activity, make the method less convenient than the radioimmunoassay and the radioreceptor assay, although a moderate number of samples can be assayed in 4 h of laboratory time. Another minor drawback is the fact that hog brain ATPase must be prepared from time to time.

Chromatographic Methods

Numerous chromatographic methods have been described for the detection of cardiac glycosides in complex mixtures, but to date only two of these approaches have been used extensively in the measurement of cardenolides in human plasma.

In 1966, Lukas and Peterson described a double isotope dilution derivative assay of serum digitoxin concentrations. This elegant, but complex method involves the addition of a digitoxin-^{3}H internal standard, dichloromethane extraction, alkali treatment to decrease lipid content, a series of extractions, a paper chromatographic step, acetylation with ^{14}C-acetic anhydride to form digitoxin triacetate (allowing 4 days for this reaction), a series of further extractions and, finally, paper chromatography followed by elution and determination of the ^{3}H and ^{14}C contents of the triacetate derivative. On the basis of ^{14}C-acetate incorporation, the digitoxin content of the final eluate can be determined and, utilizing the per cent recovery of digitoxin, its concentration in the original plasma sample calculated (Lukas and Peterson, 1966; Lukas, 1971).

This method is precise and highly specific. Unlike the assay methods described above, it does not detect digitoxin metabolites, although with suitable modifications in technique, it can be used for this purpose (Lukas, 1971). Because of the elaborate series of extractions and chromatographic procedures, this assay procedure cannot be carried out on large numbers of specimens in a single day. Upward of 2 weeks is required for a single series of determinations. A problem with this method is the great variability in recovery of digitoxin-^{3}H added to specimens at the start of the assay procedure. Average recovery was only 12%, with a range of 1%-39% (Lukas and Peterson, 1966). Another drawback is that the method cannot detect glycoside concentrations less than 1 ng/ml. This relative insensitivity constitutes a significant limitation in the application of this method to studies of digoxin. A less serious limitation is the relatively large volume (3-10 ml) of plasma required for assay.

Gas chromatography has also been applied to the measurement of plasma digoxin concentrations. This method involves the addition of a digoxin-^{3}H internal standard, dichloromethane extraction, adsorption to a florisil column, elution, thin layer chromatography, and treatment with heptafluorobutyric anhydride to form digoxigenin heptafluorobutyrate (digoxigenin HFB), further thin layer chromatography, and finally, liquid scintillation counting (to determine digoxin recovery) and passage through a gas-liquid chromatograph equipped with an electron capture detector. The HFB confers electron-capturing properties on digoxigenin (which, by itself, has little affinity for electrons), and the amount of electron capture in the area of the chromatogram at which digoxigenin HFB is encountered is proportional to the amount of digoxin in the original plasma sample. Using the per cent recovery and the gas chromatography values of known standard digoxin specimens, the amount of digoxin in the original 10 ml of plasma can be calculated. The developers of this method state that it "is reasonably simple and should present no problems, especially to workers experienced with gas-liquid chromatography." However, it requires 5 h to perform a single determination, and only a few assays can be conveniently performed in a single day (Watson and Kalman, 1971). The method also requires familiarity with, and accessibility to, a gas-liquid chromatograph with an electron capture detector. This method is quite sensitive and highly specific. Digoxin can readily be distinguished from any of its known metabolites, and in fact this method has been adapted to measure serum and urinary concentrations of many of these metabolites (Watson et al., 1972; 1973; Clark and Kalman, 1974).

Although they have not yet been applied extensively to the study of human serum or plasma, a number of high pressure liquid chromatographic methods for the study of cardiac glycosides and their metabolites have recently been described (Castle, 1975; Nachtmann et al., 1976). These methods should provide specificity comparable to that of existing chromatographic methods; moreover, these methods should also permit the simultaneous measurement of glycosides and selected metabolites. Most importantly, these methods should be more rapid and more convenient than existing chromatographic methods.

Summary

Six methods for measuring serum concentrations of cardiac glycosides have been compared. Four methods employ biochemical assay procedures: immunoassay, competitive protein binding, inhibition of red cell ^{86}Rb uptake, and inhibition of $(Na^+ + K^+)$-ATPase. These methods, in general, are sensitive and precise. They are not, however, specific in that cardioactive metabolites are usually measured together with the parent glycoside; since there is, in general, an excellent correlation between values obtained by these methods with the therapeutic responses to drugs in individual patients, the detection of cardioactive metabolites does not appear to constitute a major drawback to this group of assay methods. All four of these methods are more rapid and more convenient to perform than the currently available chromatographic techniques. Immunoassay methods require small volumes of serum, do not require an extraction step, are rapid, and can readily be automated; if careful attention is paid to the limitations of immunoassay methods and if satisfactory antisera are employed, immunoassay methods are most useful in the performance of large numbers of serum glycoside measurements.

Two methods employ chromatographic procedures: the double isotope dilution derivative method and gas chromatography. Because these procedures are cumbersome and time-consuming, they are not well-suited for use in clinical laboratories. They are, however, more highly specific than the biochemical assay procedures and, moreover, they and other chromatographic methods now being studied (notably, high pressure liquid chromatography) can readily be adapted to the measurement of metabolites. Thus, it would seem that chromatographic techniques are best suited for studies of the metabolism of cardiac glycosides.

Conclusion

In 1786, Withering wrote that he was "more and more convinced, that the Digitalis, under a judicious management, is one of the mildest . . . medicines we have, and one of the most efficacious." He also believed that "it is not necessary to create a nausea, or any other disturbance in the system" (Withering, 1946). A knowledge of the serum digitalis concentration, now so readily available, should enable a more "judicious" administration and "efficacious" use of this powerful drug without creating "a nausea or any other disturbance in the system."

References

Beiser, S.M., Butler, V.P., Jr., Erlanger, B.F.: Hapten-protein conjugates: methodology and application. In: Miescher, P.A., Müller-Eberhard, H.J. (eds.): Textbook of Immunopathology, 2nd ed. New York: Grune & Stratton 1976, p. 15

Belz, G.G., Brech, W.J., Kleeberg, U.R., Rudofsky, G., Belz, G.: Characterization and specificity of proscillaridin antibodies. Naunyn Schmiedebergs Arch. Pharmakol. 279, 105 (1973)

Belz, G.G., Stauch, M., Rudofsky, G.: Plasma levels after a single oral dose of proscillaridin. Eur. J. Clin. Pharmacol. 7, 95 (1974 a)

Belz, G.G., Rudofsky, G., Lossnitzer, K., Wolf, G., Stauch, M.: Plasmaspiegel und Elektrokardiogramm nach intravenöser Applikation von Proscillaridin und Digoxin. Z. Kardiol. 63, 201 (1974b)

Belz, G.G., Pflederer, W.: Studies on a plasma cardiac glycoside assay based upon displacement of ^{3}H-ouabain from Na^+-K^+-ATPase. Basic Res. Cardiol. 70, 142 (1975)

Bentley, J.D., Burnett, G.H., Conklin, R.L., Wasserburger, R.H.: Clinical application of serum digitoxin levels. A simplified plasma determination. Circulation 41, 67 (1970)

Berson, S.A., Yalow, R.S.: Radioimmunoassays of peptide hormones in plasma. N. Engl. J. Med. 277, 640 (1967)

Bertler, A., Redfors, A.: An improved method of estimating digoxin in human plasma. Clin. Pharmacol. Ther. 11, 665 (1970)

Bodem, G., Gilfrich, H.J.: Methoden zur Bestimmung von Digoxin und Digitoxin im Blut und ihre klinische Bedeutung. Klin. Wochenschr. 51, 57 (1973)

Brooker, G., Jelliffe, R.W.: Serum cardiac glycoside assay based upon displacement of ^{3}H-ouabain from Na-K ATPase. Circulation 45, 20 (1972)

Burnett, G.H., Conklin, R.L.: The enzymatic assay of plasma digoxin. J. Lab. Clin. Med. 78, 779 (1971)

Butler, V.P., Jr.: Digoxin: immunologic approaches to measurement and reversal of toxicity. N. Engl. J. Med. 283, 1150 (1970)

Butler, V.P., Jr.: Digoxin radioimmunoassay. Lancet 1971/I, 186

Butler, V.P., Jr.: Assays of digitalis in the blood. Prog. Cardiovasc. Dis. 14, 571 (1972)

Butler, V.P.; Jr., Beiser, S.M.: Antibodies to small molecules: biological and clinical applications. Adv. Immunol. 17, 255 (1973)

Butler, V.P., Jr., Chen, J.P.: Digoxin-specific antibodies. Proc. Nat. Acad. Sci. U.S.A. 57, 71 (1967)

Butler, V.P., Jr., Lindenbaum, J.: Serum digitalis measurements in the assessment of digitalis resistance and sensitivity. Am. J. Med. 58, 460 (1975)

Butler, V.P., Jr., Schmidt, D.H., Watson, J.F., Gardner, J.D.: Production and properties of digoxin-specific antibodies. Ann. N.Y. Acad. Sci. 242, 717 (1974)

Castle, M.C.: Isolation and quantitation of picomole quantities of digoxin, digitoxin and their metabolites by high-pressure liquid chromatography. J. Chromatogr. 115, 437 (1975)

Clark, D.R., Kalman, S.M.: Dihydrodigoxin: a common metabolite of digoxin in man. Drug Metab. Dispos. 2, 148 (1974)

Doherty, J.E.: The clinical pharmacology of digitalis glycosides: a review. Am. J. Med. Sci. 255, 382 (1968)

Doherty, J.E., Perkins, W.H.: Tissue concentration and turnover of tritiated digoxin in dogs. Am. J. Cardiol. 17, 47 (1966)

Doherty, J.E., Perkins, W.H., Mitchell, G.K.: Tritiated digoxin studies in human subjects. Arch. Intern. Med. 108, 531 (1961)

Doherty, J.E., Perkins, W.H., Flanigan, W.J.: The distribution and concentration of tritiated digoxin in human tissues. Ann. Intern. Med. 66, 116 (1967)

Duhme, D.W., Greenblatt, D.J., Koch-Weser, J.: Reduction of digoxin toxicity associated with measurement of serum levels. Ann. Intern. Med. 80, 516 (1974)

Ewy, G.A., Kapadia, G.G., Yao, L., Lullin, M., Marcus, F.I.: Digoxin metabolism in the elderly. Circulation 39, 449 (1969)

Grosse-Brockhoff, F., Hausamen, T.-U.: 200 Jahre Herztherapie mit Digitalis: William Withering und das erste Jahrhundert Digitalistherapie. Dtsch. Med. Wochenschr. 100, 1980 (1975)

Haasis, R., Larbig, D., Klenk, K.O.: Glykosidkonzentration im Serum und Urin bei Herzgesunden nach Gabe von Beta-Methyl-Digoxin. Klin. Wochenschr. 53, 529 (1975)

Härtel, G., Manninen, V., Melin, J., Apajalahti, A.: Serum-digoxin concentrations with a new digoxin derivative, β-methyl-digoxin. Ann. Clin. Res. 5, 87 (1973)

Herbert, V., Lau, K.-S., Gottlieb, C.W., Bleicher, S.J.: Coated charcoal immunoassay of insulin. J. Clin. Endocrinol. 25, 1375 (1965)

Huffman, D.H., Crow, J.W., Pentikainen, P., Azarnoff, D.L.: Association between clinical cardiac status, laboratory parameters, and digoxin usage. Am. Heart J. 91, 28 (1976)

Kaufman, J.M., Belpaire, F.M.: The influence of metabolites of digoxin and digitoxin on the [86] Rb-uptake assay. Eur. J. Clin. Pharmacol. 6, 54 (1973)

Lesne, M.: Dosage radioimmunologique de la gitaloxine et de la gitoxine. Arch. Int. Pharmacodyn. Ther. 199, 206 (1972)

Line, W.F., Siegel, S.J., Kwong, A., Frank, C., Ernst, R.: Solid-phase radioimmunoassay for digoxin. Clin. Chem. 19, 1361 (1973)

Lowenstein, J.M.: A method for measuring plasma levels of digitalis glycosides. Circulation 31, 228 (1965)

Lowenstein, J.M., Corrill, E.M.: An improved method for measuring plasma and tissue concentrations of digitalis glycosides. J. Lab. Clin. Med. 67, 1048 (1966)

Lukas, D.S.: Some aspects of the distribution and disposition of digitoxin in man. Ann. N.Y. Acad. Sci. 179, 338 (1971)

Lukas, D.S., Peterson, R.E.: Double isotope dilution derivative assay of digitoxin in plasma, urine, and stool of patients maintained on the drug. J. Clin. Invest. 45, 782 (1966)

Marcus, F.I., Kapadia, G.J., Kapadia, G.G.: The metabolism of digoxin in normal subjects. J. Pharmacol. Exp. Ther. 145, 203 (1964)

Marcus, F.I., Ryan, J.N., Stafford, M.G.: The reactivity of derivatives of digoxin and digitoxin as measured by the Na-K-AtPase displacement assay and by radioimmunoassay. J. Lab. Clin. Med. 85, 610 (1975)

Marks, B.H., Dutta, S., Gauthier, J., Elliott, D.: Distribution in plasma, uptake by the heart and excretion of ouabain-^{3}H in human subjects. J. Pharmacol. Exp. Ther. 145, 351 (1964)

Meade, R.C., Kleist, T.J.: Improved radioimmunoassay of digoxin and other sterol-like compounds using Somogyi precipitation. J. Lab. Clin. Med. 80, 748 (1972)

Medzihradsky, F., Nandhasri, P.S., Khanna, U.: Enzymatic determination of cardiac glycosides. Biochem. Med. 5, 285 (1971)

Nachtmann, F., Spitzy, H., Frei, R.W.: Rapid and sensitive high-resolution procedure for digitalis glycoside analysis by derivatization liquid chromatography. J. Chromatogr. 122, 293 (1976)

Okita, G.T., Kelsey, F.E., Talso, P.J., Smith, L.B., Geiling, E.M.K.: Studies of the renal excretion of radioactive digitoxin in human subjects with congestive failure. Circulation 7, 161 (1953)

Oliver, G.C., Jr., Parker, B.M., Brasfield, D.L., Parker, C.W.: The measurement of digitoxin in human serum by radioimmunoassay. J. Clin. Invest. 47, 1035 (1968)

Rosenthal, A.F., Vargas, M.G., Klass, C.S.: Evaluation of enzymemultiplied immunoassay technique (EMIT) for determination of serum digoxin. Clin. Chem, 22, 1899 (1976)

Schwartz, A., Matsui, H., Laughter, A.H.: Tritiated digoxin binding to $(Na^+ + K^+)$-activated adenosine triphosphatase: possible allosteric site. Science 160, 323 (1968)

Selden, R., Smith, T.W.: Ouabain pharmacokinetics in dog and man: determination by radioimmunoassay. Circulation 45, 1176 (1972)

Selden, R., Klein, M.D., Smith, T.W.: Plasma concentration and urinary excretion kinetics of acetyl strophanthidin. Circulation 47, 744 (1973)

Shatzmann, H.J.: Herzglykoside als Hemmstoff für den aktiven Kalium- and Natriumtransport durch die Erythrocytenmembran. Helv. Physiol. Pharmacol. Acta 11, 346 (1953)

Skou, J.C.: Enzymatic basis for the active transport of Na^+ and K^+ across cell membrane. Physiol. Rev. 45, 596 (1965)

Smith, T.W.: Radioimmunoassay for serum digitoxin concentration: methodology and clinical experience. J. Pharmacol. Exp. Ther. 175, 352 (1970)

Smith, T.W.: Contribution of quantitative assay technics to the understanding of the clinical pharmacology of digitalis. Circulation 46, 188 (1972)

Smith, T.W.: Digitalis toxicity: epidemiology and clinical use of serum concentration measurements. Am. J. Med. 58, 470 (1975)

Smith, T.W., Haber, E.: Current techniques for serum or plasma digitalis assay and their potential clinical application. Am. J. Med. Sci. 259, 301 (1970)

Smith, T.W., Haber, E.: Clinical value of the radioimmunoassay of the digitalis glycosides. Pharmacol. Rev. 25, 219 (1973)

Smith, T.W., Skubitz, K.M.: Kinetics of interactions between antibodies and haptens. Biochemistry 14, 1496 (1975)

Smith, T.W., Butler, V.P., Jr., Haber, E.: Determination of therapeutic and toxic serum digoxin conentrations by radioimmunoassay. N. Engl. J. Med. 281, 1212 (1969)

Smith, T.W., Butler, V.P., Jr., Haber, E.: Characterization of antibodies of high affinity and specificity for the digitalis glycoside digoxin. Biochemistry 9, 331 (1970)

Watson, E., Kalman, S.M.: Assay of digoxin in plasma by gas chromatography. J. Chromatogr. 56, 209 (1971)

Watson, E., Tramell, P., Kalman, S.M.: Identification of submicrogram amounts of digoxin, digitoxin and their metabolic products: isolation by chromatography and preparation of derivatives for assay by electron capture detector. J. Chromatogr. 69, 157 (1972)

Watson, E., Clark, D.R., Kalman, S.M.: Identification by gas chromatography-mass spectroscopy of dihydrodigoxin-a metabolite of digoxin in man. J. Pharmacol. Exp. Therap. 184, 424 (1973)

Withering, W.: An account of the Foxglove and some of its medical uses: with practical remarks on dropsy and other diseases. Birmingham England, M. Swinney, 1785. Reprinted in Med. Classics 2, 295 (1937)

Withering, W.: Letter to Hall Jackson, 1786. Cited by Caroll, D.: Introduction of digitalis into North America. N. Engl. J. Med. 235, 808 (1946)

Yalow, R.S., Berson, S.A.: Immunoassay of plasma insulin. Methods Biochem. Anal. 12, 69 (1964)

Discussion

Marcus, Tucson: I wonder if you could comment about the plasma factors as they alter the immunoassay procedure. It has been stated that one can add digoxin to plasma from various patients and can get somewhat different results. Thyroid hormone has been most recently implicated as a "plasma factor" using the iodenated digoxigenin isotope. Previously, you have mentioned that azotemia may interfere with the assay determination. Could you comment if these are really problems?

Butler: Some workers have indeed reported different results when they have added given amounts of digoxin to plasma or serum from different individuals. I think that one of the problems causing these differences with the immunoassay method is that every individual antiserum behaves somewhat differently. Thus, such differing results which some workers have obtained with certain antisera, which may be of low affinity, may not necessarily be extrapolated to results which other workers get with high affinity antisera. In our experience using antiserum of particularly high affinity and specificity, which we have used and which Dr. T. Smith used initially (and perhaps may still be using), we have not been able to detect any significant difference in the inhibition curves obtained from the addition of digoxin to normal serum from different individuals. I must say, however, that, down in the 0-0.2 ng/ml range, if we use different individual sera, we get a little bit different shape to our curve between the zero point and about 0.2 ng/ml. Above that concentration, our curves are exactly superimposable, using our high affinity antisera. I think that when one uses antisera of lesser affinity and lesser specificity, one can encounter all sorts of complications, which may represent interference from steroid hormones, problems with protein binding or the like. We simply haven't run into these problems, but I don't say they don't occur. I think it is important that one check out one's antiserum very carefully to minimize these possibilities. For example, several workers have reported that compounds such as spironolactone and dihydrodigoxin interfere with their assays. We have tested both compounds with several very good antisera and they don't seem to give any significant inhibition. I think that if one uses good antisera the problem you refer to can be minimized. I don't say that it's a non-problem, but it is something one has to be alert to.

Marcus: Your comment about azotemia?

Butler: There are several problems that azotemia may cause. We don't know very much about the significance of accumulation of cardioinactive metabolites, and I suppose that these might accumulate in azotemia to a point where they would significantly alter the immunoassay. We do know that if one uses the tritiated digoxin immunoassay system there is a significant problem in some sera with chemiluminescence, and if one does not correct for this, it can cause difficulties. This should not cause a problem if one uses the ^{125}I immunoassay method. And, of course, Shoeman and Azarnoff have reported that azotemia does cause some displacement of digitoxin from binding proteins. In our laboratory, we've analyzed only digoxin (which is not as extensively protein-bound as digitoxin) and this has not been a problem for us but I don't think I could comment on the extent of this problem with the digitoxin assay. Perhaps somebody else has had some experience with it.

Grahame-Smith, Oxford: Have you any data comparing the different assays? Would you perhaps like to say a word about that?

Butler: Several people have compared various assays in their own laboratories. We have not used any method other than the immunoassay. Several groups have compared the ^{86}Rb uptake assay with the immunoassay, and the Wisconsin group has compared their ATPase inhibition assay with the radioimmunoassay. Dr. Marcus has recently published a very interesting paper in which he's compared the radioimmunoassay with the enzymic isotope displacement assay of digoxin. Perhaps you can tell us what you found, Dr. Marcus.

Marcus: We find that the methods basically are comparable. They do detect the metabolites; they give different weights to the metabolites. We find the enzymic isotope dilution assay more cumbersome, more time-consuming, less sensitive, and less accurate.

Butler: This brings up the point that with all of the biochemical assay methods, whether it's the enzymic isotope displacement method, the radioimmunoassay, the ^{86}Rb uptake method, or the $(Na^+ + K^+)$-ATPase inhibition method, one is going to run into varying degrees of inhibition by the various metabolites. If one is interested in these various metabolites, one has to employ a chromatographic step in one's assay procedure; otherwise, one is going to get some varying results. This discussion, I was told, was to deal mainly with the clinical aspects, and I think that most of the biochemical assay methods do a good job of summing together the parent glycoside and its cardioactive metabolites, if one uses good reagents. However, as Dr. Marcus has indicated, you're going to get a little bit different weighting with different assay systems. As long as one uses one assay system in a single laboratory, it is reasonable to hope that most people will have relatively similar proportions of these various active metabolites and thus I think that one can come up with a reasonably good number to use clinically. With any immunoassay, I prefer to have people refer to the assayed substance as "immunoreactive" (the endocrinologists knew years ago that this is a good adjective) and always say that we're measuring everything which reacts with antibody. If the immunoreactive serum concentration has a good relationship to what happens clinically, I think this is useful. I think that this is true for the other methods as well, namely, that the cardioactive material expressed as digoxin in these assay methods has a good relationship to the observed clinical response to the drug.

Schaumann, Mannheim: Do you know any large-scaled comparisons with different laboratories measuring the same samples?

Butler: I'm sure that this has been done; we have anecdotally checked out results obtained by other laboratories which were developing RIA methods. Beginning in the early days, Dr. Smith did this for people all over the country and perhaps all over the world — maybe you could add something, Dr. Smith.

Smith, Boston: Dr. Vanderlinde in Albany in the State of New York Laboratory has done something quite worthwhile. He has sent aliquots of the same sample to many different laboratories and compared the results obtained with different commercial kits. As far as I know, all of the techniques that have been studied are radioimmunoassay techniques. He makes available the results of these studies comparing the various different commercial kits in a number of different laboratories under real working conditions and he finds the expected results — some of the kits give more accurate and precise results than others. These numbers are available to anyone who is interested in them.

Butler: The American College of Clinical Pathology has conducted a similar survey. I thought the question had more to do with using some of the better antisera and comparing those, because I think those would be more meaningful. Obviously, if somebody uses a poor antiserum, one is going to get some unreliable results.

Smith: It is encouraging that the results seem to be coming closer together with time. One hopes that the kit manufacturers are becoming more critical in the materials they provide with their kits.

Butler: I think that one of the earlier problems (I alluded to this in the talk), as Dr. Smith so nicely showed, the earlier one takes a bleeding from an animal, the lower the affinity and the lower the specificity for digoxin is apt to be. If one were interested in making a quick profit in developing a radioimmunoassay, we could get some very good titers of antisera within about 3 or 4 weeks, but they are just not satisfactory for clinical use. I think that most of the better manufacturers now are quite aware of this, and I have been very impressed with the antisera that we've been seeing lately in kits.

Larbig, Tübingen: Dr. Butler, do I understand you right that you are saying that the specificity of the antiserum may be dependent on the duration of the immunization period? Is this correct?

Butler: Yes, Dr. Smith showed this with some serial bleedings from some of the first rabbits we immunized that certain of the steroid hormones appear to give more interference with binding of tritiated digoxin when taken about 3 weeks after immunization than did antisera obtained after several months of immunization.

Larbig: We did immunize the rabbits with digoxin bound to human serum albumin for a period of 8 months and achieved a very sensitive antibody which reacts very poorly, for instance with spironolactone. That would go along with your statement.

Butler: I think that this would be the general experience. We've been impressed with the length of time required to raise satisfactory antibodies to some haptens.

We used the method Dr. Smith published for ouabain and, at least in our experience, it took us a very long time, in comparison with digoxin, to raise satisfactory antibodies. So I think that we were lucky picking digoxin at the start, because just after 3 weeks we had excellent titers of antibodies in all of our antisera, and it wasn't until later, when Dr. Smith studied some of these sera, that we realized some of the tremendous differences that one got in the binding characteristics with the duration of immunization. This is true of other assay systems. Jaffe and Parker and their colleagues published some results in this regard and it took them 12-16 months to get the most satisfactory antisera in the prostaglandin assay system.

Belz, Koblenz: I have a question on the practical procedure of the radioimmunoassay. It is often necessary to keep the samples frozen for some time to collect. In an experience last year, we found that after a certain time of keeping the samples at $-20°C$, the variation of the radioimmunologic determination increased more and more. It's quite interesting that we performed parallely to this an analysis with an ^{86}Rb erythrocyte assay where the variation did not increase. Do you have an explanation for this observation? I must add we used a tritium labeled digoxin for the radioimmunoassay.

Butler: That has not been our experience because we've conducted a number of studies, particularly those with Dr. John Lindenbaum, involving bioavailability studies, and we frequently go back into the freezer a year or more later to repeat analyses and we have not run into that difficulty. I have no explanation for your difficulty and I just can't really comment on it. It's certainly a problem one worries about, and the sooner one does the assay, I think the better. But the variation with time which you note has not been a problem, at least in our experience.

Dengler, Bonn: May I ask a question regarding the standardization? I think these determinations are becoming more and more available, and you made a claim of checking the specificity. What would be a minimum requirement in this respect, testing for instance against dihydrodigoxin?

Butler: I actually omitted a slide on which I had a list of some of the substances that one would want to test with. One would certainly want to test with a panel of steroid hormones of man, because, in some of the poorer antisera, these will cause certain difficulties. It would be good to test with spironolactone and dihydrodigoxin because these are compounds which are now available and which we know do interfere with certain antibody systems. A very crucial procedure is to perform inhibition studies with a panel of normal human sera to show that these don't interfere. And this, I think, would be the minimal amount. I think that most of the assay kits are going over to the use of solid phase methods which minimize the problems with desorption from the charcoal such as Meade and Kleist and Smith and Haber have described. If one is employing the coated charcoal assay system, one would want to show that, with a reasonable period of time of incubation with the charcoal, one was not getting considerable "stripping" of the tritiated digoxin from the antibody. These, I think, would be reasonable controls for the antisera. If a person is developing one's antiserum in one's own laboratory, which I think is the best way, these are minimum controls. I think that, for industrial firms that are selling the antisera, these controls should be considered mandatory.

2 A New Simple Assay for Determining Digoxin Serum Levels

K. STELLNER

When this symposium was arranged, we intended to present our solid-phase tube RIA for determining digoxin (this kit being on the market for half a year now). In the meantime, work on an enzyme immunoassay has been completed; therefore, we found it more appropriate to report on this assay, thus justifying the announcement of a new assay for determining digoxin levels. Because the ELISA will always be compared with the RIA, some information on the RIA is also given in this report. This ELISA was developed by my colleague Dr. Kleinhammer.

The assay is based on the solid-phase tube technique and the use of horseradish peroxidase as enzymic label. Enzyme labeling for quantitative immunochemical purposes has been introduced independently by Van Weemen and Engvall in 1971 and has been applied to a considerable number of different ELISAs since then, mostly for the determination of antigens.

The principle of the digoxin enzyme immunoassay is shown in Figure 2.1. Standard or sample are incubated together with an appropriate amount of digoxin-HRP-conjugate in polystyrene tubes, coated with antidigoxin antibody. Incubation time is 1 h at room temperature; Then the contents of the tubes are aspirated and discarded and the HRP activity bound to the tube wall is determined. The tubes are prepared by incubating them with a 1:8000 dilution of sheep antibody for 3 h at room temperature followed by a 30-min incubation with a 1% solution of BSA in saline. The antibody solution can be used at least twice. The coated tubes are stable for at least 1 year when stored at $-20°C$. The same tubes are used both for the RIA and the ELISA.

The preparation of the HRP-digoxin-conjugate took advantage of the experience gained during the RIA development. The same precursor — a digoxin derivative carrying a N-hydroxy-succinimidester group — used to prepare tracer and immunogen for the RIA was now coupled to HRP. The conjugates were purified by hydrophobic chromatography on PBA-Sepharose. Up to 80% of the total amount of HRP was found in the fraction eluted with ethylene glycol/sodium chloride. The conjugates show an immunoreactivity of approximately 25%. If stored in the refrigerator, they can be used for 6 months and longer.

Table 2.1 summarizes the working schedule of the digoxin enzyme immunoassay. A sample volume of 100 μl in a total incubation volume of 1.1 ml is used. After 1 h incubation at room temperature, the contents of the tubes are aspirated and dis-

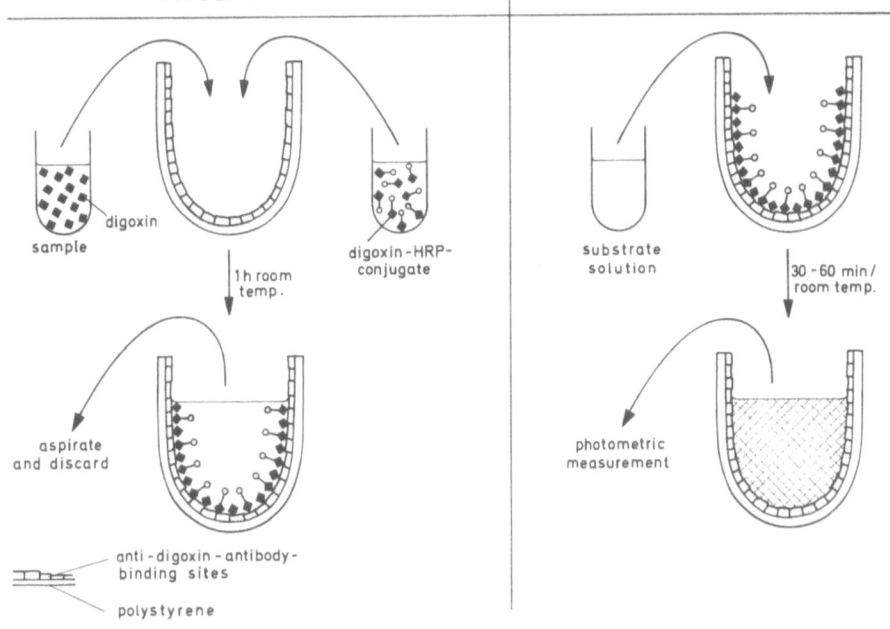

Fig. 2.1. Schematic principle of digoxin enzyme immunoassay

carded. Then the peroxidase activity is determined at pH 5 in phosphate citrate buffer using ABTS as chromogen. Incubation time for the substrate mixture is about 30-60 min. Then the extinction of each solution is read at 405 nm against the blank. Each standard or sample is done in triplicate. The standard curve is ob-

Table 2.1. Working schedule of digoxin enzyme immunoassay in antibody-coated tubes

The entire enzyme immunoassay comprises the following steps:
1. Pipette 0.1 ml of serum or standard solution into antibody-coated tubes.
2. Pipette 1 ml of digoxin-peroxydase-conjugate solution (solvent : 0.04 M phosphate buffer with 0.25% BSA) into each tube.
    — Incubate for 1 h at room temperature —
3. Aspirate and discard contents of the tubes, wash once.
4. Pipette 1 ml of substrate solution[a] into each tube.
    — Incubate for 30-60 min at room temperature —
5. Determine the extinction at 405 mm of each solution.
6. Construct standard curve and read digoxin concentrations of serum samples.

[a]Chromogen : ABTS (= 2.2'-azino-di-[3-ethyl-benzthiazoline-sulfonate (6)]).

tained with standard amounts of digoxin dissolved in serum. Under routine conditions, an O.D. at 405 nm is obtained of about 0.7 against the blank within 30 min.

A typical standard curve of the enzyme immunoassay is compared with that of a digoxin radioimmunoassay performed in antibody-coated tubes with an iodinated digoxin tracer in Figure 2.2. If we compare the 10% and 50% intercepts of both standard curves, we can see that the enzyme immunoassay is in principle as sensitive as an identically performed radioimmunoassay. The 50% intercept of approx. 2 ng digoxin/ml is equal to the upper limit of the widely accepted therapeutic digoxin concentration. Thus, in this important range, both standard curves still have an excellent steep slope.

The precision of the enzyme immunoassay was evaluated with two control sera, which were determined 24 times in triplicate. The results are shown in Table 2.2.

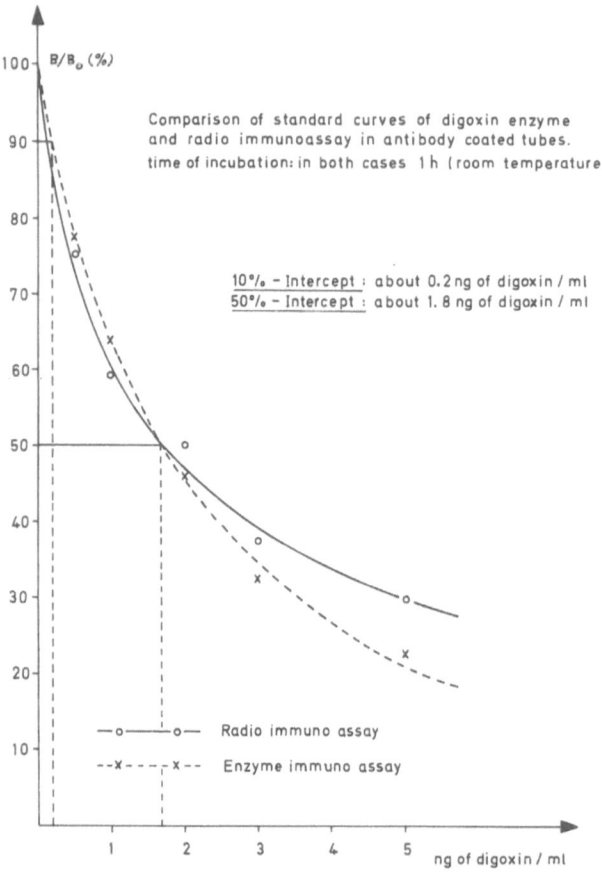

Fig. 2.2. Comparison of standard curves of digoxin enzyme and radioimmunoassay in antibody-coated tubes; time of incubation in both cases 1 h at room temperature

24

First of all one can see that the digoxin concentrations found in this study are in good agreement with the nominal values of the control sera. The intra-assay precision is characterized by a coefficient of variation of 6.5% in the therapeutic range. The corresponding interassay coefficient of variation was found to be 8.8%. These values and also the respective values of the control serum II are slightly higher than the respective coefficients of variation of the solid-phase tube radioimmunoassay.

The results of some recovery experiments are given in Table 2.3. The sera of seven healthy persons not taking cardiac glycosides were spiked individually with 1 and 2 ng digoxin per ml. The mean recovery was found to be 93% and 95% respectively. Cross-reactivities for digoxin derivatives and metabolites as well as for some other commonly used drugs were tested by comparing the concentrations of these compounds and digoxin required to produce 50% inhibition of initial binding. In both systems, there is complete cross-reaction of digoxin and the widely used β-methyl-digoxin. Cross-reactivity of digitoxin with digoxin is in the enzyme immunoassay about twice as high as in the radioimmunoassay. The last four steroids possess a negligible cross-reactivity in the enzyme immunoassay (Table 2.4).

The correlation between digoxin values determined by solid-phase tube enzyme and radioimmunoassay is quite acceptable. The equation for the regression line

Table 2.2. Intra- and interassay precision of digoxin enzyme immunoassay

Intraassay precision

	Control Serum I	Control Serum II
Mean (ng Digoxin/ml)	1.47	3.83
SD (ng Digoxin/ml)	0.096	0.27
CV (%)	6.5	7.0
n (Triplicates)	24	24

Interassay Precision

	Control Serum I	Control Serum II
Mean (ng Digoxin/ml)	1.47	3.83
SD (ng Digoxin/ml)	0.13	0.44
CV (%)	8.8	11.4
n (Triplicates)	24	24

Nominal value of control serum I   :   1.55 ± 0.4 ng/ml.
Nominal value of control serum II :   3.8 ± 0.6 ng/ml.

Table 2.3. Recovery of digoxin added to different sera by digoxin enzyme immunoassay

Serum no.	Amount of digoxin added (ng/ml)	Digoxin concentration determined (ng/ml)
1	1	0.9
2	1	1.0
3	1	0.8
4	1	0.9
5	1	0.9
6	1	1.1
7	1	0.9
		Mean: 0.93 (≙ 93% Recovery)
1	2	2.1
2	2	2.0
3	2	1.8
4	2	2.0
5	2	1.6
6	2	1.7
7	2	2.0
		Mean: 1.9 (≙ 95% Recovery)

Table 2.4. Comparison of the cross-reactivity of different substances with digoxin in the solid-phase tube digoxin enzyme and radioimmunoassay

Substance	% Cross-reactivity in enzyme immunoassay	% Cross-reactivity in radioimmunoassay
Digoxin	100	100
β-methyl-digoxin	96	102
β-acetyl-digoxin	87	96
Digoxigenin	8	31
Digoxin-Mono-Digitoxosid	96	98
Digitoxin	15	7
Prednison	< 0.01	< 0.01
Spironolactone	< 0.01	< 0.01
Cortisol	< 0.01	ND
Progesterone	< 0.01	ND

obtained by least-mean squares from the analysis of 50 sera is

RIA = 0.95 ELISA − 0.01

The correlation coefficient is 0.97. The data in this study indicate that the use of ELISA for the determination of digoxin gives results that agree well with those obtained with a commercially available RIA. We believe that this digoxin assay yields reliable values in a convenient way without the necessity of handling radio-activity.

References

Engvall, E., Perlmann, P.: Enzyme-linked immunosorbent assay (ELISA). Quanti-tative assay of immunoglobulin G. Immunochemistry $\underline{8}$, 871 (1971)
Van Weemen, B,K., Schuurs, A.H.W.M.: Immunoassay using antigen-enzyme con-jugates. FEBS letters $\underline{15}$, 232 (1971)

Discussion

Bodem, Bonn: Did you study the interference of that assay with hemolytic and lipemic plasma?

Stellner: I think this was done, but there was no interference as far as I know.

Belz, Koblenz: Is this assay available for clinical use?

Stellner: This assay will be on the market presumably in the summer of 1977.

Padeletti, Florence: Has the serum albumin concentration some effect on your standard curves?

Stellner: This has not been studied yet.

3 Chloroform-Extractable and Polar Metabolites Examined With Different Assays

U. GUNDERT-REMY, K. KOCH, and V. HRSTKA

In 1971 Dwenger and Haberland were able to demonstrate a time-dependent formation of hydrophilic metabolites of digoxin after oral application in man. A similar pattern of methyldigoxin was described by Rietbrock and Abshagen (1973) and Abshagen et al. (1974). The chemical nature of these polar metabolites were thought to be the sulfuric and glucuronic acid conjugates of the bis- and mono-glycosides and of aglucone, as first proposed by Repke et al. (Herrmann & Repke, 1962; Lauterbach & Repke, 1960; Repke, 1970). The data have been confirmed by results of other authors in animals and man (Bergmann et al., 1972; Brown et al., 1956; Cox & Wright, 1959; Doherty & Perkins, 1962; Lage & Spratt, 1965).

Our aim was to study the chloroform-extractable and polar fraction in the urine after administration of tritium-labeled digoxin with three different assays. The specimens were determined radiochemically, radioimmunologically, and with an enzymic assay, which is based on the inhibition of a membrane-bound Na-K-Mg-dependent ATPase. Furthermore, renal clearances were determined for the polar and nonpolar fractions.

Methods

Six female volunteers (37-61 years, weighing 55-75 kg) received orally 0.5 mg tritium-labeled digoxin (specific activity 200 μCi/mg). Blood was withdrawn before and in timed intervals (15, 30, 45, 60, 90, 120, 150, 180, and 240 min) after drug intake. The urine of the first 4 h was collected. The total radioactivity as well as that after chloroform extraction (three times) was determined in plasma. Quenching correction was carried out using internal standardization. In the urine, total radioactivity was estimated and radioimmunoassay also performed. To gain the chloroform-extractable fraction, 50 ml urine were extracted three times with 100 ml chloroform. The combined extracts were evaporated to dryness and redissolved with 10 ml ethanol. For the preparation of the polar metabolites, the remaining urine was extracted three times with 30 ml ether ethanol 3:1 after adding 24 g ammonium sulfate. The combined extracts were evaporated to dryness and redissolved with 10 ml ethanol. A second two-step extraction procedure was performed with ether ethanol. The combined extracts were evaporated to dryness and taken up with 10 ml ethanol. The radioactivity was determined in the ethanolic solutions. The radioimmunologic estimation was carried out with 1:10 dilution with 0.01 M phosphate buffer pH 7.4. For the enzymic assay a 1:50 and 1:100 dilution with distilled water was prepared. The results are expressed as μg digoxin equivalents. The renal clearances were quoted from the areas under the time curve (estimated using trapezoid rule) as well as the urinary excreted amounts of polar and nonpolar fractions.

Results

Plasma Curves

Plasma peak levels of total radioactivity were reached about 1 h after oral administration. In all volunteers the plasma sample taken 15 min after intake did not contain polar metabolites. Thereafter, the content of polar metabolites rose, and peak levels were seen 1-2 h after drug intake. The level of polar metabolites did not, at any time, exceed the level of the nonpolar fraction (Fig. 3.1).

Urine

The radiochemical determination of the crude urine gave a mean value of 61.1 μg digoxin equivalents (range 49.68-87.41 μg). The radioimmunologically estimated

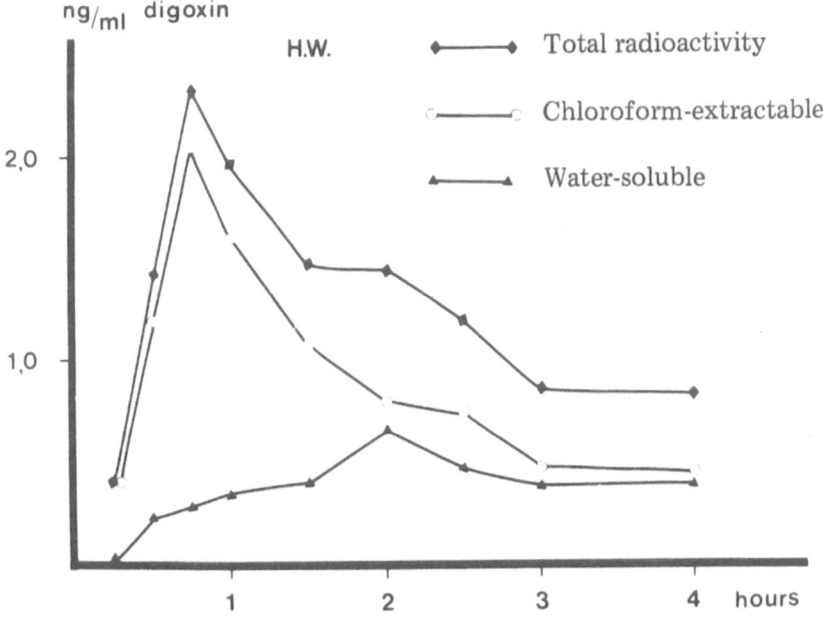

Fig. 3.1. Time course of total radioactivity, chloroform-extractable and water-soluble metabolites in the plasma after 0.5 mg ^{3}H-digoxin p.o.

content was 58.9 µg digoxin equivalents (range 49.27-81.25 µg) (Table 3.1). Volunteer E.W., data which are not included, excreted 183 µg digoxin equivalents determined radiochemically. The enzymic assay could not be performed with crude urine because of the salt content disturbing the assay.

The chloroform-extractable fraction was examined in five volunteers with three methods. From the radiochemical determination, 41.1 µg digoxin equivalents resulted as mean value whereas 49.4 µg were estimated with radioimmunoassay and 44.5 µg with enzymic assay. The values estimated with the radioimmunoassay are higher than those determined with other methods (Table 3.2). The difference between the radiochemical and immunologic values as well as the difference between the radioimmunologic and enzymic assay is significant ($p < 0.05$; Willcox-willcoxontest).

The urinary excretion of polar metabolites amounted to 13 µg digoxin equivalents on the average, determined radiochemically. Using the radioimmunologic and enzymic assay, 10.5 µg and 12.2 µg digoxin equivalents were found respectively (Table 3.3). The mean value of the radioimmunologic and enzymic assay is lower than the average value gained with the radiochemical method. However, no systematic difference could be stated.

Renal Clearances

The renal clearance of the chloroform-soluble fraction amounted to 196 ml/min on the average (H.W.'s values not included), whereas 160 ml/min are quoted for the polar fraction. In all cases except one, the renal clearance of the nonpolar fraction exceeded the renla clearance of the polar fraction (Table 3.4).

Table 3.1. Content of digoxin and metabolites in the urine (0-4 h) after 0.5 mg ^{3}H-digoxin p.o. (expressed) as µg digoxin

	Radiochemic.	Radioimmunolog.
K.A.	87.4	81.25
H.K.	49.7	44.4
H.R.-K.	49.9	49.7
A.S.	73.4	69.8
H.W.	54.7	49.3
$\bar{x} \pm s$	65.1	58.9
	16.1	14.2

Table 3.2. Chloroform-extractable metabolites in the urine after administration of 0.5 mg ^{3} H-digoxin p.o. (expressed as μg digoxin)

	Radiochemic.	Radioimmunolog.	Enzymatic.
K.A.	51.91	73.44	72.00
H.K.	32.51	36.26	30.54
H.R.-K.	37.17	40.00	39.83
A.S.	51.44	58.56	50.26
H.W.	34.94	38.52	29.76
$\bar{x} \pm s$	41.59	49.36	44.48
	± 8.36	±14.43	±15.64

Table 3.3. Water-soluble metabolites in the urine after oral administration of 0.5 mg ^{3} H-digoxin (expressed as μg digoxin)

	Radiochemic.	Radioimmunolog.	Enzymatic.
K.A.	18.71	20.59	17.78
H.K.	10.14	4.78	10.35
H.R.-K.	8.08	7.08	10.27
A.S.	13.86	14.49	11.66
H.W.	14.42	5.52	11.04
$\bar{x} \pm s$	13.05	10.49	12.22
	± 3.68	± 6.11	± 2.83

Table 3.4. Renal clearances of metabolites (quoted from the area under the curve and the urinary excretion)

	Chloroform-soluble	Water-soluble
K.A.	226	157
H.K.	145	138
H.R.-K.	203	161
A.S.	248	202
H.W.	72	410
E.W.	158	140
$\bar{x} \pm s$	196	159.6
	± 39,2	± 23,1

(without the values H.W.)

Discussion

Polar metabolites of digoxin are found in plasma and urine in accordance with results of the above mentioned authors (Abshagen et al., 1974; Dwenger & Haberland, 1971; Steiness, 1974). Using radiochemical and radioimmunologic estimations, similar values are determined as digoxin equivalents in the crude urine. A higher amount of digoxin equivalents resulted from the radioimmunologic estimation of the chloroform-extractable fraction than that found with the radiochemical and enzymic assay respectively. In the enzymic assay, the digoxin bis- and monodigitoxoside, which are extracted in the chloroform fraction (Abshagen et al., 1974; Doherty & Perkins, 1962; Dwenger & Haberland, 1971), inhibit the ATPase enzyme to the same extent as digoxin (Fig. 3.2), The affinity of digoxin to the antibody used in the radioimmunoassay and thus the higher value found with this method may be explained. Clark and Kalman (1974) as well as Greenwood and co-workers (1975) determined dihydrodigoxin as a major metabolite in the urine of patients on maintenance therapy, using gas chromatography and mass spectrometry. Of the methylenechloride and of an ethylacetate extract of the urine, 13% and 16.3% respectively were found to be dihydrodigoxin. A 3000-fold higher concentration of dihydrodigoxin was needed compared to digo-

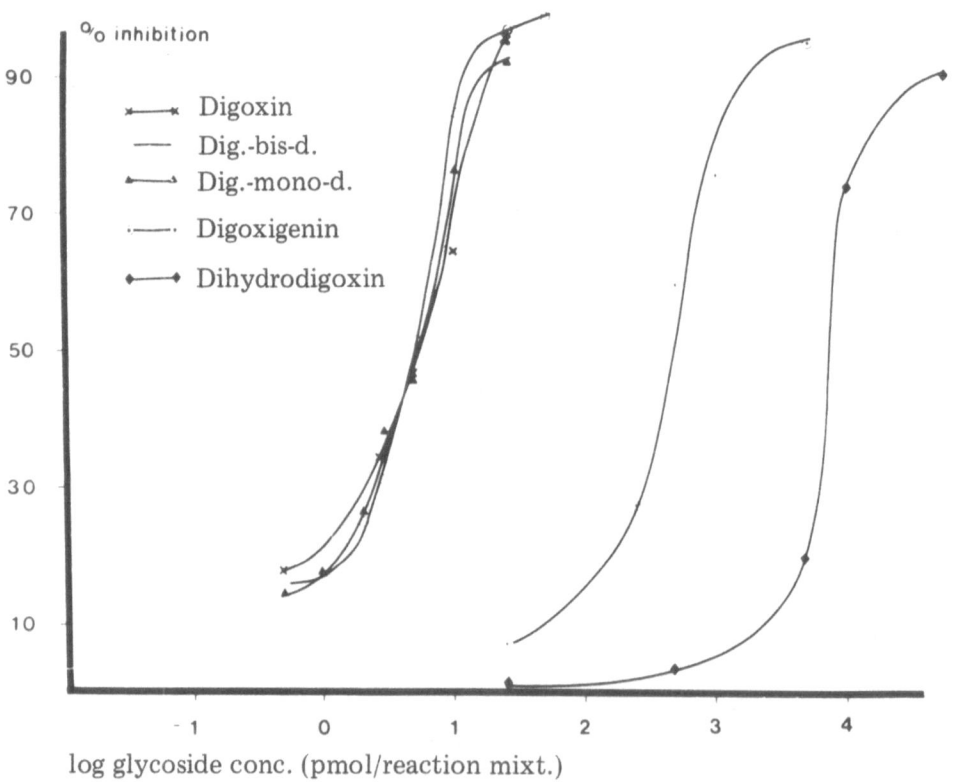

Fig. 3.2. Dose-response curves of digoxin and metabolites in the ATPase assay

xin to obtain a 50% inhibition of the ATPase in our assay (Fig. 3.2). Under the assumption that about 15% of the chloroform-extractable fraction would be dihydrodigoxin, this part of the chloroform-extractable fraction could not be estimated with the enzymic assay. Therefore, the results of the enzymic assay should be lower than the results of the radiochemical determination. Our data did not agree with this assumption because of the same digoxin equivalents found with enzymic as with radiochemical estimation. It appears, therefore, that the volunteers did not excrete a remarkable extent of dihydrodigoxin.

The examination of the polar metabolites revealed similar values of digoxin equivalents, comparing the results of the three assays. The results of the radioimmunoassay may be explained by the intact steroid moiety of the polar metabolites. Since the polar metabolites are thought to be inactive (Lüllmann et al., 1971), and since a parallel behavior is postulated between the cardioactivity and the inhibition of membrane-bound Na-K-Mg-dependent ATPase (Repke et al., 1973), the polar metabolites should not inhibit the activity of the ATPase in our assay. The results of the enzymic assay is in contrast with the above-mentioned findings. The possibility was ruled out that dissociation of the glucuronic and sulfuric acid would occur during the incubation: the incubation period was 65 min at 37°, the pH value of the reaction mixture was 7.4. Bacterial growth was minimally observed in the reaction mixture. Renal clearance of the two fractions (polar and nonpolar) are different. In 13 patients, Steiness (1974) found a digoxin clearance which exceeds the inulin clearance, indicating an active tubular secretion of digoxin. It may be speculated that the nonpolar fraction but not the polar fraction was subjected to this mechanism. Under this assumption, the difference of renal clearances could be explained.

References

Abshagen, U., Rennekamp, H., Küchler, R., Rietbrock, N.: Formation and disposition of bis- and monoglycosides after administration of ^{3}H-4'''-methyldigoxin in man. Europ.J.clin.Pharmacol. 7, 177-181 (1974)

Bergmann, K.V., Abshagen, U., Rietbrock, N.: Quantitative analysis of digoxin, 4'''-acetyldigoxin and 4'''-methyldigoxin and their metabolites in bile and urine of rats. Naunyn-Schmiedeberg's Arch.Pharmacol. 273, 154-167 (1972)

Brown, B.T., Shepeard, E.E., Wright, S.: The distribution of digitalis glycosides and their metabolites within the body of the rat. J.Pharmacol. exp. Ther. 118, 39-45 (1956)

Clark, D.R., Kalman, S.M.: Dihydrodigoxin: a common metabolite of digoxin in man. Drug Metabolism and Disposition 2, 148-150 (1974)

Cox, E., Whright, S.E.: The hepatic excretion of digitalis-glycosides and their genins in the rat. J.Pharmacol.exp.Ther. 126, 117-122 (1959)

Dengler, H.J., Bodem, G., Wirth, K.: Pharmacokinetic and metabolic studies with lanatoside C, α- and ß-acetyl-digoxin and digoxin in man. Vth International Congress on Pharmacology, San Francisco 1972

Doherty, J.E., Perkins, W.H.: Studies with tritiated digoxin in human subjects after intravenous administration. Am.Heart J. 63, 528-536 (1962)

Dwenger, A., Haberland, G.: Metabolism of ^{3}H-digoxin and some acetyl-digo-xins: time-dependent formation of hydrophilic metabolites after oral application in man. Naunyn-Schmiedeberg's Arch. Pharmacol. 270, 102-104, (1971)

Greenwood, H., Snedden, W., Hayward, R.P., Landon, J.: The measurement of urinary digoxin and dihydrodigoxin by radioimmunoassay and by mass spectroscopy. Clin.Chim.Acta 62, 213-224 (1975)

Herrmann, J., Repke, K.: Über eine neue Form der Konjugation von Geninen im tierischen Stoffwechsel. Naunyn-Schmiedeberg's Arch.exp.Path.Pharmak. 243, 333-334 (1962)

Lage, G.L., Spratt, J.L.: ^{3}H-digoxin metabolism by adult male rat tissues in vitro. J.Pharmacol.exp.Ther. 149, 248-256 (1965)

Lauterbach, F., Repke, K.: Die fermentative Abspaltung von D-Digitoxe, O-Cyma-rose und L-Thevetose aus Herzglykosiden durch Leberschnitte. Naunyn-Schmiedeberg's Arch.exp.Path.Pharmak. 238, 196-218 (1960)

Lüllmann, H., Peters, T., Seiler, K.-U.: Über die Verteilung und Biotransformation verschiedener Herzglykoside. Dtsch.med.Wschr. 23, 1018-1021 (1971)

Repke, K.: Stoffwechsel und Wirkung von Digitalisglykosiden. Öst.Apoth.-Ztg. 24, 515-522 (1970)

Repke, K.R.H., Herrmann, J., Kunze, R., Portius, H.J., Schön, R., Schönfeld, W.: Mechanism of digitalis action and the importance of the kinetics of the formation and decomposition of glycosid-receptor complex for understanding of overall pharmacokinetics of digitalis compounds. Symp. on Digitalis, Oslo 1973

Rietbrock, N., Abshagen, K.: Stoffwechsel und Pharmakokinetik der Lanataglykoside beim Menschen. Dtsch.med.Wschr. 98, 117-122 (1973)

Steiness, E.: Renal tubular secretion of digoxin, Circulation 50, 103-107 (1974)

Discussion

Nyberg, Sweden: I would like to know your definition of polar and nonpolar metabolites. For instance, a single extraction with chloroform from an aqueous solution can be expected to give a recovery of about 90%, if equal phase volumes are used. Some digoxin is then retained in the aqueous phase. Conversely, polar metabolites would be extractable to a certain extent. Thus, there is not immediately a sharp line between "polar" and "nonpolar" compounds. It depends upon the extraction procedure used.

Gundert-Remy: We extracted three times with a threefold volume of chloroform. In recovery studies, we found only 1.2% of digoxin remaining in the urine after chloroform extraction. Thus, we assumed in our study that the radioactivity which remained in the urine phase represented water-soluble metabolites. But, indeed, this procedure does not allow a strict definition of "polar metabolites".

Niebch, Frankfurt: How much of the total urinary radioactivity was extractable by chloroform and subsequently by ether ethanol?

Gundert-Remy: About 80% of the tritium excreted into the urine could be extracted with chloroform. I cannot answer by heart your question concerning the extraction step by step.

Bodem, Bonn: Did you really expect detectable quantities of dihydrodigoxin? I think Watson and Kalman found out of 151 patients only in 3 patients a high amount of dihydrodigoxin. We developed a radioimmunoassay for the determination of dihydrodigoxin and studied about 40 patients. We couldn't detect any plasma levels of dihydrodigoxin in these patients.

Gundert-Remy: There are reports (Clark and Kalman, Greenwood et al.) which show a significant urinary excretion of dihydrodigoxin under a digoxin treatment. These data, however, cannot be confirmed by the results presented in this paper.

Benthe, Hamburg: We studied the content in the urine after giving digoxin using the MS method. This method, however, is so insensitive that we could not detect below 10% of the given dose and we never found a patient who excreted more than 10% dihydrodigoxin.

Gundert-Remy: In the paper of Greenwood, I think, 47% was the highest value reported.

Klotz, Stuttgart: You collected the urine only for 4 h. What happened after 4 h? Because I think the metabolic rate will probably increase after 4 h. To get the total amount of the dose which is excreted unchanged or as any kind of metabolite one ought to collect the urine for two or three half-lives and analyze it.

Gundert-Remy: Several papers show the occurrence of water-soluble metabolites in the early hours after a digoxin application. At later times, the water-soluble fraction is very small.

4   Studies of the Metabolism of Digoxin and Digitoxin Using Double Isotope Dilution Derivative Methods[1]

D. S. LUKAS

Abstract

The double isotope dilution derivative assays for digoxin, digoxigenin, and 3-epi-digoxigenin were used to study the disposition of digoxin in three subjects maintained on the drug in standard oral tablet form. Only 21%-55% of the daily dose was excreted in the urine and feces as the chemically intact glycoside; the rest was biotransformed. Since the only acid-hydrolyzable derivative of digoxigenin that was recovered from urine and feces was digoxin itself, the genin portion of the molecule was chemically modified in the process of biotransformation. Only 0.3%-1.0% of the drug was excreted as 3-epidigoxigenin. Incubation of urine with glucuronidase and aryl sulfatase did not release additional digoxin or acid-labile derivatives of digoxigenin.

After digoxin was discontinued in two subjects, plasma concentration and daily urinary and fecal excretion of digoxin decreased exponentially during the subsequent 9 days with a half-life of 1.4 days in one subject and 1.6 days in the other; 23%-56% of the calculated body pool of the drug was cumulatively excreted in the urine and stool, and digoxin was the only acid-hydrolyzable derivative of digoxigenin recovered.

Biotransformation of orally administered digoxin was more extensive than previously reported and equalled or exceeded urinary excretion of the drug even in one subject with hepatic disease. Since only 1%-16% of the daily dose appeared in the feces, the tablet preparation was well-absorbed. The bioavailability of soluble oral preparations of digoxin may be primarily limited by a "first pass effect" manifested by enhanced hepatic uptake and metabolic conversion of the drug.

In the first application of the double isotope dilution derivative principle to analysis of cardiac glycosides in submicrogram quantities, digitoxin was converted to a readily measureable ^{14}C-triacetate derivative, and ^{3}H-digitoxin was first added to the sample to correct for subsequent analytic losses of the glycoside (Lukas and Peterson, 1964). This assay was subsequently used to study the dis-

1   Supported by United States Public Health Service Research Grants HL 14539 and RR 47 from the National Institutes of Health.

position and pharmacokinetics of digitoxin in man (Lukas and Peterson, 1966; Lukas, 1971, 1973 a, b), and in the course of those studies, in order to investigate the biotransformation of digitoxin, additional double isotope dilution derivative methods were developed for digitoxigenin, 3-epidigitoxigenin, digoxigenin, and 3-epidigoxigenin (Lukas, 1971, 1973 a, b, c).

This basic analytic method also proved to be applicable to digoxin. Since the method was published (Lukas, 1973 c), it has undergone a few modifications and preliminary trials in studies of the metabolism of digoxin. Thusfar, only a few patients have been studied, but the data are the first to be obtained by an organic chemical method specific for digoxin as well as an independent assay for digoxigenin and are the subject of this report.

Methods

Analysis of Digoxin

In the original double isotope dilution derivative assay for digoxin, ^{3}H-digoxin with a specific activity of 0.5 Ci/mmol was used as an indicator of analytic losses (Lukas, 1973 c). In the present study, randomly labeled ^{3}H-digoxin with a specific activity of 10.4 Ci/mmol was substituted as an indicator in the analysis of plasma, and 12α-^{3}H-digoxin with a specific activity of 5.2 Ci/mmol was used in the measurement of digoxin in urine and feces. The tritium-labeled glycosides were obtained from a commercial source (New England Nuclear, Boston, Massachusetts) and purified by multiple chromatographies on paper as previously described (Lukas, 1973 c). Approximately 10% of the tritium in both preparations was contained by contaminating compounds with chromatographic characteristics that were closely similar to those of digoxin.

To determine their specific activities, the pure glycosides were converted to ^{3}H-digoxin-1-^{14}C-tetraacetate by reaction with 1-^{14}C-acetic anhydride of well-characterized specific activity (nominal specific activity: 10 mCi/mmol) (Lukas and Peterson, 1966; Lukas, 1973 c). Cleavage of the glycoside bond of the randomly labeled ^{3}H-digoxin by hydrochloric acid and measurement of the specific activity of the freed digoxigenin by converting it to the 1-^{14}C-diacetate demonstrated that 59% of the tritium was contained by the digitoxose residues and 41% by the genin. Similar treatment of 12α-^{3}H-digoxin verified that all of the tritium was present in the genin.

The method was further modified by replacing the second (Lukas, 1973 c) of the five solvent systems (system C: cyclohexane, 100, dioxane, 75; methanol, 50; water, 25) used in the sequential chromatographic purification of digoxin tetra-acetate with cyclohexane, 100; dioxane, 75; methanol, 75; water, 25. This system afforded cleaner separation of the tetra-acetate from the triacetate of digoxin, which was a minor but frequent product of the acetylation reaction.

Replicate measurements of 5-500 ng of digoxin using 125,000 dpm of ^{3}H-digoxin as indicator revealed an overall analytic accuracy of 100.7 ± 1.5% (mean ± SE) with a precision of 7% (SD). For 5 ng of digoxin alone, accuracy was 101.4 ± 1.6%

and coefficient of variation 4.1%. With $12\alpha^{/3}$ H-digoxin as the indicator, 5-500 ng of digoxin was measured with an accuracy of 101.1 ± 1.5% and a coefficient of variation of 5.9%.

Plasma digoxin concentration was determined in 15 ml of plasma to which 125,000 dpm of [3] H-digoxin was added before digoxin was extracted. In the analysis of urine and stool homogenate, 150,000 dpm of 12α-[3] H-digoxin was mixed thoroughly with 100 ml of the sample, half of which was used for measurement of digoxin.

Measurement of Acid-Hydrolyzable Derivatives of Digoxigenin and 3-Epidigoxigenin in Urine and Feces

The other 50-ml portion of the urine or fecal sample was incubated for 18 h with hydrochloric acid at pH 1.0, and the digoxigenin released was measured by the double isotope dilution derivative method for this compound. Prior to acidification, a tracer quantity of [3] H-3-epidigoxigenin was added to those samples in which 3-epidigoxigenin was simultaneously measured. After extraction, digoxigenin and 3-epidigoxigenin from every sample were routinely separated by paper chromatography. The conditions of acid hydrolysis, extraction and chromatographic separations, and the double isotope dilution derivative methods for digoxigenin and 3-epidigoxigenin have previously been described in detail (Lukas, 1971; 1973 c).

The assay for digoxigenin was modified in this study by adding 12α-[3] H-digoxin instead of [3] H-digoxin to the sample before it was acidified. This maneuver afforded the advantages of measuring digoxin and acid-hydrolyzable derivatives of digoxigenin in the same sample after a single pipetting of the indicator and of correcting for possible incomplete hydrolysis of digoxigenin digitoxosides.

Enzymatic Hydrolysis of Conjugates Containing Digoxigenin

Since hydrochloric acid effectively cleaves the digitoxose-genin bond (Lukas, 1971, 1973 a; Reichstein and Weiss, 1962) digoxigenin is released for measurement in the above assays not only from digoxin and the di- and monodigitoxosides of digoxigenin but also from any conjugates of these compounds in which the conjugating group is attached to the digitoxose residues. Also, since steroid conjugates, such as aldosterone-glucuronide, can be hydrolyzed at pH 1.0 (Bougas et al., 1964), conjugates in which the conjugating group is chemically bound to the digoxigenin moiety of the compound should be detected. It is possible, nevertheless, that some of these genin conjugates are resistant to cleavage by acid and are susceptible only to enzymic hydrolysis.

To investigate this possibility, 50 ml of urine containing a tracer quantity of 12α-[3] H-digoxin, was incubated for 24 h at 37°C with 10 ml of 1.0 M acetate buffer at pH 5.0 and a partially purified preparation of succus entericus from

Helix pomatia (Sigma Chemical Co., St. Louis, Missouri). The sample contained 6000 Fishman U of β-glucuronidase and 500 μM units of aryl sulfatase per ml, and its pH was adjusted to 5.0 before incubation with a few drops of acetic acid if necessary.

After incubation, one-half of the sample was analyzed for digoxin. ^{3}H-epidigoxigenin was added to the other 30 ml, which was then acidified to pH 1.0 with hydrochloric acid, allowed to stand at room temperature for 18 h, and analyzed for digoxigenin and 3-epidigoxigenin that were released by the sequential anzymic and acid hydrolyses.

Subjects

Three subjects, whose characteristics are listed in Table 4.1, were studied during the steady state of daily maintenance on digoxin in 0.25-mg tablet form (Lanoxin, Burroughs Wellcome). Each subject had received the drug for at least the previous 6 months because of manifestations of left ventricular dysfunction due to myocardopathy in subject V, ischemic heart disease in Y, and hyperkinemia in P. Renal and hepatic functions were normal in all subjects except P, who had chronic hepatitis with esophageal varices, serum albumin of 1.4 g per 100 ml, and serum bilirubin of 3.0 mg per 100 ml. The daily oral dose was 0.25 mg in subject Y and P and 0.5 mg (1 tablet at 8:00 a.m. and 1 at 6:00 p.m.) in V.

The subjects were hospitalized and housed in a metabolic unit for at least 1 week before the studies were begun. They were given no drugs that affected the absorption or excretion of digoxin. During 4-6 days of daily maintenance on digoxin, blood was sampled daily immediately before the drug was administered and urine and feces were collected for consecutive 24-h periods, each beginning at the same hour of the morning with ingestion of the daily dose of digoxin. In subjects V and P, digoxin was discontinued; plasma was sampled and urine and feces were collected daily for 9 days after the last dose. Creatinine excretion was measured to monitor the completeness of 24-h urine collections. All samples were stored at $-20°$C until analyzed.

Table 4.1. Characteristics of subjects

	Subject		
	V	Y	P
Age, years	42	50	24
Sex	M	F	F
Weight (kg)	63	71	84
Creatinine clearance (ml/min)	135	109	115
Daily dose of digoxin (mg)	0.50	0.25	0.25

Results

Steady-State Data

The average daily excretion of digoxin during maintenance on the drug represented only 21%-55% of the daily dose (Table 4.2). Most of the excreted digoxin (71%-94%) appeared in the urine, and only 1%-16% of the dose was excreted in the stool. Fully 45%-79% (113-395 µg) of the daily dose was not recovered in the form of chemically authentic digoxin, and since the subjects were in a well-established steady state of maintenance on the drug and were physiologically stable, these fractions of the daily dose must have undergone biotransformation. Even in the subject with hepatic insufficiency, 45% of the daily dose was bio-transformed. Average plasma digoxin concentrations were in the range previously reported by others for maintenance therapy (Table 4.2).

The average daily excretion in urine and feces of compounds containing digoxigenin in acid-hydrolyzable form is shown in Table 4.3 for each of the three subjects. To facilitate comparison with digoxin excretion, the digoxigenin data were converted to nanomoles and expressed as per cent of the daily dose of digoxin, which was 640.3 nmol in subject V and 320.15 nmol in the other two subjects. In each of the subjects, the quantity if digoxigenin recovered from urine or feces after acid hydrolysis agreed closely with and in no case significantly exceeded that present in the form of digoxin. Thus, all of the digoxigenin was analytically derived from the digoxin contained by the excreta, and there was no evidence of excretion of significant amounts of the following putative metabolites of digoxin: digoxigenin didigitoxoside, digoxigenin monodigitoxoside, digoxigenin, and acid-labile conjugates of these compounds or of digoxin itself.

Table 4.2. Average daily excretion and biotransformation of digoxin during daily maintenance on the drug

| | Subject | | | | | |
| | V | | Y | | P | |
	µg	% of dose	µg	% of dose	µg	% of dose
Excretion						
Urine	99	20	94	37	114	46
Feces	6	1	39	16	16	9
Total	105	21	133	53	137	55
Biotransformation	395	79	117	47	113	45
Plasma digoxin (ng/ml)	0.94		0.89		0.58	

Table 4.3. Average daily excretion of digoxin and acid-hydrolyzable derivatives of digoxigenin in per cent of daily dose of digoxin in nanomoles

| | Subject | | | | | |
| | V | | Y | | P | |
	Digoxin	Genin	Digoxin	Genin	Digoxin	Genin
Excretion						
Urine	20	19	37	38	46	44
Feces	1	1	16	16	9	10
Total	21	20	53	54	55	54
Biotransformation	79	80	47	46	45	46

These independent analyses of acid-hydrolyzable derivatives of digoxigenin confirmed the conclusion derived from the digoxin data that 46%-80% of the daily dose of digoxin was biotransformed in the body and further indicated that in the process of biotransformation, the digoxigenin moiety of the molecule was chemically modified.

That this chemical modification of digoxigenin did not simply consist of conjugation with glucuronic acid or sulfate was evidenced by the results of the analyses of urine incubated with β-glucuronidase and sulfatase in stoichiometrically excessive concentrations. No additional digoxin was released by enzymic hydrolysis, and enzymic treatment followed by acid hydrolysis yielded no additional digoxigenin. During the 4 days for which all data were available, the average and range of daily urinary excretion of digoxin, digoxin after enzymic deconjugation, acid-hydrolyzable derivatives of digoxigenin, and acid-hydrolyzable derivatives of digoxigenin after enzymic deconjugation, all in per cent of the daily nanomolar dose of digoxin, in each of the subjects are shown in Figure 4.1. The values did not differ significantly ($P > 0.5$) in any of the subjects.

The quantities of 3-epidigoxigenin recovered after acid hydrolysis of urine and feces exceeded the blank values of 5-9 pmol/50 ml for urine and 5-10 pmol/50 ml for feces. The total quantity excreted daily, however, was small and comprised only 0.32%-1.06% of the daily dose in nanomoles (Table 4.4). Recovery of 3-epidigoxigenin was not significantly increased by prior incubation of urine with glucuronidase and sulfatase.

Data Obtained After Discontinuing Digoxin

After the administration of digoxin was discontinued in subjects V and P, plasma concentration and daily urinary and fecal excretion of digoxin decreased monoexponentially and in parallel during the ensuing 8-9 days (Figs. 4.2 and 4.3).

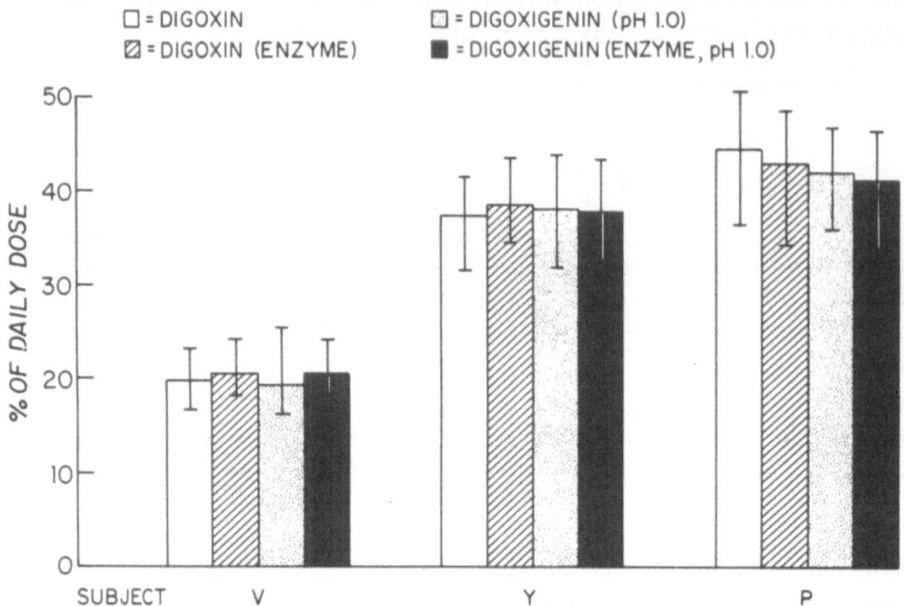

Fig. 4.1. Daily urinary excretion of digoxin and digoxigenin released by acid hydrolysis of urine at pH 1.0 in three subjects maintained on digoxin by mouth. The analyses were performed before and after the urine was incubated with glucuronidase and aryl sulfatase from Helix pomatia. The compounds were measured in nanomoles and are expressed in per cent of the daily dose. The height of each column indicates the average value for 4 days, and the vertical bar denotes the range of values

Table 4.4. Daily excretion of acid-hydrolyzable derivatives of 3-epidigoxigenin in per cent of daily dose of digoxin in nanomoles

	Subject		
	V	Y	P
Urine	0.37	0.94	0.24
Feces	0.07	0.12	0.32
Total	0.44	1.06	0.32

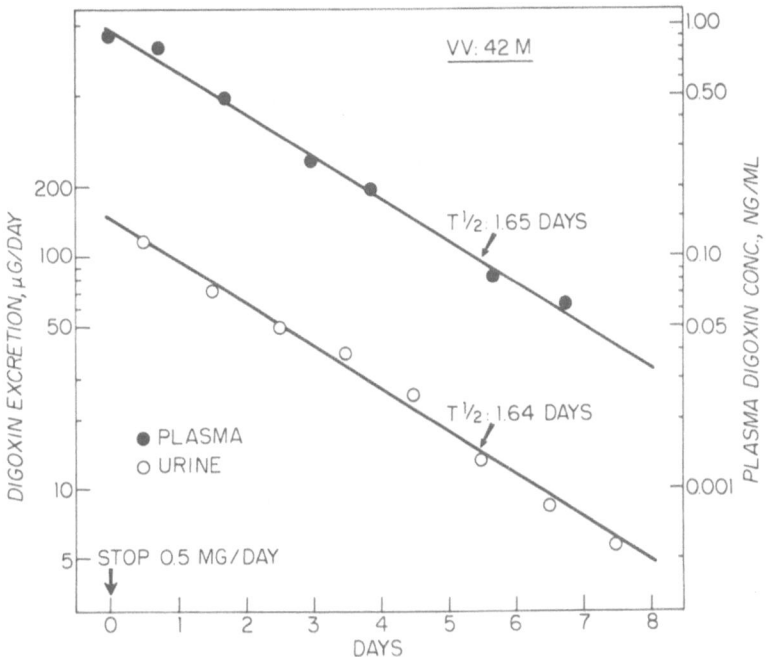

Fig. 4.2. Changes in plasma concentration and daily urinary and fecal excretion of digoxin with time after stopping daily administration of 0.25 mg of digoxin in a patient with chronic liver disease due to hepatitis. The ordinate scales are logarithmic. The half-life (T 1/2) for each parameter of persistence of the drug in the body is shown

In subject V, the half-lives were 1.65 days for plasma and 1.64 days for urine (Fig. 4.2); his stools were too infrequent and scanty in volume for reliable estimation of digoxin half-life. The half-lives of digoxin in plasma, urine, and feces of subject P were almost identical (average: 1.42 days) (Fig. 4.3).

The cumulative amounts of digoxin (integrated to infinity) that were excreted in urine and feces after the last dose of the drug are shown in Table 4.5 in micrograms and in per cent of the body pool of digoxin that was established during daily maintenance on the drug. The body pool of digoxin, as calculated from the daily dose and the half-life of the drug (Lukas, 1973 a), was 1492 μg in subject V and 658 μg in subject P. Of the body pool of digoxin 23%-56% was excreted as chemically intact digoxin, and the rest appeared to have been metabolized. In both subjects, the measurements of the disposition of digoxin from the body pool by urinary excretion, fecal excretion, and biotransformation were in very close agreement with those observed during the steady state of maintenance on the drug (Table 4.2 and 4.3).

The cumulative excretion of acid-hydrolyzable derivatives of digoxigenin in urine and feces did not exceed excretion of digoxin (Table 4.6). As in the case of the

43

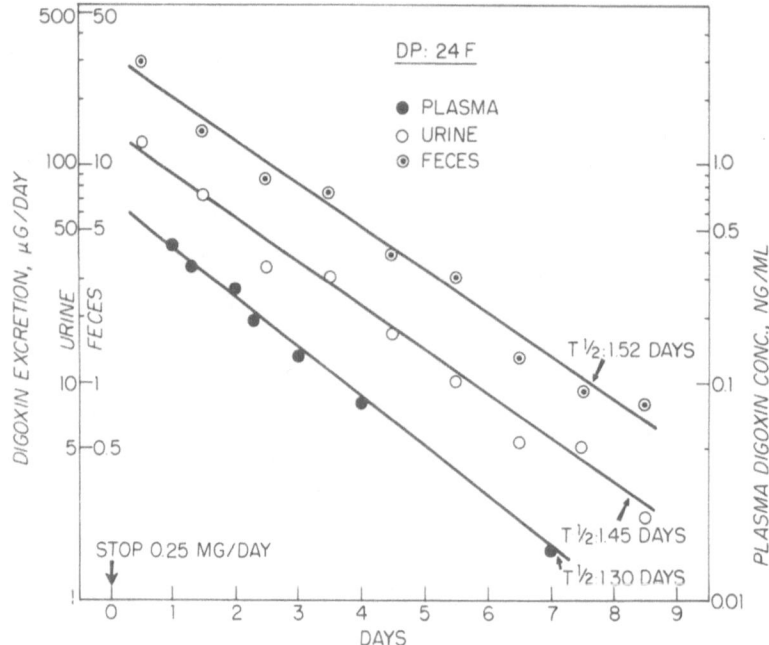

Fig. 4.3. Changes in plasma concentration and daily urinary excretion of digoxin in a 42-year-old man after daily administration of 0.5 mg of digoxin was discontinued. The ordinate is logarithmic. The half-life (T 1/2) for each parameter of persistence of the drug in the body is shown

Table 4.5. Cumulative excretion and biotransformation of digoxin in micrograms and per cent of body pool of digoxin after stopping daily administration of drug

	Subject			
	V (pool: 1492 μg)		P (pool: 658 μg)	
	μg	% of pool	μg	% of pool
Excretion				
Urine	308	21	314	47
Feces	27	2	61	9
Total	335	23	365	56
Biotransformation	1157	77	293	44

Table 4.6. Cumulative excretion of digoxin and acid-hydrolyzable derivatives of Digoxigenin after stopping daily administration of drug

| | Subject | | | |
| | V | | P | |
	Digoxin	Genin	Digoxin	Genin
Urine (nmol)	394	364	389	361
Feces (nmol)	35	36	86	86
Total (nmol)	429	400	475	447
% of body pool	23	21	56	53

steady-state studies, all of the digoxigenin was excreted in the form of digoxin; thus, there was no evidence of excretion of other digitoxosides or acid-labile derivatives of digoxigenin.

Excretion of 3-epidigoxigenin in urine and feces also declined after digoxin was discontinued, but since samples from only 3 separate days were analyzed for 3-epidigoxigenin and the amounts were small, cumulative excretion of this compound was not quantified.

Discussion

The specifity of the double isotope dilution derivative method for digoxin is achieved by subjecting the glycoside to multiple procedures designed to isolate it in pure form, first in its native chemical state and then after it has been converted to a unique derivative (Lukas, 1973 c). In the analysis for derivatives of digoxigenin, specificity is enhanced by submitting the compounds to two chemical reactions: acid hydrolysis and conversion of the liberated digoxigenin to digoxigenin diacetate.

It should be acknowledged, however, that completely unambiguous proof of the specificity of these methods when they are applied to samples obtained from subjects given digoxin cannot be provided until all of the biotransformation products of the glycoside have been unequivocally characterized. It is entirely possible for a metabolite to invade the zones of chromatographic migration of the parent glycoside, especially in the presence of heavy residues extracted from urine and feces, and for it to be acetylated to a derivative that subsequently cannot be completely separated from the acetate of the parent compound even by multiple chromatographies in different solvent systems.

In the present study, confidence in the specificity of the data was enhanced by the fortuitous, quantitative agreement between the measurements of digoxin and the assays of acid-hydrolyzable derivatives of digoxigenin. Although the results will require confirmation by studies of additional subjects, they do focus on a number of issues.

The present data indicate that digoxin is more extensively biotransformed in the body than previously estimated. Studies of the disposition of orally administered ^{3}H-digoxin have generally concluded that 85%-90% of the dose is excreted in its original chemical form and that only 10%-15% is metabolically altered (Doherty, 1968, 1973; Marcus et al., 1966). In our subjects, approximately 50% of the drug was chemically modified, and the rate of biotransformation of digoxin equalled or exceeded urinary excretion of the intact glycoside.

In a previous study, normal half-lives for digoxin were found in three patients with cirrhosis of the liver and were regarded as further evidence of the minor role played by the liver, as compared to the kidneys, in the disposition of the drug (Marcus and Kapadia, 1964). In our subject with hepatic cirrhosis, the normal half-life for digoxin was equally attributable to preservation of her capacity to biotransform digoxin and to the ability of her kidneys to excrete the drug.

The end-products of the metabolic conversion of digoxin were not identified. Neither urine or feces contained significant quantities of the di- or monodigitoxoside of digoxigenin, digoxigenin, conjugates of these compounds, or of digoxin itself. Since all of the digoxigenin released by acid hydrolysis of urine and feces and by sequential enzymic and acid hydrolyses of urine was derived from digoxin, it appears that the genin portion of the molecule had undergone one or more chemical conversions.

Simple epimerization at C-3 of the genin, as our studies show, represented a quantitatively minor reaction. The possibility of metabolic attack on the lactone ring has received some support from the identification by other investigators of significant amounts of dihydrodigoxin in the urine of some patients receiving digoxin (Luchi and Gruber, 1968; Watson et al., 1973). The existence of a conjugate resistant to enzymic and acid hydrolysis remains to be excluded.

Our previous studies led to remarkably similar conclusions concerning the disposition of digitoxin. We found that after a single 1.0-mg dose and during steady-state maintenance on digitoxin, 50%-75% of the drug is biotransformed and that the excretory end-products of metabolic conversion do not consist of digitoxosides of either digitoxigenin (other than digitoxin) or digoxigenin, free digitoxigenin or digoxigenin, or acid-labile conjugates of any of these compounds (Lukas, 1971; 1973 a, b). Vöhringer and Rietbrock, however, have reported that small quantities of a tritium-labeled compound with the chromatographic mobility of digitoxigenin monodigitoxoside were released by glucuronidase and sulfatase from urine of subjects to whom ^{3}H-digitoxin had been administered (Vöhringer and Rietbrock, 1974).

It has been tacitly assumed that the bioavailability of digoxin in the standard tablet preparation (Lanoxin, Burroughs Wellcome), which has been estimated as equivalent to 50%-70% of the intravenous preparation, is mainly limited by incomplete intestinal absorption (Greenblatt et al., 1973; Huffman et al., 1974;

Marcus et al., 1976). Our data, however, demonstrate that only 1%-16% of the daily dose was recovered from the feces, and even this fraction probably did not arise entirely from incomplete absorption of the daily dose since fecal excretion of digoxin persisted after administration of the glycoside was discontinued. At least 84%-99% of the daily dose, therefore, appeared to have been absorbed by our subjects.

It seems possible that obligatory passage of digoxin through the liver before it enters the peripheral plasma rather than incomplete intestinal absorption primarily limits the bioavailability of soluble oral preparations of the drug. During its initial passage through the liver, hepatic uptake and chemical transformation of digoxin may be enhanced by mechanisms similar to those producing a "first pass effect" with other drugs. Biotransformation of ingested digoxin may begin with cleavage of digitoxose residues from the compound by gastric acid and intestinal bacteria, but the extent of such hydrolysis has been reported to be small (Beermann et al., 1972), and the feces of our subjects did not contain measureable quantities of digoxigenin digitoxosides other than digoxin itself.

A final point concerns the pharmacokinetic behavior of digoxin. After prolonged daily maintenance on the drug was stopped, all parameters of persistence of the drug decreased in simple exponential fashion over a period that encompassed five to six half-lives of the drug. Thus, there was no evidence that significant amounts of digoxin had been sequestered in a slowly exchanging body compartment for the drug. The existence of such a compartment for metabolites of digoxin, however, was not excluded.

References

Beermann, B., Hellström, K., Rosen, A.: The absorption of orally administered 12α-³H-digoxin in man. Clin.Sci. 43, 507 (1972)

Bougas, J., Flood, C., Little, B., Tait, J.F., Tait, S.A.S., Underwood, R.: Dynamic aspects of aldosterone metabolism. In: Aldosterone. Baulieu, E.E., Robel, P., (eds.) Philadelphia: F.A. Davis, 1964, p. 25

Doherty, J.E.: The clinical pharmacology of digitalis glycosides: A review. Am.J.Med.Sci. 255, 382 (1968)

Doherty, J.E.: Digoxin: present knowledge of pharmacokinetics and pharmacodynamics. In: Symposium on Digitalis. Storstein, O., (ed.) Oslo: Gyldendal Norsk Forlag 1973, p. 419

Greenblatt, D.J., Duhme, D.W., Koch-Weser, J., Smith, T.W.: Evaluation of digoxin bioavailability in single-dose studies. N.Engl.J.Med. 289, 651 (1973)

Huffman, D.H., Mannion, C.V., Azarnoff, D.L.: Absorption of digoxin from different oral preparations in normal subjects during steady state. Clin.Pharmacol.Ther. 16, 310 (1974)

Luchi, R.J., Gruber, J.W.: Unusually large digitalis requirements. A study of altered digoxin metabolism. Am.J.Med. 45, 322 (1968)

Lukas, D.S.: Some aspects of the distribution and disposition of digitoxin in man.

In: Drug Metabolism in Man. Vesell, E.S., (ed.) Ann.N.Y.Acad.Sci. <u>179</u>, 388 (1971)

Lukas, D.S.: The pharmacokinetics and metabolism of digitoxin in man. In: Symposium on Digitalis. Storstein, O., (ed.) Oslo: Gyldendal Norsk Forlag 1973 a, p. 84

Lukas, D.S.: The role of the liver in the chemical transformation of digitoxin. In: Symposium on Digitalis. Storstein, O., (ed.) Oslo: Gyldendal Norsk Forlag 1973 b, p. 192

Lukas, D.S.: Double isotope dilution derivative assay of digitoxin, digoxin, and their genins. In: Symposium on Digitalis. Storstein, O., (ed.) Oslo: Gyldendal Norsk Forlag 1973 c, p. 18

Lukas, D.S., Peterson, R.E.: Determination of digitoxin in plasma by double isotope dilution derivative assay. J.Clin.Invest. <u>43</u>, 1942 (1964)

Lukas, D.S., Peterson, R.E.: Double isotope dilution derivative assay of digitoxin in plasma, urine, and stool of patients maintained on the drug. J.Clin.Invest. <u>45</u>, 782 (1966)

Marcus, F.I., Kapadia, G.G.: The metabolism of tritiated digoxin in cirrhotic patients. Gastroenterology <u>45</u>, 517 (1964)

Marcus, F.I., Burkhalter, L., Cuccia, C., Pavlovich, J., Kapadia, G.G.: Administration of tritiated digoxin with and without a loading dose. A metabolic study. Circulation <u>34</u>, 865 (1966)

Marcus, F.I., Dickerson, J., Pippin, S., Stafford, M., Bressler, R.: Digoxin bioavailability: Formulations and rates of infusions. Clin.Pharmacol.Ther. <u>20</u>, 253 (1976)

Reichstein, T., Weiss, E.: The sugars of the cardiac glycosides. Adv.Carbohyd. Chem. <u>17</u>, 65 (1962)

Vöhringer, H.F., Rietbrock, N.: Metabolism and excretion of digitoxin in man. Clin.Pharmacol.Ther. <u>16</u>, 796 (1974)

Watson, E., Clark, D.R., Kalman, S.M.: Identification by gas chromatography-mass spectroscopy of dihydrodigoxin — a metabolite of digoxin in man. J.Pharmacol.Exp.Ther. <u>184</u>, 424 (1973)

Discussion

Kuhlmann, Berlin: What was your recovery in urine and feces after 7 days, and have you measured the urinary and fecal excretion over a longer period of time to detect the terminal excretion half-life which may reflect the excretion from a deep compartment?

Lukas: We measured cumulative excretion of digitoxin for 8-9 days in these two subjects and extrapolated to infinity; so the data were obtained over a period that exceded 7 days. Total body stores were theoretic body stores, derived from application of the usual pharmacokinetic principle relating dose and half-life to body stores of the drug. As we showed, the fraction of the body pool that was excreted after the drug was stopped was identical with the fraction of the daily dose that was excreted during daily, steady-state maintenance. These data were obtained by measuring chemically intact digoxin. Also, measurements of acid, hydrolyzable derivatives of digoxigenin expressed in per cent of the body stores or per cent of the daily dose were in close agreement and showed that all of the digoxigenin recoverable from urine and feces was in the form of digoxin. I want to emphasize that we have not ruled out excretion of a conjugate that is resistant to hydrolysis. There are some conjugates of steroids that resist enzymic and acid hydrolysis.

Storstein, Norway: I think it's very important that Dr. Lukas has reported on drug metabolism on maintenance dosage, because the findings after a single dose may be quite different from those obtained on a maintenance dosage. I have studied digitoxin metabolism both after a single dose and on maintenance dosage (Clin.Pharm.Ther. 21:125, 1977) by using thin layer chromatography and enzymic cleavage of conjugation bonds to glucuronic and sulfuric acid in combination with the 86 Rb method. In this way, 16-24 metabolites were separated and quantitated. Unchanged digitoxin is the main cardioactive substance in serum from patients on maintenance dosage with digitoxin and after a single dose. The amount of hydroxylated metabolites, however, differs between the two groups. In patients on maintenance dosage, we find hardly any digoxin (less than 1%), but after a single dose, we find 12% as digoxin 24 h after the dose. The metabolic pattern after a single dose is changing with time (Clin.Pharm.Ther. 21:255, 1977) so that it should always be defined by observation time. Around 30% were metabolites conjugated to glucuronic and sulfuric acid.

Marcus, Tuscon: Dr. Lukas, did you mention whether or not digoxin metabolites were present in the plasma?

Lukas: We measured only digoxin in the plasma and did not try to measure hydrolyzable compounds of digoxigenin in plasma. I might point out that we have measured acid-hydrolyzable compounds of digitoxigenin and digoxigenin in plasma of patients receiving digitoxin. The only compound we found was digitoxin itself; we did not detect measurable quantities of other digitoxosides of digitoxigenin or digitoxosides of digoxigenin in the plasma.

Dengler, Bonn: Dr. Lukas, do I interpret you correctly when I conclude that whatever metabolite you have it will be detectable with the RIA? Because very many studies show that in urine you can recover between 60% and 65% if you measure over a period of — let's say — 10 days.

Lukas: Yes, I think that the studies of Drs. Greenblatt, Smith, and Koch-Weser show that after intravenous administration of digoxin, 76% of the dose can be recovered in the urine. However, their data for oral digoxin showed that 50% or even less of the single dose was excreted in the urine. Azarnoff and associates in steady-state maintenance studies recovered 40%-50% of the daily dose in the urine. In his bioavailability studies which call attention to the critical issue of how quickly to administer an intravenous digoxin standard, Dr. Marcus recovered approximately 50% of an oral dose as radioimmunoassayable digoxin in urine. I made no measurements of radioimmunoassayable digoxin in my studies for comparison with the measurements made by the double isotope dilution derivative method.

Grahame-Smith, Oxford: You made the point — if I understood you properly — that probably bioavailability may in fact be clouded by metabolism. The bioavailability problem blew up originally, because tablets were made differently, and then when manufacture of the tablets was restored to the original quality, the problem in terms of plasma levels disappeared. Therefore, bioavailability problems exist pharmaceutically as well as being concerned with biotransformation. At the clinical level, it was the tablet problem rather than the biotransformation problem that was the real problem. Would you agree with that?

Lukas: I certainly agree. I referred to soluble oral preparations of digoxin in my talk, and I should have underlined the word, soluble, for emphasis.

Marcus: Dr. Lukas, am I correct in understanding that you have not been able to find the bis- and monoderivatives of digoxin in urine as an excretory part? I mention this because I know that others have reported to have found this by paper and thin layer chromatography. Gault studied patients with normal and chronic renal disease on maintenance doses and found bis- and monodigitoxosides of digoxin in small amounts.

Lukas: I was very careful not to use "detectable amounts," because it's conceivable that I missed small amounts of these compounds since I measured the total mass of acid-labile compounds of digoxigenin. Of course the situation in uremia may be different, but to be frank I will not be happy with the identification of these compounds until whatever is identified as a mono- or bisdigitoxoside is really shown to contain one or two molecules of digitoxose as well as the genin in its authentic chemical form. So I'd like to see some basic principles of qualitative and quantitative organic chemical analysis applied to the characterization of these metabolites.

Smith, Boston: I am delighted to hear Dr. Lukas' presentation. I think there has been a kind of "emperor's new clothes" syndrome for some time in that we have continued to teach that digoxin is essentially quantitatively excreted unchanged in the urine of patients with normal renal function, despite the fact that our own studies — and I think nearly everyone else's — have consistently demonstrated recovery of about 40%-50% of administered doses either in single dose or steady-state studies. The immunoassayable digoxin which is measured does include some metabolic products in the urine. So I'm most interested to hear these results and look forward to further characterization of these potentially important metabolic products. I might add that such studies may prove to be even more important in patients with chronic renal failure than in patients with normal renal function. Dr. Richard Selden and I, a few years ago, demonstrated in experimental animals (and also obtained some inferential evidence in humans) that ouabain appears to be excreted in feces, or at least appears in bowel contents, in animals with complete interruption of hepatobiliary tract drainage. It appeared to us that ouabain, as in the case of some tricyclic antidepressant compounds, gets into the gut by pathways apart from the biliary tract. I wonder if you would comment on the possibility of this in the case of digoxin, especially in view of your interesting results from your patients with chronic hepatic insufficiency.

Lukas: I really have no information on this issue. I struggled with our data on the disposition of digitoxin, which showed that an appreciable quantity of the drug appeared in the stool in its original chemical form. Our gastroenterologic group suggested that the intestine might excrete digitoxin or that maybe simple shedding of intestinal mucosal cells, which contain a lot of digitoxin, is responsible for the appearance of digitoxin, which is a well-absorbed drug, in the feces.

5 Occurence and Chemical Nature of Polar Water-Soluble Digoxin Metabolites

H. F. BENTHE

Digoxin is excreted primarily by the kidney as an unchanged glycoside. Only in the first hours after oral absorption is there a chloroform-insoluble metabolite fraction detectable in the urine, this phenomenon being first described in 1972 by Dwenger-Haberland (Dwenger and Haberland, 1972). The polar fraction in urine increases to a maximum 4 h after ingestion of the glycoside. At this time, half of the renally excreted amount is not extractable with chloroform. Ten hours after, this fraction decreases to a very low level. The purpose of this study is to describe the time-dependent occurrence of the polar fraction after digoxin, and to compare it with the behavior of digitoxin. Further, we have carried out some analytic work in the polar metabolites of digoxin.

Methods and Materials

Experiments were performed on healthy male volunteers, aged 41-60 years. Three persons received orally 21-22-^{3}H-digitoxin ($\sim$100 μCi) (Haberland and Maerten, 1969) plus 1.4 mg inactive drug and six persons 12-α-^{3}H-digoxin ($\sim$100 μCi) plus 1.6 mg inactive drug. The glycosides were administered in a volume of 4 ml 30% vol/vol ethanol plus 100 ml water. The administration was always 3 h after the last meal.

Urine collections began 30 min after dosing and continued in 1-h intervals up to 12 h, thereafter in longer intervals, terminating after 72 h; 0.2 ml of each urine sample was added to scintillation fluid and directly counted. Following this, the whole urine sample was divided into smaller aliquots, each extracted three times with twice the volume of ethyl acetate. The extract was evaporated to dryness, redissolved in 10 ml methanol, and aliquots of the extract and the nonextractable fraction counted. The complete water-soluble residue was applied to an Amberlite®️ XAD-2 column. After collection of a high polar H_2O fraction, the main ^{3}H activity could be eluated by ethanol (Fig. 5.1). The ethanol fraction was cleaned up on Sephadex®️ LH-20 several times.

After evaporating to dryness, an aliquot was applied to TLC plates whereas most of the residue was dissolved in 5 ml acetate buffer (pH 5.1) and incubated with glucuronidase sulfatase for 48 h at 37°C. Tritium activity was determined, and the whole solution extracted three times with chloroform. The evaporated chloroform

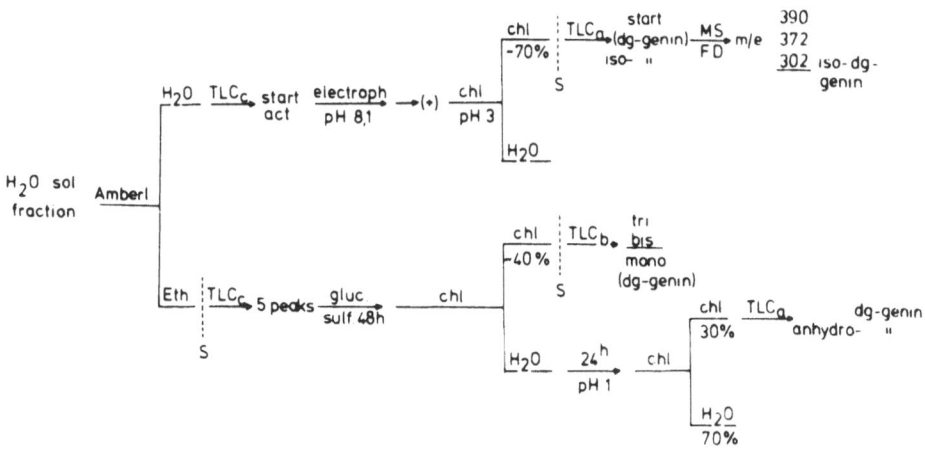

Fig. 5.1. Scheme of extraction and chromatographic partition of the water-soluble fraction in the urine. TLC a, b, c = thin layer chromatography in different solvent systems; electroph. = paper electrophorese, (+) anodic migration, chl = chloroform, gluc-sulf = glucuronidase arylsulfatase, s = clean up on Sephadex LH-20 column

layers were redissolved in methanol and aliquots used for measuring radioactivity and TLC. Aliquots of the remaining aqueous layers were taken for counting.

For further elucidation of the polar fraction, a concentrated aliquot was applied with a pyrophosphate-HCl buffer pH 8.1 to a paper electrophoresis system; radioactivity was located by scanning. TLC was performed on silica gel plates 0.25 mm (Merck). Solvent systems: 1. chloroform methanol 92:8; 2. ethyl acetate; 3. chloroform-methanol-water 64:31:5. The radioactive zones were located with the Berthold scanner II and compared with reference substances after staining with trichloracetic acid. Mass spectrometry was performed on a Varian MAT-311-A instrument equipped with a field desorption electron impact combination ion source.

Results

As already described by Dwenger and Haberland (1972), the water-soluble digoxin metabolites in urine are excreted within the first 24 h. After reaching a maximum between the 2nd and 6th h, the fraction decreases rapidly to a very low level, whereas the total ^{3}H excretion increases further. Figure 5.2 shows the time-dependent relation within the interval from 0-8 h and 0-24 h. Between 8 and 24 h after dosing, the total amount of excreted radioactivity increases averagely from 20%-30% of the dose, whereas the water-soluble fraction only shows small increments within the same time interval.

In different persons, the amount of water-soluble products varied in a range from 6%-13% of the dose. However, there was a remarkable variation in the same person, as seen in Figure 5.2. In the first experiment, 10% of the dose was excreted in form

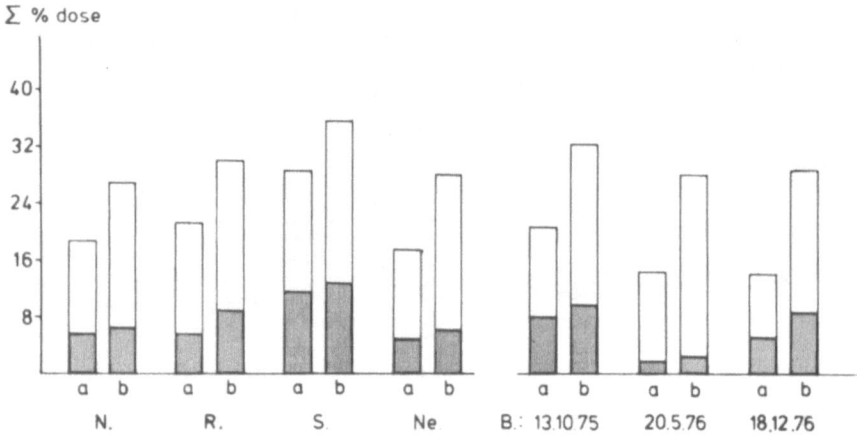

Fig. 5.2. Total amount of ^{3}H activity excreted (open bars) and H$_2$O-soluble fraction (stripped bars) within different time intervals: 0-8 h (a), 0-24 h (b), expressed in percent of dose; left panel: exp. in four healthy volunteers, right panel: three exp. in the same person at different times

of water-soluble metabolites, in the second one only 2.4%, and in the third 8.4%, whereas the total amount of excreted radioactivity in the urine remained nearly constant in the different experiments. For further differentiation, we calculated the excreted rate of renal activity and that of water-soluble products. As seen in Figure 5.3, there was a rapid formation of digoxin metabolites declining to zero at 24 h after oral administration. In contrast to digoxin, the amount of renally excreted digitoxin and its metabolites was much smaller, but there existed a constant relationship between chloroform and water-soluble products over the period of the study (Fig. 5.4). The relative time course of the water-soluble fraction in urine afte digoxin can be described by a very simple Bateman function (Fig. 5.5). This is surprising, since the appearance of the hydrophilic metabolites in the urine provides several steps: absorption, metabolic degradation, and renal elimination.

For further analytic work, we followed the scheme in Figure 5.1. The complete water-soluble residue of each urine sample was applid to Amberlite columns, resulting in partition of a high "polar fraction" by eluating with H$_2$O and a fraction eluated by ethanol (96%). The amount of the high polar fraction increased slowly, the relationship between polar fraction and ethanolic fraction was time dependent, beginning with a quotient 0.2:1, and increasing to 1:1 10 h after administration (Fig. 5.5).

The chromatographic (TLC) investigation of the ethanol fraction is illustrated in Figure 5.6. It could be supposed that the pattern represents glucuronic and sulfate conjugates, but no further separation was carried out. After incubation with glucuronidase arylsulfatase for 48 h, chloroform extraction yields two phases. The chloroform-soluble fraction could be characterized by TLC as bisdigitoxoside mainly; smaller amounts of tri- and monodigitoxosides were detectable. Only a

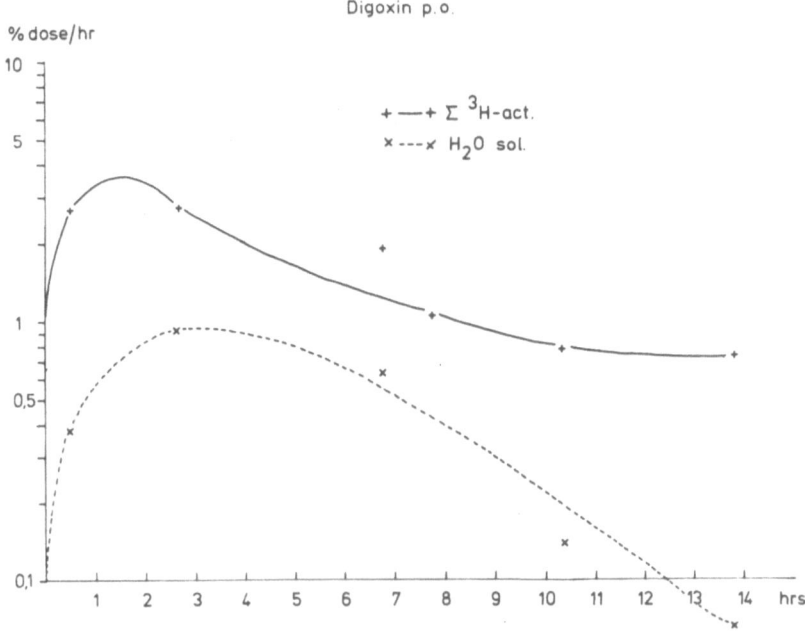

Fig. 5.3. Rate of renal ^{3}H excretion after orally administered 12-α-^{3}H-digoxin
+ --- + total amount of radioactivity
x --- x H$_2$O-soluble fraction

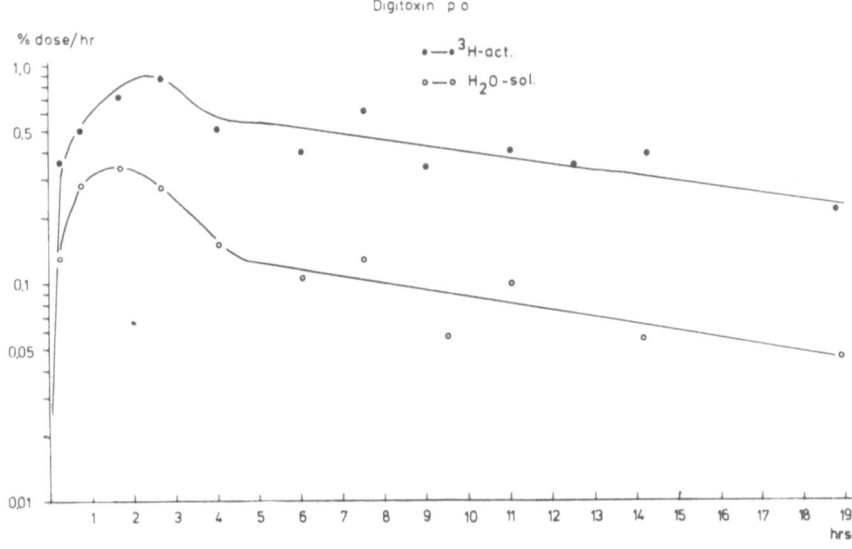

Fig. 5.4. Rate of renal ^{3}H excretion after orally administered ^{3}H-digitoxin
● --- ● total amount of radioactivity
o --- o H$_2$O-soluble fraction

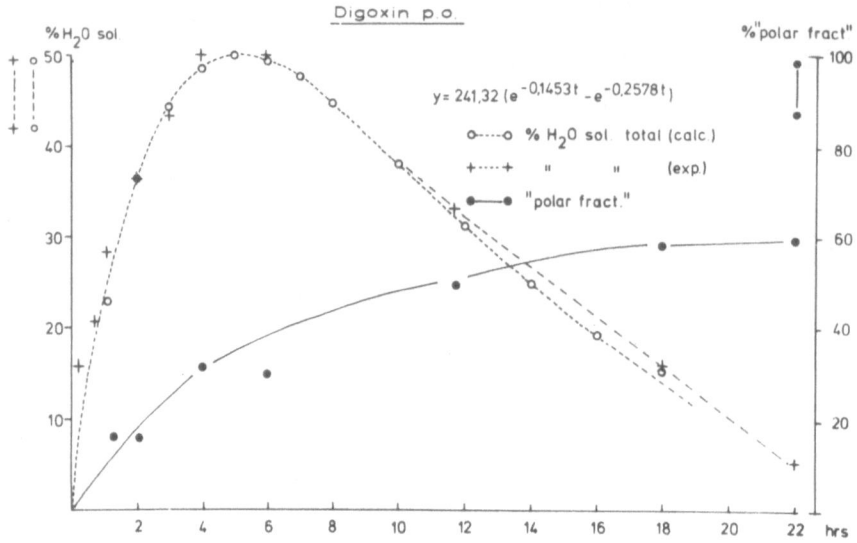

Fig. 5.5. Time-dependent occurrence of H_2O-soluble metabolites after a single dose of digoxin. Left ordinate: + --- + experimental data, o --- o calculated data (Bateman function)

Right ordinate: polar fraction expressed in per cent of the total amount of H_2O-soluble products

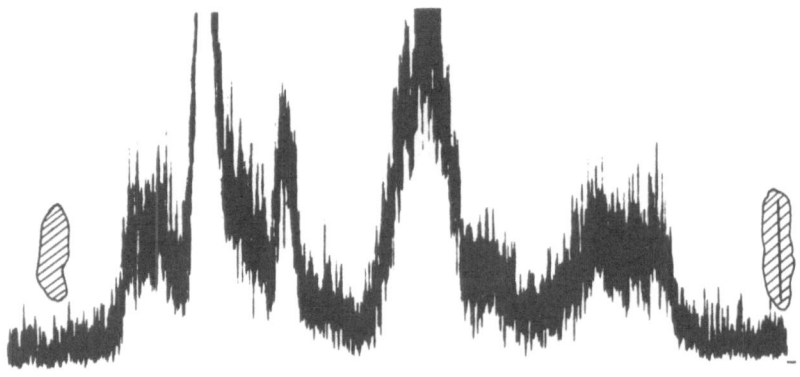

Fig. 5.6. TLC (solvent c) of H_2O-soluble fraction after separation of Amberlite[®] eluated by ethanol, Dg = digoxin as reference substance

part (30%) of the chloroform-insoluble fraction could be hydrolyzed by 1-n-hydrochloric acid. Analysis by TLC (solvent a) showed that peaks of activity were found in the corresponding areas of digoxigenin and anhydrodigoxigenin. There remained an unknown residue (~70%) nonacid hydrolyzable to chloroform-soluble deratives (Fig. 5.1).

Applied to TLC (solvent c), the radioactivity of the polar fraction remained at the start region, and it had to be proved if this compound is of ionogenic nature. Analysis of this fraction achieved by paper electrophoresis and scanning the perogram showed that the predominant peaks of activity migrated in anodic direction. After acidifying (pH ∼3), nearly 70% of the polar fraction became extractable with chloroform. Analyzed by TLC (solvent a), the main peak of radioactivity corresponded to isodigoxigenin (Fig. 5.7). Thereafter, the total amount of chloroform extracts was cleaned up on Sephadex LH-20, and this chromatographic procedure repeated several times until most of the pigments had disappeared. Finally, the combined fractions were evaporated to dryness, redissolved in methanol, and investigated by MS.

All spectra showed the ions m/e 390, 372, and 302; the ion m/e 390 is the molecular ion of digoxigenin. But in contrast to digoxigenin, there is only a weak signal at 354, whereas m/e 302 is of highest intensity (Fig. 5.8). This could be identified as a characteristic fragmentation peak of isodigoxigenin, due to the combined loss of acetate and carbonyl (Fig. 5.9).

Discussion

The total amount of renally excreted radioactivity after ingestion of ^{3}H-digitoxin and ^{3}H-digoxin, respectively, differs remarkably. After digitoxin on the average 9%, and after digoxin 28%-35% of the dose are detectable in the urine on the 1st day (Dwenger and Haberland, 1972; Kuhlmann et al., 1974; Lukas and Peterson, 1966;

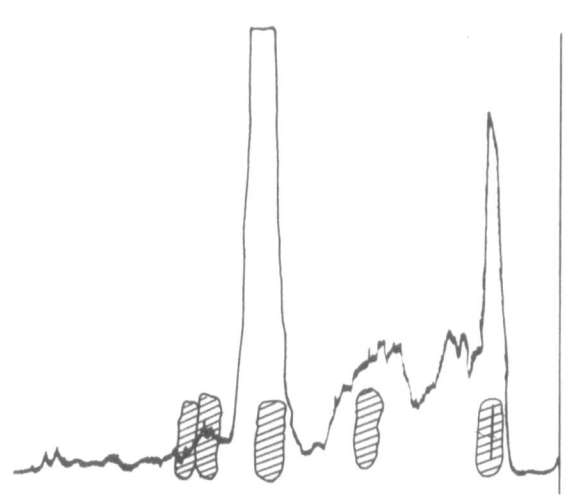

Fig. 5.7. TLC (solvent a) of chloroform-soluble products of the acidified polar fraction. Reference substance: digoxigenin, isodigoxigenin, anhydrodigoxigenin

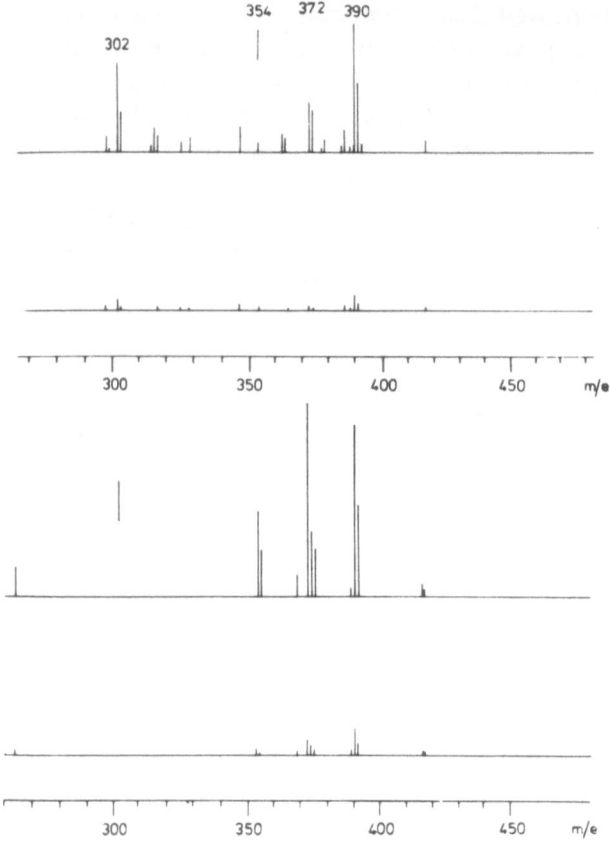

Fig. 5.8. Lower part: mass spectrum of digoxigenin ($M^+ = 390$)
Upper part: mass spectrum of chloroform-soluble products of the acidified polar
fraction. Note the fragment ion m/302, not present in the spectrum of digoxigenin

Dg-genin

Dg-genin-acid
"polar fraction"

$M^\cdot - 60$

$M^\cdot - 28$

Iso-dg-genin

pH~3

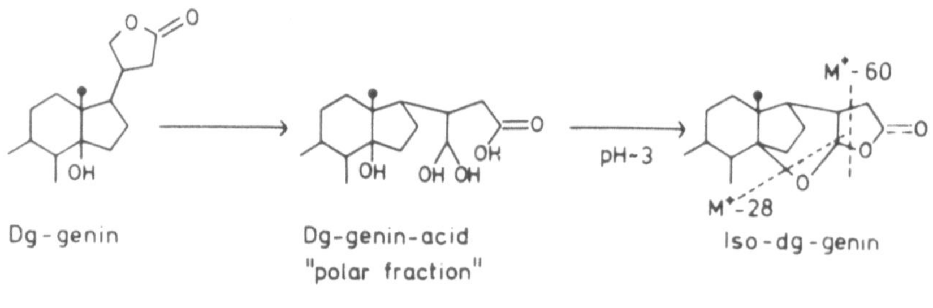

Fig. 5.9. Diagram illustrating the formation of digoxigeninacid (polar fraction),
relactonizing by acid and MS fragmentation pattern delivering the ion m/e = 302
($M^+ = 82$)

Marcus, 1973; Marcus et al., 1966; Zilly et al., 1975). The part of the nonchloroform-soluble metabolites varied in the same range. In the case of digitoxin, 26% of the daily excreted amount is of polar nature (Vöhringer and Rietbrock, 1974), whereas after digoxin this level was only reached during the 1st day; thereafter the polar fraction declined to a scarcely detectable level. The same relationship was obtained comparing the excretion velocity.

We assume a high digoxin blood concentration to be necessary for the formation of polar metabolites. This high concentration is only reached during the first hours after absorption, whereas the plasma concentration of digitoxin remains ten or more times greater. Since the protein binding of a drug does not prevent degradation by metabolism, there will be at all times a sufficient gradient of diffusion to enter the metabolizing compartment of the hepatic cell. The time-dependent course of the total water-soluble fraction in urine after digoxin is following the simple Bateman function with the maximum between 2 and 6 h after ingestion (Fig. 5.5).

By column chromatography, a high polar fraction could be separated from the total H_2O-soluble products. This fraction increased much slower, reaching a peak level after 24 h (Fig. 5.5). The proportion of the polar fraction increased from 20% during the 1st hour to 60% after 24 h. Qualitative analytic examination provides indirect evidence that the high polar fraction of digoxigenic acid seems to exist, formed by a lactonase activity in metabolic degradation.

Comparing the quantitative relationship, it could be summarized that the total amount of H_2O-soluble products in the urine after a single oral dose of digoxin fluctuated about 15%. About 30% of these products consisted of a high polar fraction formed by the occurrence of digoxigenic acid. Part of the ethanolic fraction could be identified as conjugates of glucuronides and sulfates of bisdigitoxosides. However, in both fractions there remained a nonacid hydrolyzable residue not delivering chloroform-soluble fragments.

References

Dwenger, A., Haberland, G.: Metabolism of ^{3}H-digoxin and some acetyldigoxins: time dependend formation of hydrophylic metabolites after oral application in man. Naunyn Schmiedeberg's Arch. Pharmakol. 273, 154-167 (1972)

Haberland, G., Maerten, C.: Ein spezifischer Deuterium- und Tritium-Austausch in Cardenoliden und Cardenolid-Glykosiden. Naturwissenschaften 56, 516 (1969)

Kuhlmann, J., Abshagen, U., Rietbrock, N.: Pharmacokinetics and metabolism of digoxigeninmonodigitoxosid in man. Eur. J. Clin. Pharmacol. 7, 87-94 (1974)

Lukas, D., Peterson, R.E.: Double isotope dilution derivative assay of digitoxin in plasma, urine and stool of patients maintained of the drug. J. Clin. Invest. 45, 782-795 (1966)

Marcus, F.J.: Metabolism of digoxin in normal man and factors influencing the body distribution. In: Symposium on Digitalis, Oslo 1973, p. 112

Marcus, F.J., Peterson, A., Salel, A., Scully, J., Kapadia, G.G.: The metabolism of tritiated digoxin in renal insufficiency in dogs and man. J. Pharmacol. Exp. Ther. 152, 372-382 (1966)

Vöhringer, H.F., Rietbrock, N.: Metabolism and excretion of digitoxin in man. Clin. Pharmacol. Ther. 16, 796-806 (1974)

Zilly, W., Richter, E., Rietbrock, N.: Pharmacokinetics and metabolism of digoxin- and β-methyl-digoxin 12-^{3}H in patients with acute hepatitis. Clin. Pharmacol. Ther. 17, 302-309 (1975)

Discussion

Dengler, Bonn: Dr. Benthe, I may not have gotten the figure, can you calculate or at least give some estimates of the amount of isodigoxin excreted in your experiments?

Benthe: No, we can calculate only averagely the amount, because we lost a lot of activity in each clean-up step, and I think about 30% of the water-soluble residue consists of a metabolite with an open lactone ring configuration.

Belz, Koblenz: I think it will be important to know if the polar metabolites are active in respect to the biologic properties. We had the possibility to check quite a lot of chemically synthetized polar digoxin and digitoxin metabolites, glucuronides, and sulfates (Fig. 1). On the abscissa you see the glycoside concentration which is necessary to induce half maximal inhibition of ^{86}Rb uptake of human erythrocytes IC_{50}, M), and on the ordinate, you see the concentration which is necessary to induce a doubling of the contractile force of guinea pig papillary muscle ($C_{+100\%}$, M). Substance No. 1 reflects digoxin, and No. 2 digoxin glucuronide. You see there is not a great difference in the biologic activity of these two substances. Let us now have a look at the genins (substance 5: digoxigenin, substance 6: digoxigenin glucuronide). The inactivation produced by binding to glucurone acid increases to a larger extent if we approach the genins. Another interesting fact — only mentioned additionally — is the very good correlation between the influence on the active cation transport and on the contractile force of the heart.

Schaumann, Mannheim: If I remember correctly, Rietbrock claimed that practically the whole water-soluble fraction consisted of glucuronides and sulfates of digoxigenin monodigitoxoside. But that is not in agreement with your results.

Benthe: No, we found mainly the conjugates of bisdigitoxide.

Kuhlmann: Digoxigenin monodigitoxoside could be found as the main conjugation product of glucuronic acid in rats (Abshagen et al., Naunyn-Schmiedeberg's Arch., 1973) and after administration of β-methyldigoxin and digoxigenin monodigitoxoside in humans (Rietbrock et al., Europ. J. clin. Pharmacol. 9, 105, 1975; Kuhlmann et al., Europ. J. clin. Pharmacol., 1974).

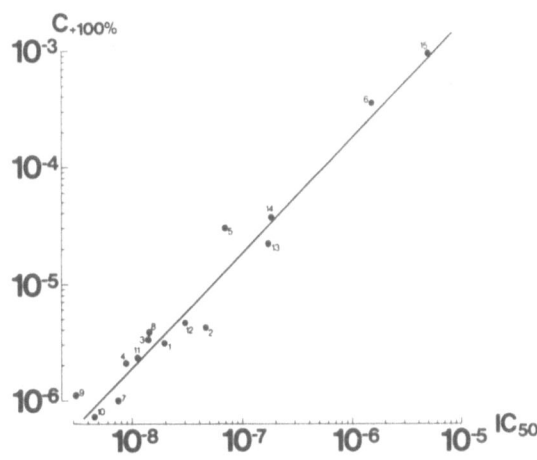

Fig. 1. Influence of polar and nonpolar digoxin and digitoxin metabolites on ^{86}Rb uptake of human erythrocytes and contractility of isolated guinea pig papillary muscle
Substances: 1 = digoxin; 2 = digoxin glucuronide; 3 = digoxigenin bisdigitoxoside; 4 = digoxigenin monodigitoxoside; 5 = digoxigenin; 6 = digoxigenin glucuronide; 7 = digitoxin; 8 = digitoxin glucuronide; 9 = digitoxin bisdigitoxoside; 10 = digitoxin monodigitoxoside; 11 = digitoxigenin monodigitoxoside glucuronide; 12 = digitoxigenin; 13 = digitoxigenin glucuronide; 14 = digitoxigenin sulfate; 15 = epidigitoxigenin glucuronide

I would like to ask if you can explain the high amount of H_2O-soluble fraction during the first hours? Is it due to the high glycoside uptake by the liver?

Benthe: We have done no experiments during maintenance therapy. I think an explanation could be that only a short time after absorption, the digoxin concentration will be high enough to enter the metabolizing compartments of the liver where the water-soluble products are formed. As I said we have no data about the relationship of water-soluble metabolites under maintenance therapy.

Kuhlmann: In our steady-state experiments in dogs the H_2O-soluble fraction in urine and feces is constant also after cessation of the multiple doses.

Kramer, Göttingen: Concerning the excretion of polar metabolites during the first hours in your patients, I have one question. How did you exclude that your digoxin preparation administered by the oral route did not contain some polar metabolites which were excreted with a higher renal clearance than digoxin itself?

Benthe: I think we can exclude this possibility from the setup of our experiments.

Flasch, Hamburg: We also examined a number of polar derivatives of digoxin and digitoxin, especially glucuronides and sulfates, some of which are discussed as possible metabolites of the two glycosides. Cardenolide glycosides are prepared by the reaction with acetobromglucose, secondly the hydroxymethyl group of the glucose moiety is oxidized in presence of a platinium catalyst to the carboxyl group of the final glucuronic acid. Sulfates are prepared by direct reaction of the cardenolides with chlorosulfonic acid.

In Table 1 you see the solubilities of the conjugates in water and chloroform and the octanol/water partition coefficients (P). Great differences in the physico-chemical character could be seen in comparing the values of digoxin and digoxin-16'-glucuronide: digoxin is about six times more soluble in chloroform than in water, the water solubility of the glucuronide is 10^5 times higher than the chloroform solubility. The differences in the other pairs of glycoside/conjugate are similar.

The affinity of the highly water-soluble glycoside conjugates to digoxin antibodies is of some interest for radioimmunologic digoxin estimation (Fig. 2). In the graph you see the concentration of antibody-bound digoxin-^{3}H dependent upon the concentration of cross-reacting digoxin conjugate: the glucuronides of digoxin and digitoxin compete with the labeled digoxin to the antibody nearly in the same manner as digoxin itself. In contrast, digoxigenin-3.12-disulfate shows a marked increase in cross-reactivity (Table 2) caused by the structural change in the genin part of the molecule.

These findings are in agreement with the results of Dr. Gundert-Remy.

Table 1. Solubilities and distribution coefficients of several cardenolide conjugates

Cardenolide	Water solubility g/l	Chloroform solubility g/l	P n-octanol/ water
Ouabain	11.1	0.002	0.01
Digoxin	0.4	0.25	18
Digoxin-16'-glucuronide[a]	36.9	< 0.0002	0.02
Digitoxin	0.008	14	70
Digitoxin-16'-glucuronide[a]	33.4	0.0004	1.4
Digitoxigenin-mono-Digitoxoside	0.092	107	390
Digitoxigenin-mono-Digitoxoside-Glucuronide[a]	—	—	0.05
Digitoxigenin	0.064	67	250
Digitoxigenin-glucuronide[a]	36.4	0.0005	ca. 0.1
Digitoxigenin-sulfate[a]	65.1[b]	0.0004	0.62
Epidigitoxigenin-sulfate[a]	6.7	0.0002	0.73

[a] During determination of P, Na salt was used instead of water in 0.05 m phosphate buffer pH 7.4.

[b] K salt 27.9.

Table 2

Antigen	Molar antigen concentration for a 50% suppression			Cross-reactivity %
Digoxin	8.5	·	10^{-9}	100
20.22-dihydrodigoxin	2.5	·	10^{-7}	3.4
Digoxin-16'-glucuronide	1.7	·	10^{-8}	50.0
Digoxigenin	9.5	·	10^{-9}	89.5
Digoxigenin-3-glucuronide	1.0	·	10^{-8}	85.0
Digoxigenin-3.12 disulfate	2.6	·	10^{-7}	3.3
Digitoxin	9.0	·	10^{-8}	9.4
Digitoxin-16'-glucuronide	1.2	·	10^{-7}	7.1
Digitoxigenin-mono-Digitoxoside	1.4	·	10^{-7}	6.1
Digitoxigenin-mono-Digitoxoside-4'-Glucuronide	1.6	·	10^{-7}	5.3
Digitoxigenin	1.0	·	10^{-7}	8.5
3-epidigitoxigenin	4.0	·	10^{-7}	2.1
Epidigitoxigenin-3-sulfate		$> 10^{-6}$		

Antigen concentrations, which cause a 50% suppression of the digoxin-^{3}H by digoxin antibody (reduction of the digoxin-^{3}H binding from 45% to 22.5%).

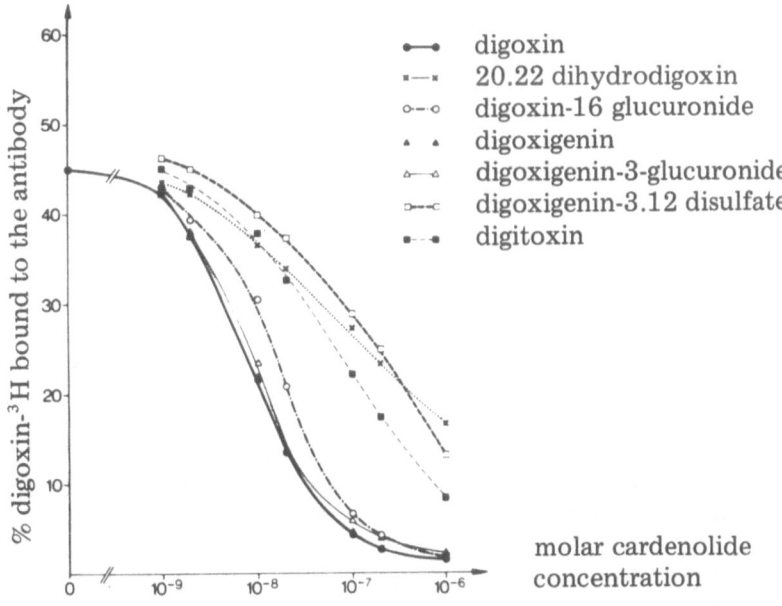

Fig. 2. The binding curves for digoxin-^{3}H to digoxin antibody in the presence of different cardenolide metabolites

6 Pharmacokinetics and Metabolism of Digitoxin in the Human

H. F. VÖHRINGER and N. RIETBROCK

The present knowledge of pharmacokinetics and metabolism of digitoxin in man, derived from single dose (Caldwell et al., 1971; Doherty, 1968; Kramer et al., 1970; Lahrtz et al., 1969; Okita et al., 1953, 1955; Vöhringer and Rietbrock, 1974; Weissler et al., 1966) as well as from multiple dose studies (Jelliffe, 1967; Lukas, 1971, 1973; Peters et al., 1975; Solomon et al., 1971; Storstein, 1974; Wirth et al., 1976) using different methods, can be characterized as follows:

1. The elimination of digitoxin with a half-life of 6-8 days in plasma and urine is very slow.
2. The metabolism of digitoxin in man is assumed to occur with a cleavage of digitoxose side chains, with a β-hydroxylation of digitoxin to digoxin, and with a formation of polar compounds. However, there is controversy in the literature as to exactly how far digitoxin is quantitatively metabolized. Therefore, in this paper new data on digitoxin kinetics are presented during maintenance therapy.

Methods and Material

Five volunteers with normal renal and hepatic function were orally digitalized with a loading dose of 0.6 mg digitoxin (Digimerck®) for 2 days and a maintenance dose of 0.1 mg per day. On the 7th, 8th, and 9th days a tracer dose of 30 μCi random labeled ^{3}H-digitoxin with a specific activity of 1 mCi/0.038 mg (Nen, Boston, USA) was additionally administered p.o. A venous blood sample was drawn every 24 h after the last dose, while specimens of urine and feces were collected at daily intervals from day 8 until 11 after the tracer dose was given.

The plasma concentrations of digitoxin were measured by radioimmunoassay (GammaCoat Radioimmunoassay Kit of Clinical Assay Inc., Cambridge, USA). The extraction procedure, TLC, and determination of radioactivity for the samples of blood, urine, and feces were the same as described previously (Vöhringer and Rietbrock, 1974). The TLC was performed on silica gel plates (Merck, Darmstadt, West Germany), 0.25 mm layer, flow distance 15 cm. Solvent system I: diisopropylether/methanol (9:1), five times; solvent system II: methylethylketone/xylene (1:1), two times on formamide/acetone precoated TLC plates (Storstein, 1976).

Results

Figure 6.1 a shows a rapid increase of the glycoside plasma concentration after digitalization with 0.6 mg for 2 days followed by 0.1 mg per day. After 72 h a mean steady-state plasma level of 22 ng/ml is reached in four subjects. During steady state, the plasma concentrations vary with a mean variation coefficient of 15%. The higher plasma level of digitoxin in subject III may be due to the low body weight of 48 kg compared to 68.7 ±3.1 kg in the other four subjects. In Figure 6.1 b, the tritium level per liter plasma is shown as percent of the daily stored radioactivity in the body. The uniform course of radioactivity in plasma with a mean variation coefficient of 8%, measured over a period of 4 days, implies that the measurements of tritium concentrations in urine and feces can be calculated as measurements of the glycoside concentrations during steady-state equilibrium. Thus, if the specific activity in plasma calculated for each day is transferred to the total elimination of tritium in urine and feces, the total excreted amount of the glycoside is obtained (Fig. 6.1 c). The five subjects, whose daily dose of digitoxin was 0.1 mg, excreted within 4 days a mean total amount of 224 μg in urine and 130 μg in feces or 56 μg per day in urine and 33 μg in feces. Two-thirds of the daily digitoxin dose was excreted via urine and one-third via feces. These findings are consistent with the results obtained after a single-dose study in healthy subjects.

Metabolism of Digitoxin in Man

Nearly one-fifth to one-fourth of the daily tritium concentration in plasma, urine, and feces was not extractable with chloroform (Fig. 6.2). The same results are obtained by extraction with methylene chloride. The $CHCl_3$-insoluble fraction in urine was analyzed by separation on a Al_2O_3 column according to Barlow and Kellie (Barlow and Kellie, 1959). This procedure revealed three eluation fractions which were incubated with an enzyme preparation of β-glucuronidase and arylsulfatase. However, only one fraction eluted with ethanol /2% ammonium hydroxide (1:1) from the Al_2O_3 column could be cleavaged to 90% after incubation with 5 mg β-glucuronidase (Helix pomatia). The thin layer chromatography of the cleavage products (solvent system I) shows that dgt-mono can be regarded as a main conjugation partner of glucuronic acid in urine along with smaller amounts of the epimer of dgt-g.

The thin layer chromatographic analysis of the $CHCl_3$-soluble fractions in plasma, urine, and feces are illustrated in Figure 6.3 and 6.4. In plasma, digitoxin is found in all collecting periods as the major part of the total $CHCl_3$-soluble fraction. The other small radioactive area appears to be attached to dgt-bis, whereby this finding could only be detected in solvent system I. In urine, traces of hydroxylated products and dgt-bis are present, but the unchanged digitoxin is the major urinary compound. A similar composition of metabolites and drug is found in feces, with one difference that additionally the monodigitoxoside of digitoxigenin is present. All metabolites exhibited the same chromatographic behavior as the authentic standards.

65

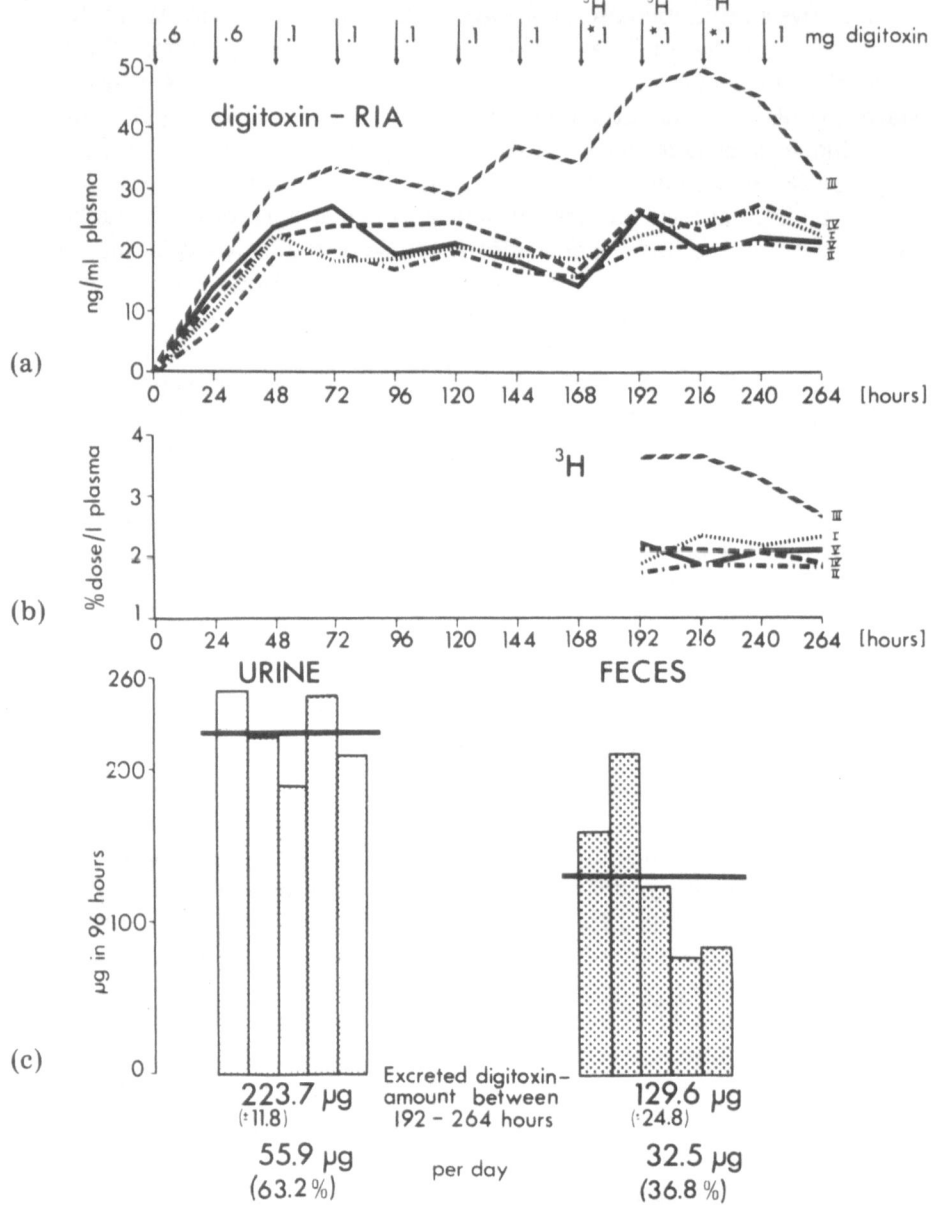

Fig. 6.1. Plasma concentrations of digitoxin (a) and tritium (b) and cumulative excretion of the glycoside in urine and feces (c) within 96 h in five healthy subjects. Loading dose: 1.2 mg; maintenance dose 0.1 mg per day; tracer dose 30 μCi per day

PLASMA	URINE	FECES
17.85 ± 1.6	28.42 ± 2.5	26.05 ± 3.1

TLC – separation of CHCl₃– insoluble fraction

URINE

Incubation with glucuronidase

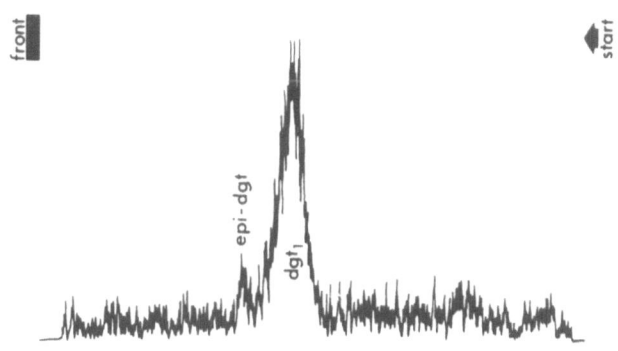

Fig. 6.2. CHCl₃-insoluble fraction in plasma, urine, and feces in percent of the total concentration during steady state (mean ± SEM, n=5). Solvent system: diisopropylether/methanol 9:1 (5x)

In summarizing the thin layer chromatographic findings, the most important aspect is that unchanged digitoxin is the predominant compound in plasma, urine, and feces. The stepwise removal of the sugar side chains is shown to yield dgt-bis and, in feces, dgt-mono. There is also evidence that 12-β-hydroxylation from digitoxin and its metabolites to digoxin and its metabolites occurs in man, but the quantitative significance of this reaction is very small. At least 6%-7% of the daily excreted glycoside is associated with hydroxylated compounds.

Conclusion

1. The disposition of digitoxin in healty subjects can be characterized by two elimination routes: 63% of the daily administered dose are eliminated via urine and 33% via feces, respectively.

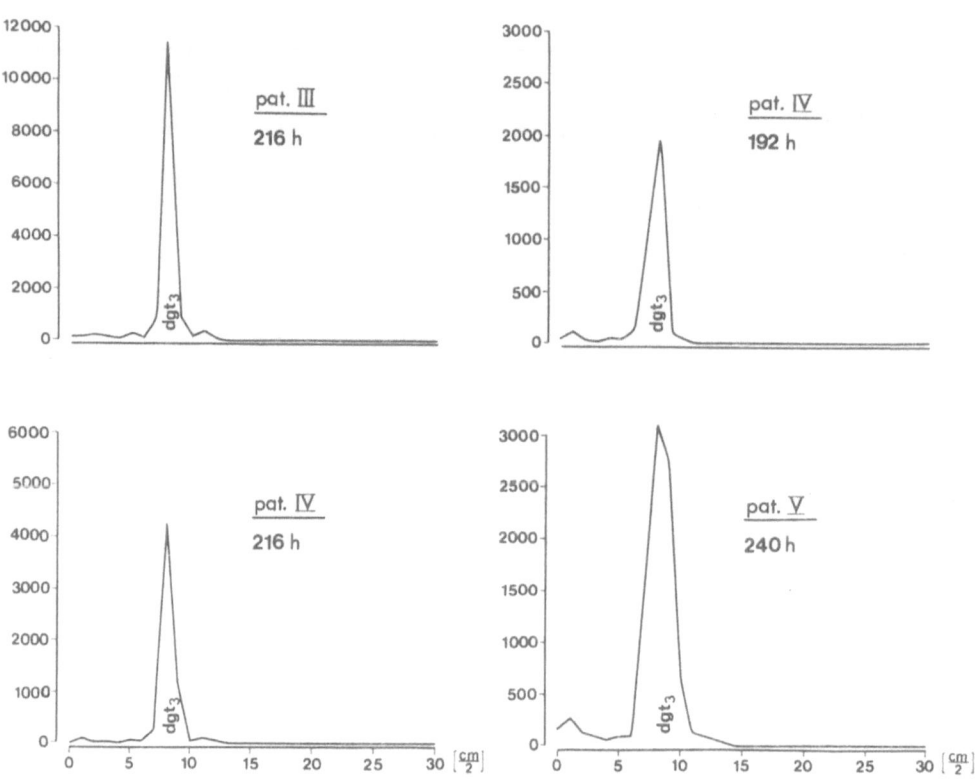

Fig. 6.3. TLC: separation of $CHCl_3$-soluble fraction in plasma during different collecting periods

2. In plasma, as well as in urine and feces, the unchanged substance digitoxin accounts for 50%-60% of the plasma concentration and of the daily eliminated amount.
3. The main metabolites of digitoxin are polar products, which could be detected in urine as conjugation compounds of dgt-mono and glucuronic acid. Since dgt-mono in feces is found as a second metabolite, it may be concluded that the conjugation reaction to polar products occurs mainly in the step of dgt-mono.
4. The limited degradation of digitoxin in man suggests that the pharmacologic effects are mediated predominantly by digitoxin itself.

diisopropylether/methanol 9:1 (5x)   ethyl methyl ketone/xylene 1:1 (2x)

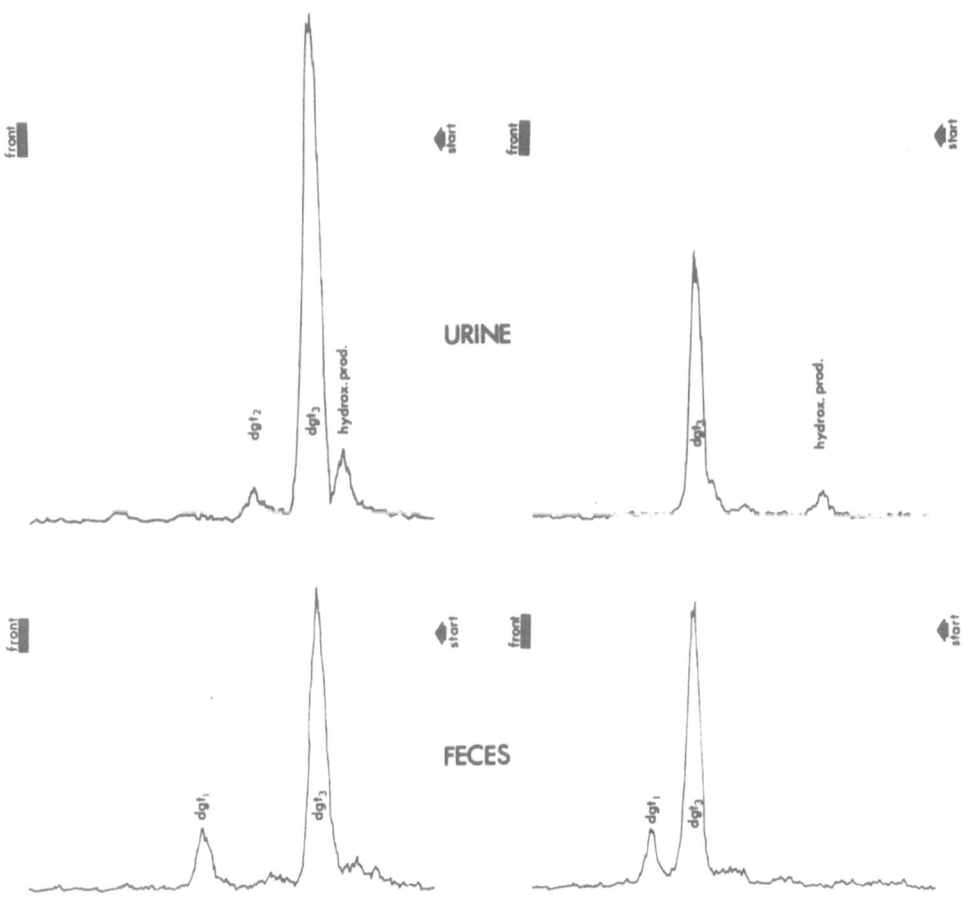

Fig. 6.4. TLC: separation of CHCl₃ -soluble fraction in urine and feces

Special abbreviations used

dg	Digoxin
dgt (dgt₃)	Digitoxin
dgt-bis (dgt₂)	Digitoxigenin bisdigitoxoside
dgt-mono (dgt₁)	Digitoxigenin monodigitoxoside
dgt-epi	3-epidigitoxigenin
dgt-g	Digitoxigenin
TLC	Thin layer chromatography

References

Barlow, J.J., Kellie, A.E.: A quantitative method for the chromatographic separation of 17-oxo steroid sulphates from 17-oxo steroid glucuronides: with observations on the behaviour of conjugated corticosteroids on the same system. Biochem.J. 71, 86-91 (1959)

Caldwell, J.H., Bush, Ch.A., Greenberger, N.J.: Interruption of the enterohepatic circulation of digitoxin by cholestyramine. II. Effect on metabolic disposition of tritium-labeled digitoxin and cardiac systolic intervals in man. J.Clin. Invest. 50, 2638-2644 (1971)

Doherty, J.E.: The clinical pharmacology of digitalis glycosides: A review. Am.J. Med.Sci. 255, 382-414 (1968)

Jelliffe, R.W.: A mathematical analysis of digitalis kinetics in patients with normal and reduced renal function. Math.Biosci. 1, 305-325 (1967)

Kramer, P., Horenkamp, J., Wilms, B., Scheler, F.: Das Kumulationsverhalten verschiedener Herzglykoside bei Anurie. Dtsch.Med.Wochenschr. 95, 444-453 (1970)

Lahrtz, H.G., Reinold, H.M., van Zwieten, P.A.: Serumkonzentration und Ausscheidung von ³H-Digitoxin beim Menschen unter normalen und pathologischen Bedingungen. Klin.Wochenschr. 47, 695-700 (1969)

Lukas, D.S.: Some aspects of the distribution and disposition of digitoxin in man. Ann.N.Y.Acad.Sci. 179, 338-361 (1971)

Lukas, D.S.: The pharmacokinetics and metabolism of digitoxin in man. In: Storstein, O. (ed.) Symposium on digitalis. Oslo: Gyldendal Norsk Forlag 1973, pp. 84-102

Okita, G.T., Kelsey, F.E., Talso, P.J., Smith, L.B., Geiling, E.M.K.: Studies of the renal excretion of radioactive digitoxin in human subjects with cardiac failure. Circulation 7, 161-168 (1953)

Okita, G.T., Talso, P.J., Curry, J.H., Smith, F.D., Geiling, E.M.K.: Metabolic fate of radioactive digitoxin in human subjects. J.Pharmacol.Exp.Ther. 115, 371-379 (1955)

Peters, U., Hengels, K.J., Hausamen, T.U., Grosse-Brockhoff, F.: Einfluß von Rifampicin auf den Metabolismus des Digitoxins. Verh.Dtsch.Ges.Inn.Med. 81, 1675-1676 (1975)

Solomon, H., Reich, S., Gaut, Z., Pocelinko, R., Abrams, W.: Induction of the metabolism if digitoxin in man by phenobarbital. Clin.Res. 19, 356 (1971)

Storstein, L.: Studies on digitalis. I. Renal excretion of digitoxin and its cardioactive metabolites. Clin.Pharmacol.Ther. 16, 14-24 (1974)

Storstein, L.: Studies on digitalis. IV. A method for thin-layer chromatography (TLC) separation and determination of digitoxin and cardioactive metabolites in human blood and urine. J.Chromatogr. 117, 87-96 (1976)

Vöhringer, H.F., Rietbrock, N.: Metabolism and excretion of digitoxin in man. Clin.Pharmacol.Ther. 16, 796-806 (1974)

Weissler, A.M., Snyder, J.R., Schoenfeld, C.D., Cohen, S.: Assay of digitalis glycosides in man. Am.J.Cardiol. 17, 768-780 (1966)

Wirth, K.E., Frölich, J.C., Hollifield, J.W., Falkner, F.C., Sweetman, B.S., Oates, J.A.: Metabolism of digitoxin in man and its modification by spironolactone. Eur.J.Clin.Pharmacol. 9, 345-354 (1976)

Discussion

Flasch, Hamburg: You told us that about 20%-30% of the ^{3}H activity you found in urine was not extractable with chloroform. How much of this fraction can be split with sulfatase or glucuronidase, i.e., is assumed to be conjugates, and how much of this water-soluble fraction belonged to unidentified products?

Vöhringer: I don't know the exact answer to this question. In our procedure of analyzing the chloroform-insoluble fraction, we have lost radioactivity during the different extraction steps. A complete extraction of the chloroform-insoluble metabolites in urine with ether/ethanol (3:1) would be found at pH 1. This cannot be done with cardiac glycosides. I cannot say how much digitoxin monodigitoxoside was found. It can only be stated that this metabolite was the main conjugation partner of glucuronic acid. I was not successful yet in splitting polar compounds in the feces.

Scholz, Hannover: Most examinations about the disposition of cardiac glycosides, as your study, are done in healthy volunteers. Is there any difference or is it irrelevant whether you are doing the experiments in healthy young volunteers or in those older people normally suffering from cardiac insufficiency? Are there differences in the kinetics or the metabolism of digitoxin in a person of your age, for instance, or in a 60-year-old person who really suffers from congestive heart failure?

Vöhringer: You are quite correct; this cannot be extrapolated. On the other hand, I do not know about any differences in kinetics or metabolism of digitoxin between healthy volunteers and cardiac patients.

Lukas: This is a very important question, indeed. We studied a patient with very severe liver disease, whose urine and feces were a veritable gold mine of pure digitoxin; 85%-90% of her daily dose of the drug was eliminated in that form. So you are perfectly correct when you imply that some difficulty with renal or hepatic function might, indeed, change the metabolism of a cardiac glycoside.

Amlie, Norway: We have made a study on the pharmacokinetics of digitoxin after one single intravenous dose in six patients with chronic active hepatitis (CAH). Figure 1 shows the elimination half-life of digitoxin in the CAH patients compared to a control group. Figure 2 shows the metabolites of digitoxin in serum and urine 24 h after the intravenous dose. The patients with CAH had significantly more hydrolyzed metabolites than the controls.

Storstein, Norway: We did our studies in cardiac patients who were taking digitoxin for maintenance treatment. We found that all the cardioactive metabolites were conjugated to glucuronic and sulfuric acid, and thereby rendered inactive. The inactive DT metabolites, that is the conjugates with digitoxin and the

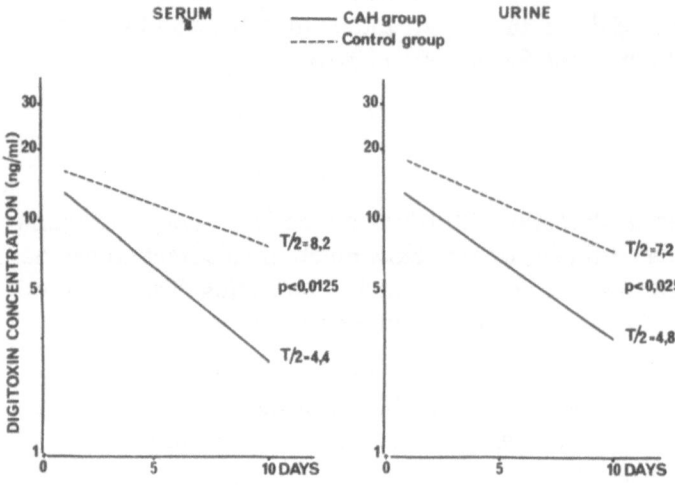

Fig. 1

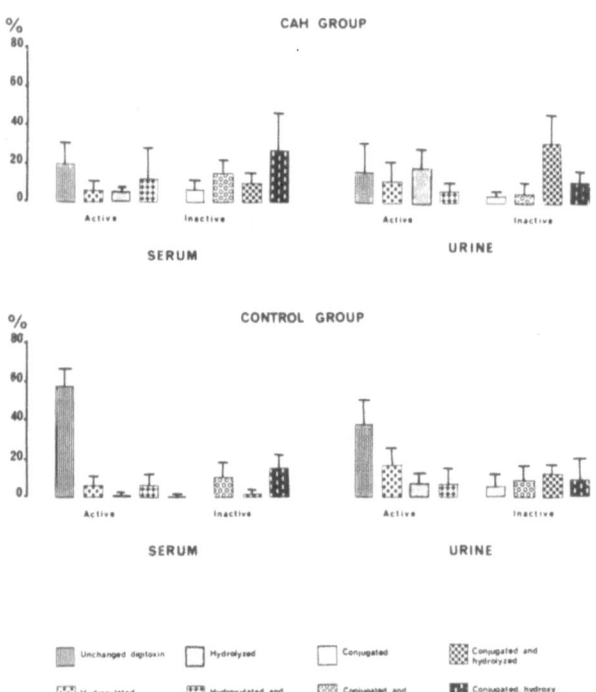

Fig. 2

hydrolyzed metabolites of digitoxin, (DT-2, DT-1, and DT-0) predominate and accord for around 90%.

Ohnhaus, Bern: I think you have to be very careful in differentiating patients in cardiac failure, because there are different kinds of cardiac failures. Also you have to analyze the creatinine clearance and you have to have information about the hepatic function in these patients.

Haberland, Hamburg: We studied the metabolism of digoxin in a patient with severe liver disease and did not observe any difference in comparison to healthy individuals.

Lukas: Dr. Vöhringer, I was interested in the fact that you had given a loading dose of 1.2 mg, which appeared to overshoot the steady-state mark, as indicated by the subsequent decline of plasma concentrations during maintenance in all except one of your subjects.

Vöhringer: But they also came up. The mean coefficient of variation was calculated interindividually to be 15%. The plasma glycoside levels were determined using a GammaCoat radioimmunoassay. The mean variation coefficient of this method is between 5% and 10%. Indeed, I think the plasma concentrations in our experiment vary within normal limits.

Lukas: May I point out that on the basis of our pharmacokinetic data, we would have chosen a loading dose of about 0.7-0.8 mg to approximate the body pool of digitoxin that is eventually attained in a subject during steady-state maintenance on 0.1 mg per day.

Vöhringer: This is right, but the steady state is a dose-dependent relation and if you look in the literature concerning the digitalization for patients with and without renal impairment, the loading dose is always 1.2 mg and the maintenance dose 0.1 mg. With this dosage regimen, you will get less cardiac toxicity by a sufficient pharmacodynamic effect than if you increase the dose.

v. Bergmann, Bonn: If I understand you correctly, you have used the randomly labeled digitoxin. Have you recrystallyzed your compound and looked how stable the label was? And a second question refers to the water-soluble metabolites. Did you find any tritium water in the urine?

Vöhringer: The tritium water in urine was less than 1%. To the first question: the stability of the tritium label was not exactly examined throughout the experiment.

7 Dihydrodigitoxin, a Metabolite of Digitoxin in Humans

G. BODEM and E. v. UNRUH

Summary

A gas chromatographic-mass spectroscopic technique was used to identify dihydrodigitoxin, a metabolite of digitoxin, in the plasma of healthy volunteers and patients with renal failure. Digitoxin and dihydrodigitoxin were extracted from plasma and derivatized with heptafluorbutyric anhydride. In normal subjects, only minimal concentrations of dihydrodigitoxin in plasma could be determined (1 ng/ml) after an intravenous bolus injection of digitoxin. Under a chronic treatment with a daily dose of 0.1 mg digitoxin in three out of seven individuals, detectable dihydrodigitoxin plasma levels were observed (0.7, 1.5, 1.7 ng/ml) (Table 7.1). On the other hand, in seven patients with renal failure, high dihydrodigitoxin plasma concentrations (8.9 ± 0.9 ng/ml) were shown which were in a similar range as those of the parent compound (8.7 ± 2.2 ng/ml) under maintenance treatment with digitoxin.

Pharmacokinetics and metabolism with radioactively labeled cardiac glycosides were examined for the first time in the 1950s and 1960s. In the meantime, methods have become available which also make the determination of concentrations of nonlabeled digitalis glycosides in blood and urine possible. Rubidium uptake method and radioimmunoassay increased our sophistication about the behavior of cardiac glycosides during long-term treatment. Nevertheless, there are many clinical questions which still have to be answered because of the lack of specific assays.

A gas chromatographic method for measuring digoxin and dihydrodigoxin in blood and urine has been designed by Watson and co-workers (Watson et al., 1973). It was shown that dihydrodigoxin is more common than any other degradation product of digoxin. There are no reports yet about the formation of dihydrodigitoxin in the metabolism of digitoxin. Therefore, the present study was designed to investigate the transformation of digitoxin to dihydrodigitoxin in patients using a gas chromatographic-mass spectroscopic technique.

Methods

Patients

Five healthy volunteers, aged 29-37 years, participated in the study. A dose of 1 mg digitoxin (Digimerck®) was injected over a time period of 5 min intravenously. Blood samples were obtained in 24 h intervals for 10 days. Also, in six patients with heart failure who were on a daily oral maintenance dose of digitoxin (Digimerck®), a blood sample was drawn immediately before the next dose was taken. In addition, plasma of seven patients with renal failure (plasma creatinine concentration: Table 7.2) under chronic oral digitoxin treatment (Digimerck®) was analyzed.

Assay

To correct for losses during analysis, 50,000 dpm ^{3}H-digitoxin (15 Ci/mM; New England Nuclear, Frankfurt, Dreieichenhein) were added to 10 ml of plasma prior to extraction and an equal amount was taken as a standard for liquid scintillation counting. The plasma sample was extracted once with six volumes of methylene chloride by stirring for 25 min at room temperature. The methylene chloride was run to a conical glass tube and evaporated under a stream of nitrogen. The residue was redissolved in 3 ml methanol-methylene chloride (1:1) and transferred onto a column (diameter: 1.4 cm; length: 22 cm) packed with florisil (80/100 mesh).

Prior to use, the column was washed with 20 ml of methylene chloride. The effluent was removed. The elution was performed with 20 ml of ethylacetate-methylene chloride-methanol-acetone (1:3:3:4). This solution was evaporated under nitrogen and the residue was transferred using 50 μl methanol-chloroform (1:1) to a silica gel TLC plate (20 x 20 cm; silica gel 60, 0.25 mm layer, Merck, Darmstadt). TLC then was carried out in the solvent system chloroform-acetone (13:7) for three times to a height of 15 cm. Reference substances were chromatographed in separate lanes.

Digitoxin was located by scanning of the thin layer plate in a Berthold scanner (Frieseke a. Hoepfner, mod. LB-2560). The reference compounds were identified using a spray technique described by Kaiser (Kaiser, 1955). The area corresponding to digitoxin was scrapped off the TLC plate and stirred in 10 ml methanol-chloroform (1:1) for 20 min and then centrifuged for 5 min at 5000 xg. The supernatant was evaporated and the residue reconstituted with 2 ml of benzene. The HBF derivative was formed by reacting this solution with 10 μl of heptafluorbutyric anhydride (Pierce Chemical Comp., Rockford, U.S.A.) for 1 h at 90°C. Then this reaction mixture was evaporated under nitrogen. The residue was applied to TLC plates (20 x 20 cm; silica gel 60, 0.25 mm layer, Merck, Darmstadt) using 50 μl benzene. The plates were preimpregnated with methylene chloride-methanol (1:1). The plates were developed in a solution of methylene chloride-methanol-benzene (45:45:5) to a height of 17cm. Digitoxin HBF was chromatographed in a separate lane and was located by ultraviolet absorption. The area (1 x 3 cm) was removed from the thin layer plate and stirred in 20 ml methylene chloride-methanol (1:1). After centrifugation as described earlier, the supernatant was evaporated and the residue dissolved in 50 μl benzene. Five μl standard solution was added and 2 μl were injected into the gas chromatograph. At the same time, one-half of the final sample was transferred into 10 ml of scintillator fluid (Unisolve, Zinser, Frankfurt) for counting (Isocap 300, Ser.Nr. 2290, Nuclear Chicago). The gas chromatograph was a "Varian-Aerograph Series 2700" with a ^{63}Ni electron capture detector (Varian, Darmstadt). Silanized glass columns (90 cm x 2 mm inside diameter) were packed with OV-17 (Varian, Darmstadt). The carrier gas was cleaned nitrogen. The injector temperature was 260°C. The column was operated at 248°C. The detector was maintained at 305°C.

For the preparation of the internal standard, 2 mg of paramethoxy prenylamine (Hoechst, Frankfurt) was dissolved in 2 ml of benzene and reacted with 20 μl trifluoroacetic anhydride (Merck, Darmstadt) for 50 min at 90°C. The solution was evaporated and the residue redissolved in 300 μl benzene. The calculations of the plasma digitoxin levels were done after correction of the losses during the extraction procedure relating to the standard peak as described by Watson and co-workers (Watson et al., 1973) for the gas chromatographic determination of digoxin.

For the mass spectroscopic examinations, a LKB-2091-GC-MS combination (LKB Instrument GmbH, Düsseldorf) was used. GC-conditions were as follows: 90 cm x 4 mm inside diameter glass columns packed with OV-17 on Gaschrom, 100-120 mesh; helium flow, 30 ml/min; temperature program 240°-270°C/min; injector temperature, 260°C; molecular separator temperature, 250°C. The operating conditions of the mass spectrometer were: electron energy, 70 eV; ion source temperature, 250°C; trap current, 50 μA; and an accelerating voltage of 3.5 kV.

Results

The minimal concentrations which could be determined using the described method were 0.5 ng/ml for both digitoxin and dihydrodigitoxin. The overall recovery of the assay for ^{3}H-digitoxin added to the plasma was 42.1 ± 0.6%. The RF values of digitoxigenin, digitoxigenin monodigitoxoside, digitoxigenin bisdigitoxoside, and digitoxin were 0.9, 0.71, 0.55, and 0.19, respectively, in the chosen TLC system. Dihydrodigitoxin showed the same RF value as digitoxin. Measurable concentrations of digitoxigenin, digitoxigenin monodigitoxoside, or digitoxigenin bisdigitoxoside could not be found in four patients with normal plasma creatinine levels, nor in three patients with renal failure under a chronic digitoxin treatment.

Figure 7.1 illustrates the plasma level decay curve of digitoxin in five healthy volunteers after intravenous application of 1 mg Digimerck®. The curve declines continually with a plasma half-life of 5.0 ±1.3 days. Dihydrodigitoxin was not detected in three volunteers; two individuals had low levels, which were, however, always below 1 ng/ml even when plasma was analyzed at different times after the administration of digitoxin. Under a daily oral maintenance therapy of 0.1 mg for at least 4 weeks, the digitoxin plasma levels were 13.2 ± 3.2 ng/ml in seven patients without signs of impaired renal function. Dihydrodigitoxin was observed in three patients in low concentrations, which amounted maximally to one-sixth of the digitoxin concentration.

Patients with renal failure treated with the same oral digitoxin dose under maintenance conditions showed significantly lower plasma levels (8.7 ± 2.2 ng/ml) than the group of patients without retention of BUN (13.2 ± 3.2 ng/ml). Dihydrodigitoxin on the other hand was detected in all these patients in relatively high concentrations (8.9 ± 0.9 ng/ml). In several patients with low kidney functions (Table 7.2; No.: 202, 203, 204), the plasma levels of dihydrodigitoxin were even higher than those of digitoxin. Figures 7.2 and 7.3 demonstrate representative chromatograms, Figure 7.2 that of a patient with no signs of a renal disease (no metabolite to be found), and Figure 7.3 that of a patient with renal failure (dihydrodigitoxin).

The mass spectra of the derivatives were determined under the same conditions as the samples from the patients. The existence of digitoxin heptafluorbutyrat

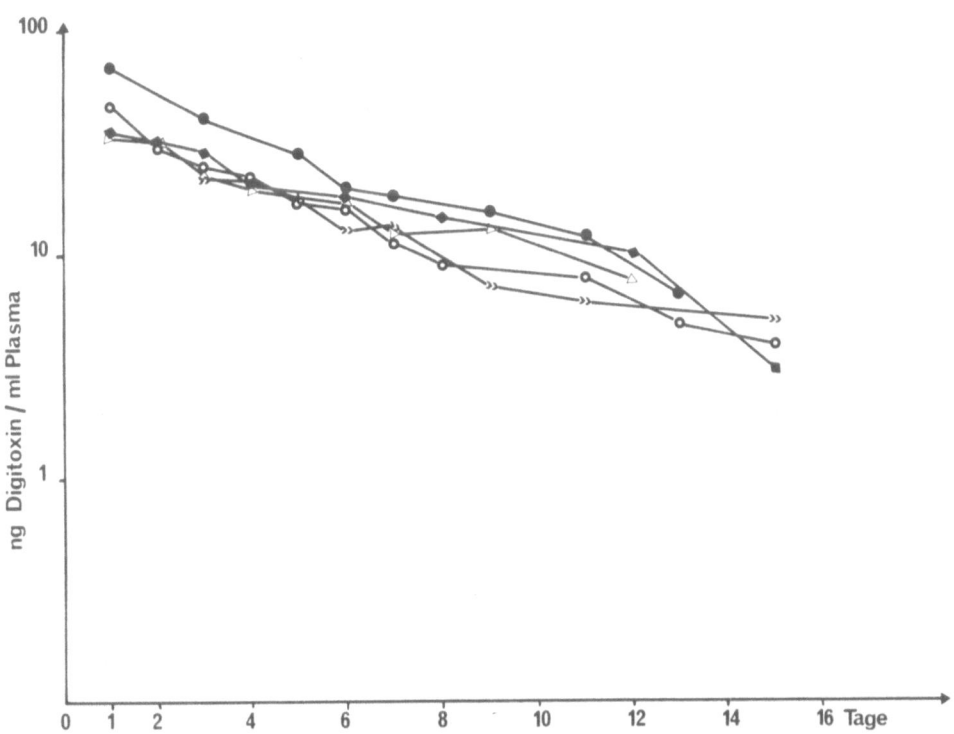

Fig. 7.1. Digitoxin plasma level decay curves of five healthy individuals

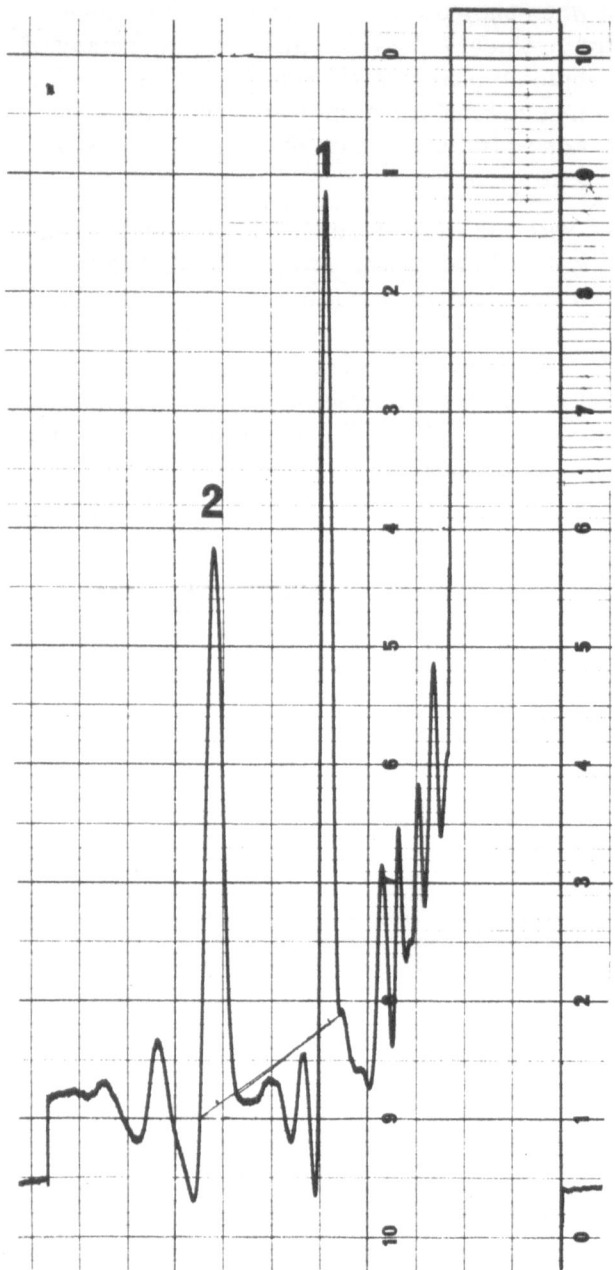

Fig. 7.2. Representative chromatogram of a patient without signs of a renal disease under a maintenance therapy with 0.1 mg digitoxin daily

Peak 1:   Standard
Peak 2:   Digitoxigenin HFB

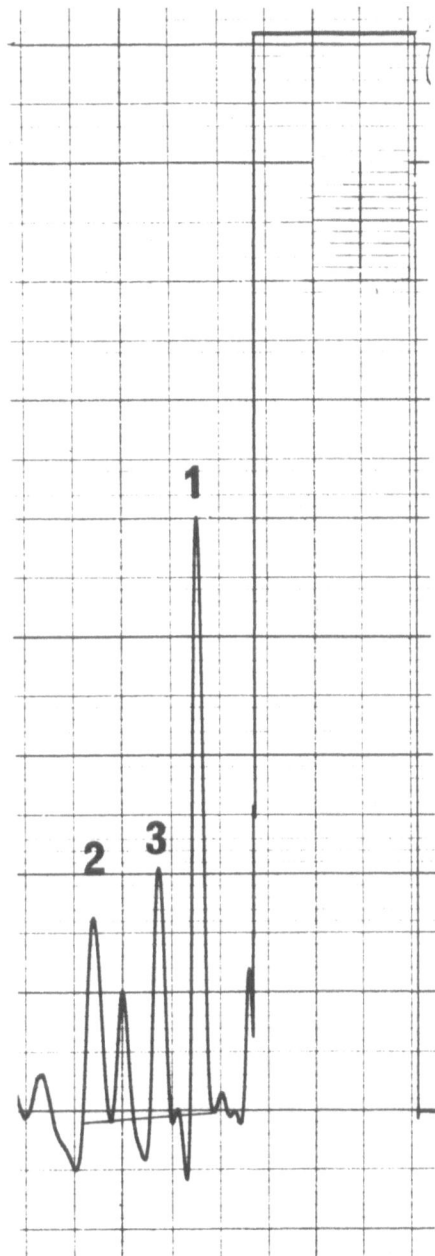

Fig. 7.3. Representative chromatogram of a patient with renal insufficiency under an oral maintenance therapy with 0.1 mg digitoxin daily
Peak 1: Standard
Peak 2: Digitoxigenin HFB
Peak 3: Dihydrodigitoxigenin HFB

and dihydrodigitoxin heptafluorbutyrat was proved by the characteristic ions at m/e 323 and 338, and m/e 325 and 340, respectively. The signal at m/e 338 or 340 was under the worst conditions still 50 times that of the noise and was not impaired by the background.

Table 7.1. Serum levels of digitoxin and dihydrodigitoxin in seven patients without signs of renal insufficiency under a daily maintenance therapy with 0.1 mg digitoxin

Protokoll No.	Digitoxin (ng/ml)	Dihydrodigitoxin (ng/ml)
101	31.0	<0.5
102	11.0	<0.5
103	11.0	<0.5
104	15.8	1.7
105	7.0	<0.5
106	9.8	1.5
107	7.1	0.7
M	13.2	—
SEM	3.2	—

Table 7.2. Serum levels of digitoxin and dihydrodigitoxin in seven patients with renal insufficiency under a daily maintenance therapy with 0.1 mg digitoxin

Protocol No.	Creatinine in Serum	Digitoxin (ng/ml)	Dihydrodigitoxin (ng)ml)
201	5.3	10.2	6.7
202	8.7	6.4	7.4
203	6.3	4.2	10.0
204	6.6	0.8	7.4
205	4.8	6.9	6.4
206	5.7	16.7	11.7
207	8.4	15.5	12.4
M	—	8.7	8.9
SEM	—	2.2	0.9

Discussion

The pharmacokinetics of digitoxin in humans have been the subject of several studies of the last 10 years. The results obtained with different methods of analysis look similar in patients with normal renal function. Only with the double isotope dilution derivative assay were shorter plasma half-lives found than with radioactive substances or using the rubidium assay. In the plasma and the urine mainly, the parent compound and only low amounts of metabolites were detected. The transformation of digitoxin to dihydrodigitoxin was minimal.

In the present study, the plasma half-live measured by gas chromatography was 5.0 ± 1.3 days and, therefore, in about the range found with the double isotope dilution derivative assay (Lukas, 1973). Both methods are highly specific, whereas in studies carried out with the other techniques it cannot be ruled out that even after prepurification with TLC degradation products of the given glycoside and additional administered drugs may influence the method. The advantage of GC has to be seen in the fact that an exact separation of the parent substance from dihydrodigitoxin is possible. Dihydrodigitoxin is a metabolite which shows only a very low cardiotonic activity. Watson and co-workers (Watson et al., 1973) observed in a previous study with digoxin a significant transformation to dihydrodigoxin in about 1.5% of the examined patients. Digitoxin as compared to digoxin has a longer plasma half-live. Therefore, it had to be examined if higher concentrations of dihydrodigitoxin can be determined after the administration of digitoxin. In healthy volunteers, however, only very low plasma levels were found. After a single dose of digitoxin dihydrodigitoxin plasma concentrations were never higher than 1 ng/ml.

Under an oral maintenance therapy of at least 4 weeks with a constant daily dose of digitoxin, only a small amount of dihydrodigitoxin could be measured in the plasma. In three out of seven patients, the plasma levels of the metabolite were in the measurable range. In patients with renal failure, however, significantly higher plasma concentrations of dihydrodigitoxin, which in some cases were even higher than those of the parent compund, could be found (Table 7.2).

There have to be considered two possible causes for the high plasma levels of dihydrodigitoxin in renal failure:
1. An increased transformation of digitoxin to the less cardioactive metabolite dihydrodigitoxin
2. An extremely slow elimination of dihydrodigitoxin in this disease

Pharmacokinetic studies with dihydrodigitoxin in healthy individuals or patients have not yet been made; nevertheless, there are strong indications that the metabolism of digitoxin in renal failure is increased, which seems to be supported by the observation that the plasma levels of digitoxin are lower (Grosse-Brockhoff, 1976) and the half-lives not longer in uremic patients (Storstein, 1973; Vöhringer et al., 1976).

References

Grosse-Brockhoff, F.: Digitalistherapie bei der Niereninsuffizienz. Therapie
Woche <u>30</u>, 4796 (1976)

Kaiser, F.: Die papierchromatographische Trennung von Herzgiftglykosiden.
Chem. Ber. <u>88</u>, 556 (1955)

Lukas, D.S.: The pharmacokinetics and metabolism of digitoxin in man. In:
Storstein, O. (ed.): Symposium on Digitalis. Oslo: Gyldendal Norsk Forlag
1973, p. 84

Storstein, L.: The influence of renal functions on the pharmacokinetics of digitoxin. In: Storstein, O. (ed.): Symposium on Digitalis. Oslo: Gyldendal
Norsk Forlag 1973, p. 158

Vöhringer, H.F., Rietbrock, N., Spurny, P., Kuhlmann, J., Hampl, H., Baethke, R.:
Disposition of digitoxin in renal failure. Clin. Pharmacol. Ther. <u>19</u>, 387 (1976)

Watson, E., Clark, D.R., Kalman, S.M.: Identification by gas chromatography-
mass spectroscopy of dihydrodigoxin. J. Pharmacol. Exp. Ther. <u>184</u>, 424
(1973)

Discussion

Lukas: Dr. Bodem, did you determine the half-time of digitoxin in your patients
with renal failure?

Bodem: No. It is just not possible to draw blood several times in uremic patients.
For each assay you need 25 ml of plasma.

Lukas: That is one of the reasons why we do not have very much data on the
plasma half-life of digitoxin in patients with renal failure using the double isotope dilution derivative assay. The assay requires 10-15 ml of plasma.

Kramer, Göttingen: Dr. Bodem, I think I have some difficulties in understanding
your data concerning the plasma concentrations determined for dihydrodigitoxin
in uremic patients which were — as far as I recall — in some patients almost as
high as for digitoxin. Thus, I think we have to assume that there was a 50%-de-
gradation of digitoxin to dihydrodigitoxin, unless the elimination rate is much
lower and the plasma half-life of this degradation product is much longer than
that of digitoxin. So, I wanted to ask you whether you have done any studies
on the plasma half-life of dihydrodigitoxin in uremic patients, or whether you
are aware of such studies performed by other authors?

Bodem: In fact, I don't know any data about the determination of dihydrodigitoxin in man, as yet. Especially I don't know about studies on the half-life of dihydrodigitoxin in renal failure or in normals. Again, it will be a problem to determine
half-lives in renal failure because you need a great amount of plasma for these
examinations, and you have to draw blood several times to construct a blood
level decay curve. Concerning your attempts to interpret my data, I think you
also have to take into account that there might be a different distribution pattern
for the dihydrometabolite.

Kramer: May I just make a remark concerning the problem of uremic patients. We return the red blood cells to the patients just taking the plasma with a very simple technique which was proposed by some Polish authors.

Belz, Koblenz: I think I can help Dr. Bodem in the question of whether dihydrodigitoxin may be cardioactive or not. We have analyzed the influence of dihydrodigoxin on the ^{86}Rb uptake of human erythrocytes. This substance has a potency which is about 50 times less than that of digoxin. I would not expect a great difference between dihydrodigitoxin and dihydrodigoxin.

Kuhlmann, Berlin: We have made investigations in dogs with tritiated dihydrodigoxin and we have measured a plasma half-life of 8-10 h and we have found only low concentrations in the various tissues 24 h after a single dose of 0.0125 mg/kg.

Benthe, Hamburg: I can confirm the assumption that the dihydrodigoxin will not be cardioactive since the uptake of the myocard is small in comparison to digoxin.

Bodem: You are speaking about dihydrodigoxin. Do you have any data about dihydrodigitoxin as well?

Benthe: No. I would also like to ask you if you studied the metabolites of the water-soluble fraction in the urine of the renal failure patients, because dihydrodigitoxin is a very instable compound and the lactone structure opens easily. So, I would expect a high amount of water-soluble substances in the urine of these patients.

Bodem: We did not do any urinary examinations at all. In the plasma, we concentrated on the extracted portion in the plasma. The patients did not get the radioactively labeled drug, and this would be necessary at the moment to study the metabolism of the aqueous phase.

Schaumann, Mannheim: If I understood you correctly your high percentage of dihydrodigitoxin was not time dependent, suggesting an equilibrium between both and not a long half-life. Do you have an idea whether the dihydrodigitoxin is formed in the liver, or by bacteria in the gut, and whether a retransformation from dihydrodigitoxin to digitoxin is conceivable?

Bodem: I can say hardly anything to this question. Indeed, in the study with the bolus injection, the proportion of dihydrodigitoxin and digitoxin remained constant. I cannot say anything about the patients under a maintenance therapy. We did the evaluation under these conditions only once. I have no idea where dihydrodigitoxin is formed. It might be the gut. But at the moment I think that is speculation.

Grahame-Smith: One of the points that has struck me so far this morning is that in terms of pharmacokinetics we have been talking mainly about half-lives, but one of the factors that determines pharmacokinetic behavior is the volume of distribution, and if you have polar and nonpolar metabolites and particularly in renal failure, the volume of distribution is likely to change really very greatly.

I am just wondering whether the volume of distribution changes. Could this explain in any way the high level of dihydrodigitoxin that you have?

Bodem: That could be possible. We did not determine the volume of distribution of dihydrodigitoxin, as I already mentioned. I am sure it will be different from that of digitoxin.

Grahame-Smith: And this might apply in renal failure, compared with normal.

Benthe, Hamburg: It is well-known that during renal impairance biliary excretion of digitoxin is enhanced. Can you exclude the possibility that the dihydrodigitoxin is formed in the gut and is absorbed and you measured it in the plasma?

Bodem: This is an interesting point. But I do not believe that all the dihydrodigitoxin we measured is formed in the gut because we could determine it in two patients already 1 h after an intravenous injection.

Lukas: Dr. Bodem, you have been measuring plasma concentrations, and I think it would be very useful to know what you or others have found about the binding of dihydrodigitoxin to the plasma proteins.

Bodem: Sorry, there we have no data available and I don't know about results of other authors.

Lukas: So, information concerning the free concentration of dihydrodigitoxin in plasma and the inferences that one might draw regarding the size of the body pool of dihydrodigitoxin are limited. Nevertheless, your finding of high total concentrations of dihydrodigitoxin in the plasma of uremic patients is of exceptional interest.

Marcus: I may be able to answer Dr. Grahame-Smith's question. Dr. Klaus Gierke and I are investigating the metabolism of digoxin and the bisdigitoxoside metabolism before and after azotemia. We have found that there is a decreased volume of distribution of digoxin and the bis-compound after azotemia; also, there appears to be a smaller volume of distribution of the bis-compound in comparison with digoxin. Therefore, it may be that the dihydro-compound of digitoxin may have a smaller volume of distribution than digitoxin.

8 Enterohepatic Circulation of Digitoxin Metabolites in the Dog[1]

G. Ch. Oliver, L. A. Santini, G. Griffin, and R. Ruffy

Introduction

In the last 2 decades, the enterohepatic circulation of digitoxin and its metabolites has been the object of numerous studies in both animals and man. Several investigators have concluded that the enterohepatic circulation plays an important role in the metabolism and fate of digitoxin in various species (Okita et al., 1955; Katzung and Meyers, 1965, 1966; Caldwell and Greensberger, 1971; Caldwell et al., 1971). However, available information is fragmentary, and many questions remain unanswered. Controversy exists over the extent to which the prolonged biologic half-life of digitoxin can be attributed to its enterohepatic recycling (Caldwell and Greensberger, 1971; Beerman et al., 1971; Storstein, 1975). In addition, the fate of water-soluble, noncardioactive metabolites which appear abundantly in the bile shortly after the oral or parenteral administration of pure digitoxin (Katzung and Meyers, 1965, 1966) is virtually unknown. This report describes observations made on the fate of water-soluble metabolites of digitoxin immediately following their intraduodenal administration to anesthetized dogs.

Methods

Collection of Water-Soluble Metabolites of Digitoxin

Twelve fasted mongrel dogs weighing between 18 and 23 kg were anesthetized with intravenous pentobarbital (30 mg/kg), intubated, and ventilated with a Harvard animal respirator. Throughout the procedure, 5% dextrose in lactated Ringer's solution was infused via an external jugular vein.

An upper midline laparotomy was performed, and the common bile duct was identified and dissected to its point of entrance into duodenum. At this level, the duct was ligated, partially transected, and cannulated with a No. 14 gauge polyethylene catheter just proximal to the ligation. The cystic duct was ligated to exclude the gallbladder from the biliary tree. The catheter was brought out through the midline and the abdomen closed. At this point, 1 mg of nonradioactive digi-

---

1 Supported in part by N.I.H. Grant 5 T 01 HL 06011.

toxin (Eli Lilly), mixed with 1 mc of tritiated digitoxin (New England Nuclear), was given intravenously and bile was collected for 6-8 h.

The bile collected from the 12 dogs was pooled, and the entire collection was extracted four times with ten volumes of chloroform. A sample of the aqueous fraction was subjected to thin layer chromatography on Gelman SG paper. Developing solvents were cyclohexane:acetone 60:40 and acetone:benzene 20:80. Digitoxin was chromatographed simultaneously for reference. A saturated solution of antimony trichloride was used as a stain. After localization of the digitoxin standard, the chromatogram was cut into 1-cm strips each of which was counted in a liquid scintillation counter. No radioactivity was found in the extract at a point corresponding to the migration of the digitoxin standard, indicating complete removal of digitoxin.

Administration of Water-Soluble Metabolites

Three mongrel dogs weighing between 18 and 23 kg were anesthetized, intubated, and ventilated as previously described. A 5% dectrose in lactated Ringer's solution was infused throughout the procedure via an external jugular vein, at a rate of 100 ml/h. Through an upper midline laparotomy, the bile duct was cannulated as described above. The splenic vein was ligated and cannulated with a similar catheter which was advanced into the portal vein. A Foley catheter was introduced into the bladder through a cystostomy.

Baseline samples of bile, urine, and jugular venous and portal blood were collected. Each dog was then given radiolabeled water-soluble metabolites of digitoxin collected as previously described by direct injection into the second portion of the duodenum. The radioactive dose administered ranged from 3.75×10^8 dpm to 8.34×10^8 dpm. Serial blood, urine, and bile samples were collected for 7 h thereafter.

Sample Analysis

Volumes of all samples were measured and an aliquot of each added to a liquid scintillation cocktail. Bile samples were bleached with a freshly prepared saturated solution of benzoyl peroxide (Fisher), and incubated in a water bath for 1 h before being added to the cocktail. Samples were counted on an Isocap/300 liquid scintillation counter (Nuclear Chicago) and corrected for quenching using internal standardization.

Blood and urine samples with high total radioactive counts were selected for chloroform extraction as described previously. The chloroform layer was then evaporated to dryness in a scintillation vial, and the residue dissolved in 2 ml of ethanol 95%. After addition of the scintillation cocktail, each sample was counted and corrected for quenching.

Results

Figure 8.1 shows the average radioactivity of portal venous blood, jugular venous blood, bile, and urine of all three dogs. Radioactivity appeared promptly in portal venous and jugular venous plasma, being readily detected in the first sample obtained 15 min following administration of the metabolites. The radioactivity of jugular venous plasma was essentially identical to that of portal blood particularly after the first hour. Initially, radioactivity of portal venous blood exceeded that of jugular venous blood suggesting entry into the vascular department via the portal vein. After a sharp rise which occurred within the first hour, the radioactivity increased less rapidly throughout the remainder of the experiment. Radioactivity appeared equally rapidly in bile and urine. The rate of excretion tended to increase throughout the time interval studied.

The rate of excretion of total radioactivity (biliary plus urinary excretion) increased through the experiment (Figure 8.2) indicating a progressive increase in the intestinal absorption of the metabolites over the 7 h. Table 8.1 shows the cumu-

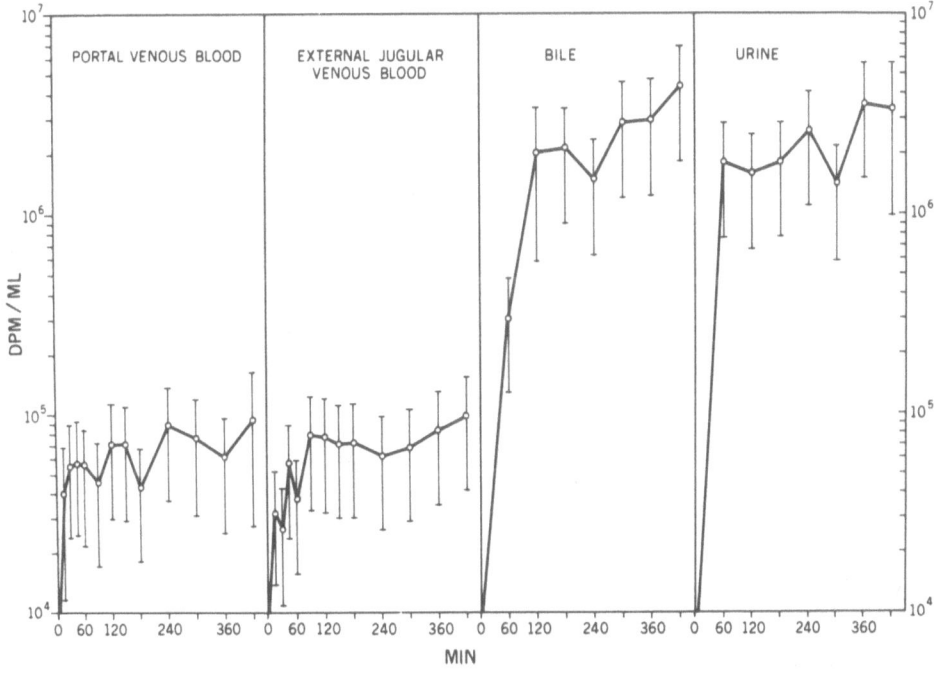

Fig. 8.1. Average and SEM for radioactivity in portal venous and jugular venous blood, bile, and urine. Radioactivity appears promptly in portal venous blood and slightly later in jugular blood. The concentration has apparently not reached a peak in any of the sampled sites by the end of 7 h. Although biliary and urinary concentrations are similar, most radioactivity is excreted via the urinary route, because of the greater volume of urine flow compared with bile (see Table 8.1)

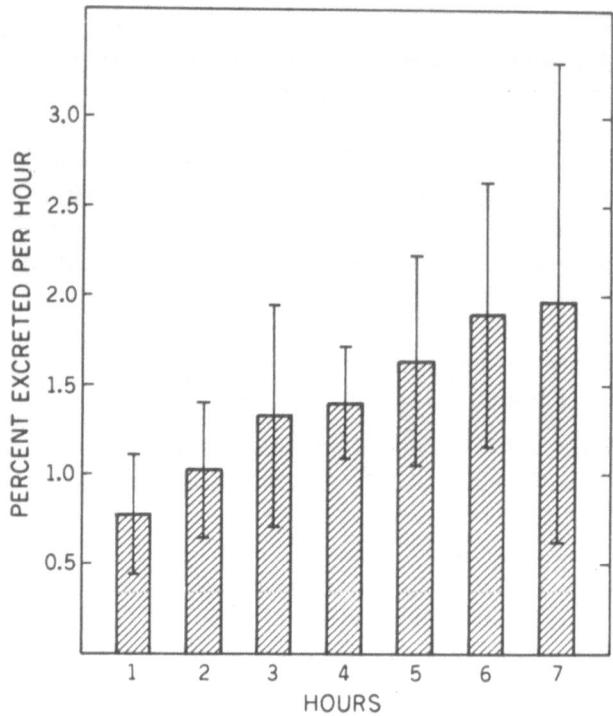

Fig. 8.2. Hourly total (urine plus bile) excretion of radioactivity. This Figure shows clearly that the hourly excretion was still rising at the end of 7 h

Table 8.1. The total (7 h) biliary and urinary excretion of radioactivity for three dogs is shown, along with the mean and standard deviation. There is considerable variation between animals. Of note is that in only 7 h 10% of the total administered radioactivity is excreted (see text)

	Dog I	Dog II	Dog III	Mean	SD
Total 7 h biliary excretion (% of total dpm administered)	5.8	4.5	2	4.1	1.9
Total urinary excretion (% of total dpm administered)	6.3	8	3.7	6	2.2
Total radioactive excretion (% of total dpm administered)	12.1	12.5	5.7	10.1	3.8

lative excretion of radioactivity for each dog. There was marked biologic variation from one animal to the other.

Chloroform extracts of all portal venous and jugular venous plasma and urine specimens tested failed to show radioactivity in the chloroform phase. Thus, during the period studied, no evidence was found of biotransformation of water-soluble metabolites into digitoxin. All radioactivity detected was nonchloroform-soluble and presumably represented water-soluble metabolites.

Discussion

It is generally believed that digitoxin, a lipid-soluble substance, is essentially completely absorbed by the gut (Beerman et al., 1971). The oral and parenteral doses required to produce a given biologic effect is the same, lending further support to this belief (Moe and Farah, 1965). Following intragastric or intraduodenal administration, digitoxin can be promptly detected in portal venous blood, and presumably enters the blood stream through this route (Oliver et al., 1971). In contrast, water-soluble substances are absorbed less well, and it has been generally accepted that the water-soluble metabolites of digitoxin are absorbed poorly by the gut, if at all (Katzung and Meyers, 1965; Beerman et al., 1971).

Our study was aimed at determining the fate af water-soluble metabolites of digitoxin after their delivery to the proximal portion of the small intestine. We have been able to demonstrate their presence in abundance in the aqueous phase of chloroform extracts of portal and peripheral blood collected as soon as 15 min after their administration.

Okita et al. showed in 1955 that the liver, biliary tract, and proximal portion of the small intestine contained a high proportion of metabolites and little unchanged digitoxin in three human subjects given the drug shortly before their death (Okita et al., 1955). Analysis of the distal intestinal content showed a marked decrease in the metabolite/digitoxin ratio. From these observations, Okita proposed, for the first time, an enterohepatic circulation of digitoxin and its metabolites.

Ten years later, Katzung and Meyers showed in the dog that diversion of the biliary stream from the gut led to a marked increase in the rate of disappearance of digitoxin from the body (Katzung and Meyers, 1965). They concluded that Okita was correct in his hypothesis of an enterohepatic circulation of digitoxin but felt that water-soluble metabolites could not be absorbed. They added the assumption that the water-soluble metabolites are hydrolyzed in the gut to a lipid-soluble derivative of digitoxin (or even digitoxin itself) and then absorbed. These authors also showed that the water-soluble metabolites recovered in bile could be hydrolyzed to products chromatographically indistinguishable from hydrolysates of digitoxin (Katzung and Meyers, 1966). Subsequent investigators have generally accepted the proposed biotransformation (Caldwell and Greensberger, 1971; Okita, 1967).

Our data does not confirm this hypothesis. We have found that at least part of the metabolites are recycled as water-soluble compounds. Furthermore, the extent of the absorption is considerable with approximately 10% of the metabolites absorbed and excreted in only 7 h (Table 8.1). As Figure 8.2 indicates, the excretion had not leveled off at this time and clearly would have exceeded 10% had collection been continued for several more hours. Despite chloroform extraction of numerous plasma and urine samples, we were unable to detect any lipid-soluble compounds. We conclude that if biotransformation does occur, it does not appear to take place during the first 7 h following intestinal administration of the metabolites. The possibility remains, however, that biotransformation may take place beyond 7 h. Longer observation is needed to demonstrate such biotransformation, and such studies are currently in progress in our laboratory.

Summary

Following administration of tritiated digitoxin to 12 dogs, bile was collected and lipid-soluble material including digitoxin was removed by repeated chloroform extraction. The digitoxin-free aqueous phase, containing water-soluble metabolites of digitoxin, was administered intraduodenally to three other dogs, who had total biliary diversion. The water-soluble metabolites were absorbed rapidly and to a significant extent by the gut. Chloroform extracts of urine and portal and jugular plasma failed to show radioactivity. We found no evidence for biotransformation of water-soluble digitoxin metabolites back into digitoxin or other lipid-soluble substances during the first 7 h after their intraduodenal administration.

References

Beerman, B., Hellström, K., Rosén, A.: Fate of orally administered ^{3}H-Digitoxin in man with special reference to the absorption. Circulation 43, 852 (1971)

Caldwell, J.H., Greensberger, N.J.: Interruption of the enterohepatic circulation of digitoxin by cholestyramine. I. Protection against lethal digitoxin intoxication. J. Clin. Invest. 50, 2626 (1971)

Caldwell, J.H., Bush, C.A., Greensberger, N.J.: Interruption of the enterohepatic circulation of digitoxin by cholestyramine. II. Effect on metabolic disposition of tritium-labeled digitoxin and cardiac systolic intervals in man. J. Clin. Invest. 50, 2638 (1971)

Katzung, B.G., Meyers, F.H.: Excretion of radioactive digitoxin by the dog. J. Pharmacol. Exp. Ther. 149, 257 (1965)

Katzung, B.G., Meyers, F.H.: Biotransformation of digitoxin in the dog. J. Pharmacol. Exp. Ther. 154, 575 (1966)

Moe, G.C., Farah, A.E.: Digitalis and allied cardiac glycosides. In: the Pharmacological Basis of Therapeutics. Goodman, L., Gilman, A. (eds.) New York: MacMillan Company 1965, p. 665

Okita, G.T.: Species difference in duration of cardiac glycosides. Fed. Proc. 26, 1125 (1967)

Okita, G.T., Talso, P.J., Curry, Jr., J.H., Smith, Jr., F.D., Geiling, E.M.K.: Metabolic fate of radioactive digitoxin in human subjects. J. Pharmacol. Exp. Ther. 115, 371 (1955)

Oliver, G.C., Cooksey, J., Witte, C., Witte, M.: Absorption and transport of digitoxin in the dog. Circ. Res. 29, 419 (1971)

Storstein, L.: Studies on digitalis. III. Biliary excretion and enterohepatic circulation of digitoxin and its cardioactive metabolites. Clin. Pharmacol. Ther. 17, 313 (1975)

Discussion

Jahrmärker, München: Can those metabolites slow down the further degradation of digitoxin?

Oliver: You pose a very interesting question. It is possible that there is some type of negative feedback in which the metabolites themselves influence the degree to which digitoxin is metabolized. However, I know of no data to support this interesting hypothesis.

Lukas: Do you agree with the data of Beerman and Rosén that approximately 4% of digitoxin undergoes the enterohepatic circulation per day?

Oliver: The percent of digitalis recirculated is time dependent if one uses the usual method of calculation as proposed by Okita et al. If you choose to determine the percentage of recirculation in 1 h you get one number. If you decide to calculate percent recirculation over a longer time such as 10 h, you will get a different number. It is a time-dependent function and therefore any figure of the percentage of the compound recirculated has to be interpreted in terms of the time in which the determination was made. It is a difficult concept to deal with. Secondly, calculations are often made in biliary fistula animals which I think further complicates the entire issue of what percentage of the compound is recirculated. If there is biotransformation, exclusion of the metabolites from the gut by biliary fistula will influence the calculation of percent recirculation. Finally, there is a speces difference between animals. The dog is a very extensive metabolizer of digitoxin compared with the human. In short, I do not know whether I do or I do not agree with their particular figure. I think we need a better way of measuring the degree of participation of digitoxin in the enterohepatic circulation.

Marcus: Dr. Oliver, the limitation in your preparation is that it is an anesthesized animal with marked diminution of gut activity. Under more physiologic circumstances, I wonder whether there might be a recirculation of these polar metabolites into the gut, following degradation of digitoxin by bacteria and then, by enterohepatic recirculation of the digitoxin. Have you any thoughts on this?

Oliver: That is a fair question. Indeed, we have some preliminary evidence that if one prolongs the period of observation beyond 7 h, there may be some con-

91

version of metabolites back into digitoxin. It certainly does not contradict, however, the fact that the metabolites themselves are absorbed. I did not emphasize that the degree of absorption is really quite substantial. Within the time period studied, an excess of 10% of the total radioactivity was absorbed. The figures I showed indicate that the peak concentration of these substances had not been reached.

Dengler, Bonn: Although I realize your very sophisticated experimental setup, I have a question regarding the bile flow. If you remove some bile before flowing to the gut you increase bile flow to an extent that is sometimes doubled. Have you any idea what the drainage of bile in your case does on the bile flow?

Oliver: I am sorry, I don't know.

Lukas: Dr. Oliver, Beerman and Rosén concluded from their calculations, which are indeed somewhat difficult to interpret, that perhaps the most important factor in prolonging the half-life of digitoxin is the great ability of the renal tubules to reabsorb the drug as it passes down the nephron. Do you agree with that conclusion?

Oliver: Well, I think it is possible, I am not prepared yet to buy that as the total explanation. It certainly seems to be true that if you give humans resins which bind digitoxin, one can reduce the half-life of digitoxin in that fashion. If the enterohepatic circulation had no effect, one would not expect the resins to have much effect.

Larbig, Tübingen: Dr. Oliver, what in your opinion would then be the major determinant for the long-standing action of digitoxin? It is apparently not enterohepatic circulation. Is it just the low renal clearance?

Oliver: I think the long action is affected by a number of factors. I have not ruled out by any means the possibility that there is conversion of the metabolites back into digitoxin. In fact, I think it probably is true. Dr. Marcus is quite correct in stating that in the anesthesized animal model one would not be expected to see the gut at its maximal efficiency. I think we still have to find out whether the enterohepatic circulation, renal excretion, or protein binding is the most important factor.

9 β-Methyl-Digoxin, a New Lipophilic Digoxin Derivative

W. SCHAUMANN

β-Methyl-digoxin was synthesized in 1967 by Kaiser (1971) in the search for
a glycoside combining the complete absorption of digitoxin with the duration
of action of digoxin. It has been on the market in Germany and many other
countries since 1971.

Physicochemical Properties and Absorption

As a rule there is an inverse relationship between the apolarity of a glycoside, as
defined by the distribution coefficient between water and a mixture of carbon
tetrachloride and isopropanol (Benthe, 1975), and its solubility in water. This
holds for the sequence digitoxin-digoxin-lanatoside C, but not for β-methyl-digoxin which, although it is highly apolar, is more soluble in water than either of
them (Table 9.1). The high water solubility favors a rapid dissolution of β-methyl-
digoxin if given in solid form. The rate of dissolution is one of the factors which
determine the bioavailability.

Apart from the rate of disintegration of the tablets and of dissolution of the
active ingredient, the bioavailability of a drug is largely determined by the rate
of absorption. The rate constants in Table 9.1 were obtained by injecting known
amounts of ^{3}H-labeled glycoside into an intestinal loop and assaying the remaining
radioactivity after 20 or 60 min. There is a good correlation between the apolarity of the glycosides investigated and their rates of absorption from a solution
in rats and guinea pigs (Table 9.1).

In man, absorption can be measured by comparing the serum concentrations or
the urinary glycoside excretion after i.v. and oral administration. Rapid and
complete absorption of β-methyl-digoxin from solutions was found in single-
dose investigations with ^{3}H-labeled substance (Larbig et al., 1971; Carbonin et
al., 1971; Rennekamp et al., 1972; Beermann, 1972; Wirth et al., 1972). Absorption from commercial preparations can only be determined by radioimmunoassay (RIA). There was no difference in the time course of the glycoside concentrations after oral administration of 0.4 mg β-methyl-digoxin in the form of
Lanitop® Liquidum or tablets (Fig. 9.1). The area under the curve was somewhat greater and the urinary glycoside excretion smaller after administration of
the tablets than after administration of the solution (Fig. 9.2). Single-dose inves-

Table 9.1. Water solubility, apolarity, and rate of absorption of digitalis glycosides

	Solubility in water mg/liter	Apolarity[a]	Rate constants for absorption, min⁻¹	
			Rat[b]	Guinea pig[c]
Digitoxin	13	10.9	—	0.036
β-Methyl-digoxin	460	6.0	0.022	0.014
Digoxin	40	2.1	0.007	0.008
Lanatosid C	86	—	—	0.0035

[a] Distribution coefficient between CCl₄ + Isopropanol and water (Benthe, 1975).
[b] Adapted from Rietbrock et al. (1972a).
[c] Adapted from Schaumann et al. (1972).

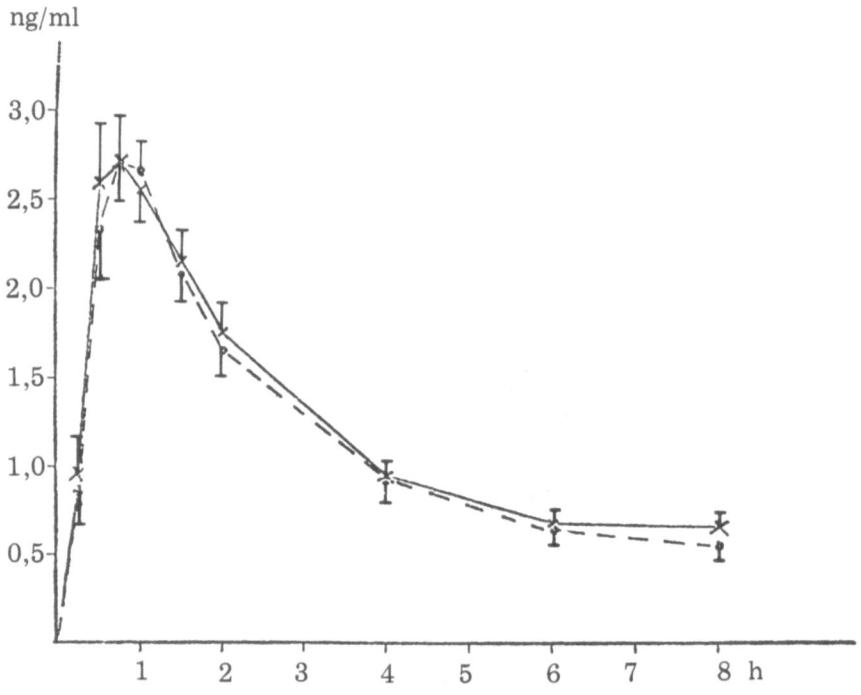

Fig. 9.1. Glycoside concentrations in the serum after 0.4 mg β-methyl-digoxin orally. o --- o Lanitop liquidum, x --- x Lanitop tablets. Cross-over investigation in 12 healthy fasting volunteers. $\bar{x}$ ± SEM

tigations being of limited value, the minimum serum glycoside concentrations under steady-state conditions during treatment with 0.2 mg β-methyl-digoxin daily in the form of Lanitop tablets or Lanitop Liquidum were compared in a cross-over investigation in 24 healthy volunteers. Treatment was initiated by giving 0.2 mg β-methyl-digoxin twice daily for 2 days followed by 0.2 mg every morning for 8 days. Then the other formulation was given for another 7 days. Blood samples were collected on the mornings 24 h after the last three doses of tablets or solution before the next daily dose. All samples from one individual were assayed by RIA on the same day. The mean of the three consecutive determinations for each formulation was used for statistical evaluation. The figures in Table 9.2 show that there was no significant difference between the average serum concentrations during both phases of treatment and that the mean of the individual differences was not significantly different from O. A statistical analysis of the results showed that a difference of > 0.15 ng/ml can be excluded with a probability of p > 0.99 (Hrstka, Kleeberg and Zilly, unpublished investigations). These investigations show that β-methyl-digoxin is as well absorbed from tablets as from a solution.

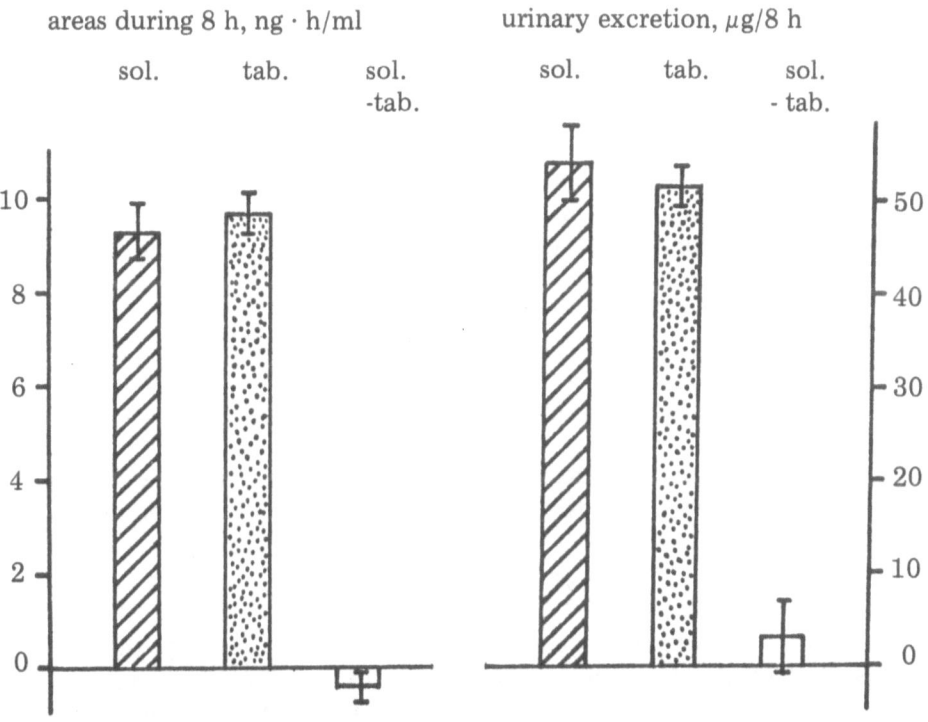

Fig. 9.2. Bioavailability of β-methyl-digoxin from Lanitop tablets and Lanitop liquidum. Cross-over experiment in 12 healthy fasting volunteers receiving 0.4 mg β-methyl-digoxin in either form

///////// Lanitop liquidum   ::::::::: Lanitop tablets

Table. 9.2. Comparison of the bioavailability of β-methyl-digoxin from Lanitop tablets and Lanitop liquidum in healthy volunteers under maintenance treatment. Minimum serum concentrations in ng/ml during administration of 0.2 mg β-methyl-digoxin daily; means ± SEM (Hrstka, Kleeberg, and Zilly; unpublished investigations)

Solution	1.479 ± 0.155
Tablets	1.430 ± 0.143
Solutions — tablets	+ 0.049 ± 0.065

The determination of absorption from tablets by RIA gave equivocal results. In five healthy volunteers under steady-state conditions, Rietbrock et al. (1976) calculated an absorption of only 65% and 75% from the serum concentrations and the urinary excretion. Haertel et al. (1973), on the other hand, saw no increase in the steady-state serum concentrations when they switched four patients from an oral to the same i.v. maintenance dose of β-methyl-digoxin. Johnson et al. (1976) obtained 87% absorption from the cumulative urinary excretion of β-methyl-digoxin after i.v. and oral administration. In a single-dose study in 18 healthy volunteers, Boerner et al. (1976) found 70% absorption, whereas there was no difference between the minimum serum concentrations during i.v. and oral maintenance therapy in 18 patients in a cross-over investigation. The experience gained from the treatment of patients showed that, as a rule, identical doses of β-methyl-digoxin should be given orally and intravenously (König and Ohly, 1970; Storz, 1970; Doering et al., 1973; Steinorth and Schweers, 1973).

Equivalent Concentrations and Doses of β-Methyl-Digoxin and Digoxin

In animal experiments, equal concentrations of β-methyl-digoxin and digoxin have the same positive inotropic and cardiotoxic effects (Tofannetti et al., 1971; Schaumann and Koch, 1974a; 1974b). In man, identical glycoside concentrations are found in serum of patients under maintenance therapy with either glycoside (Strobach et al., 1972; Larbig, 1975; Larbig and Haasis, 1975; Weiss et al., 1975). Equal serum concentrations of both glycosides may, therefore, be expected to have the same activity. No distinction was made between β-methyl-digoxin and digoxin in studies correlating side-effects with serum glycoside concentrations (Haasis and Larbig, 1975; Risler et al., 1975).

The question is, what doses of digoxin and β-methyl-digoxin are necessary to achieve identical serum concentrations in man? After i.v. injection, Rietbrock and Abshagen (1973) found appreciably higher serum concentrations in five volunteers given β-methyl-digoxin than in two subjects who received the same

dose of digoxin. This was confirmed by Zilly et al. (1975). However, in the
latter study, digoxin gave remarkably low serum concentrations. Larbig and
Haasis (1975) found no difference in serum glycoside concentrations after
i.v. injection of 0.5 mg β-methyl-digoxin or digoxin in seven healthy volunteers.
In investigations by Marinow et al. (1977), the area under the serum concentration curve during and 30 h after the infusion of 0.4 mg β-methyl-digoxin was
13% greater than in another group of volunteers receiving the same dose of digoxin. From a cross-over investigation in 20 patients receiving identical maintenance doses of β-methyl-digoxin and digoxin, they concluded that the minimum
glycoside concentrations at equilibrium would be 16% higher during treatment
with β-methyl-digoxin. Both studies together indicate that the average serum
concentration $\bar{c}$ during i.v. maintenance therapy with β-methyl-digoxin would be
15% higher than with digoxin. If D is the daily injected or absorbed maintenance
dose and Cl_{tot} is the total body clearance,

$$\bar{c} = \frac{D}{Cl_{tot} \times 24} \text{ and } Cl_{tot} = \frac{D}{\bar{c} \times 24}$$

With the data of Marinow et al. (1977), it follows from these equations that the
total clearance of digoxin is 15% greater than that of β-methyl-digoxin.

After oral administration, the difference between the equivalent doses of β-methyl-
digoxin and digoxin is greater because of the better absorption of β-methyl-digoxin.
From the results of their open large-scale clinical trial, Steinorth and Schweers
(1973) concluded that oral maintenance doses of 0.3 mg β-methyl-digoxin and

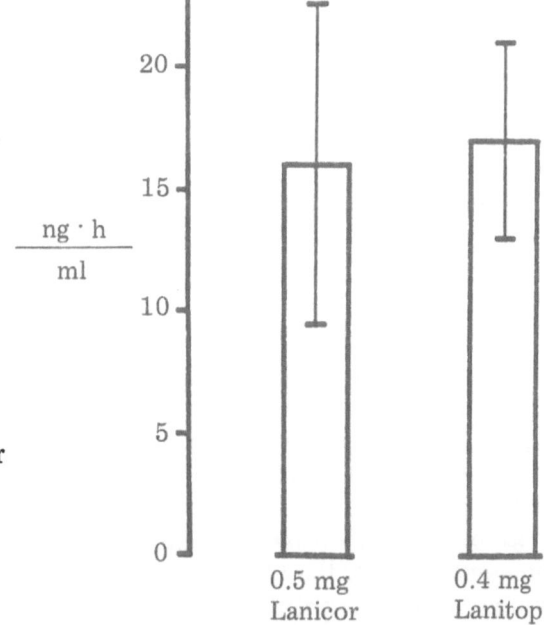

Fig. 9.3. Variation of the areas under
the serum glycoside concentration/
time curves during 32 h after intake
of 0.5 mg digoxin as Lanicor (N =
20) and 0,4 mg β-methyl-digoxin as
Lanitop (N = 17). $\bar{x} \pm$ SD

97

0.5 mg digoxin would be equiactive. This ratio was confirmed by pharmacokinetic data (Larbig, 1975; Johnson et al., 1976; Kongola et al., 1976). The variation was greater for digoxin than for β-methyl-digoxin. This was confirmed in an unpublished study carried out in our department for Clinical Pharmacology: the variation in the areas under the serum concentration curves was less after administration of β-methyl-digoxin than after administration of digoxin (Fig. 9.3). The lower variation is explained by the more complete and thereby more reliable absorption of β-methyl-digoxin.

Tissue Distribution

A distinction should be made between the rate of penetration into the tissue and the tissue/medium ratio at equilibrium. The distribution coefficients (DCs) shortly after an injection are mainly determined by the rate of penetration, the DCs under steady-state conditions by the ratios of the inflow/outflow rates. The DCs measured by Schaumann and Koch (1974b) 1 h after the injection of β-methyl-digoxin, digoxin, and digitoxin are essentially determined by the rates of penetration. For all three glycosides, the DCs between tissue and plasma water decreased in the order kidney > liver > heart > diaphragm > erythrocytes > perirenal fat > brain. The DCs for all tissues were greater for digitoxin than for β-methyl-digoxin and digoxin.

After repeated i.v. injection of cardiac glycosides in cats (Flasch and Heinz, 1976) and dogs (Kuhlmann et al., 1976), a higher accumulation was found in the brain than in other tissues. This was confirmed by Dietmann et al. (1978). The DCs between the right ventricle and the plasma in cats was the same 24 h after a single injection as after 4 days at steady state, whereas there was a twofold increase in the DCs of cerebrum and cerebellum. β-Methyl-digoxin and digoxin are equally bound to serum albumin in man (Kramer et al., 1974; Kongola et al., 1976).

Lack of Correlation Between Cerebral Glycoside Content and Side-Effects

Kuhlmann et al. (1976) assumed a correlation between the tissue concentrations of various glycosides and their cerebral side-effects. The slow penetration into the brain and the different DCs of β-methyl-digoxin and digoxin made it possible to test this hypothesis (Dietmann et al., 1978). Unanesthetized cats tolerated a loading dose of 30 μg/kg β-methyl-digoxin followed by three daily injections of 7.5 μg/kg without signs of intoxication (Fig. 9.4). The concentration in the brain was much higher 24 h after the last injection than 3 h after a single dose of 100 μg/kg, which regularly induced vomiting. The threshold vomiting doses of β-methyl-digoxin and digoxin were identical, although β-methyl-digoxin penetrated more rapidly into the brain than digoxin (Schaumann and Koch, 1974b). The dose of β-methyl-digoxin leading to intoxication by repeated injections was somewhat higher than that of digoxin (Schaumann and Wegerle, 1971), although much higher concentrations of β-methyl-digoxin than of digoxin are found in the

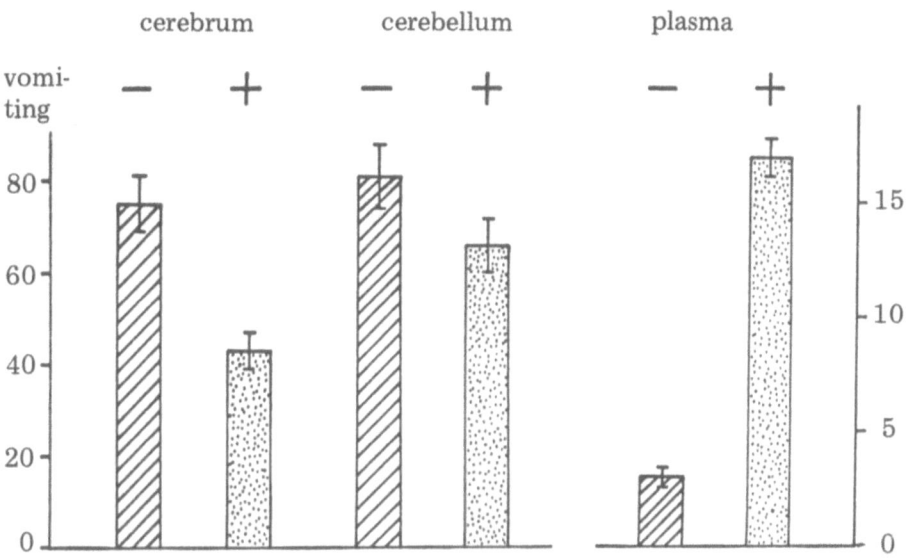

Fig. 9.4. Lack of correlation between cerebral concentrations of β-methyl-digoxin and vomiting in cats

▨▨▨▨▨ 24 h after μg/kg loading dose and 4 × 7.5 μg/kg/day
▧▧▧▧▧ 3 h after a single dose of 100 μg/kg. Left ordinate: tissue concentration in ng/g. Right ordinate: plasma concentration in ng/ml. - and + indicates the absence and presence of vomiting

brain after repeated injections (Flasch and Heinz, 1976). There is no appreciable difference in the emetic doses of β-methyl digoxin and digoxin in dogs although β-methyl-digoxin in this species, too, penetrates more readily into the brain (Kuhlmann et al., 1976). In patients with CNS side-effects, the same serum glycoside concentrations were found in those treated with β-methyl-digoxin and digoxin (Haasis and Larbig, 1976a), although the DC between most parts of the brain and the serum is higher for β-methyl-digoxin than for digoxin (Haasis and Larbig, 1976b). The DC between serum and cerebrospinal fluid was identical for β-methyl-digoxin and digoxin in man (Somogyi et al., 1978a).

In unanesthetized cats, an i.v. loading dose of 70 μg/kg β-methyl-digoxin or digoxin followed by four injections of 15 μg/kg at 48-h intervals induced a severe, but constant intoxication with constant and identical glycoside concentrations in the plasma (Dietmann et al., 1978). According to the results of Flasch and Heinz (1976), the cerebral concentrations of β-methyl-digoxin in these investigations must have been several times higher than those of digoxin. All these investigations show that the severity of cerebral side-effects of β-methyl-digoxin and digoxin is much better correlated with their concentrations in the serum than in the brain.

Metabolism and Elimination

β-Methyl-digoxin is partly demethylated to digoxin (Kramer et al., 1970; Rietbrock et al., 1972b; Rietbrock and Abshagen, 1973; Abshagen et al., 1974). Since there is very little difference in the properties of both glycosides once they are absorbed, demethylation is without practical importance. Hydrolysis of the methylated digitoxose (Rietbrock et al., 1974) leads to the metabolic pathway of digoxin. β-Methyl-digoxin and digoxin are partially transformed into chloroform-insoluble metabolites (Rietbrock et al., 1972; Rietbrock and Abshagen, 1973; Abshagen et al., 1974); it has not yet been established whether or not these are cardioactive.

The rate constant β for the elimination of a drug after equilibration with the tissue depends on the volume of distribution V_{ss} and the total body clearance Cl_{tot}.

$$\beta = \frac{Cl_{tot}}{V_{ss}}$$

β was determined in several studies with ^{3}H-labeled β-methyl-digoxin or digoxin. On average, a half-life of 42 h was found for both glycosides (for references, see Marinow et al., 1977). From the rate of urinary excretion measured by RIA, Johnson et al. (1976) found after a single dose half-lives of 39 h for β-methyl-digoxin and 35 h for digoxin. From the rate of decline of the glycoside concentrations in the serum of healthy volunteers after interruption of a maintenance treatment, Larbig and Haasis (1976) calculated average half-lives of 47.5 h for β-methyl-digoxin and 47.3 h for digoxin. The duration of action in patients with atrial fibrillation was practically identical for both glycosides (Storz, 1970). There are no cross-over studies comparing the V_{ss} of β-methyl-digoxin and digoxin in the same individual.

In healthy volunteers, the renal clearance of digoxin is about 1.5 times greater than that of β-methyl-digoxin (Larbig and Haasis, 1976; Marinow et al., 1977; Kongola et al., 1976). As with digoxin, the rate of elimination of β-methyl-digoxin is decreased considerably in anuric patients (Kramer et al., 1970; Larbig et al., 1974). The difference in the renal clearance of β-methyl-digoxin and digoxin is greater than that in the total clearance as calculated by Marinow et al. (1977). Johnson et al. (1976) found in a cross-over study a higher percentage of injected digoxin than of β-methyl-digoxin in the urine. This leads to the conclusion that more β-methyl-digoxin than digoxin must be eliminated extrarenally. Of the total radioactivity recovered after i.v. injection of ^{3}H-labeled glycosides, 35% of β-methyl-digoxin (Rietbrock et al., 1975) and 13% of digoxin (Doherty and Perkins, 1962) were found in the feces. Sumner et al. (1976), on the other hand, found an extrarenal digoxin clearance of 28% of total clearance.

In patients with acute hepatitis, Zilly et al. (1975) found higher serum concentrations of β-methyl-digoxin than in other patients without liver disease. Somogyi et al. (1978b) compared the minimum serum concentration of β-methyl-digoxin and digoxin intraindividually in 20 patients each during and after acute hepatitis. The average serum concentrations of both glycosides were in the therapeutic range and remained constant after recovery. No elevated serum concentrations were found in patients with liver cirrhosis under maintenance therapy with β-methyl-digoxin (Somogyi et al., 1978c). The maintenance dose of β-methyl-digoxin like that of digoxin should be adjusted to the renal function. It should not be reduced in patients with liver disease.

References

Abshagen, U., Rennekamp, H., Küchler, R., Rietbrock, N.: Formation and Disposition of Bis- and Monoglycosides after Administration of ^{3}H-4'''-Methyl-digoxin to Man. Eur. J. Clin. Pharmacol. 7, 177-181 (1974)

Beermann, B.: The Gastrointestinal Uptake of Methyldigoxin-12α-^{3}H in Man. Eur. J. Clin. Pharmacol. 5, 1-6 (1972)

Benthe, H.F.: Organverteilung verschiedener Herzglykoside. Digitalistherapie — Beiträge zur Pharmakologie und Klinik. Berlin-Heidelberg-New York: Springer-Verlag, 1975, pp. 19-34

Boerner, D., Olcay, A., Schaumann, W., Weiss, W.: Absorption of β-Methyl-Digoxin Determined after a Single Dose and under Steady State Conditions. Eur. J. Clin. Pharmacol. 9, 307-314 (1976)

Carbonin, P.U., Zecchi, P. Bellocci, F., Ruffa, S., Loperfido, F., Pharmakokinetik von Methyl-Digoxin-H^3 nach oraler und intravenöser Gabe beim normalen Menschen. Atti del XXXII Congresso della Società Italiana di Cardiologia. Taormina, 30.5.-2.6.1971

Dietmann, K., Hrstka, E., Koch, K., Schaumann, W.: β-methyl-digoxin: VIII. Relation of Cerebral Side-Effects in Cats to Concentrations in the Plasma and the Brain Naunyn-Schmiedeberg's Arch. Pharmacol. (1978) (in press)

Doering, W., König, E., Kronski, D., Hall, D.: Bestimmung der Kenngrößen von β-Methyldigoxin mit Einschwemmkatheterverfahren und nicht-invasiven Methoden. Dtsch. Med. Wochenschr. 98, 2274-2280 (1973)

Doherty, J.E., Perkins, W.H.: Studies with Tritiated Digoxin in Human Subjects after Intravenous Administration. Am. Heart J. 63, 528-536 (1962)

Flasch, H., Heinz, N.: Konzentration von Herzglykosiden im Myokard und im Gehirn. Arzneim. Forsch. 26, 1213-1216 (1976)

Haasis, R., Larbig, D.: Serumglykosidkonzentration und Digitalisintoxikation. Dtsch. Med. Wochenschr. 100, 1768-1773 (1975)

Haasis, R., Larbig, D.: Vergleichende Untersuchungen der Serum-Glykosidkonzentrationen bei Glykosidintoxikationen mit extrakardialen Nebenwirkungen nach Einnahme von Beta-Methyldigoxin, Beta-Acetyldigoxin und Digoxin. Verh. Dtsch. Ges. Inn. Med. 82, 1702-1704 (1976a)

Haasis, R., Larbig, D.: Radioimmunologische Bestimmung der Glykosidkonzentrationen im menschlichen Gehirngewebe. Verh. Dtsch. Ges. Kreislaufforschg. 42, 275-277 (1976b)

Härtel, G., Manninen, V., Melin, J., Apajalahti, A.: Serum-digoxin Concentrations with a New Digoxin Derivative, β-Methyl-Digoxin. Ann. Clin. Res. 5, 87-90 (1973)

Johnson, B.F., Bye, C.E., Jones, G.E., Sabey, G.A.: The Pharmacokinetics of Beta-Methyl-Digoxin Compared with Digoxin Tablets and Capsules. Eur. J. Clin. Pharmacol. 10, 231-236 (1976)

Kaiser, F.: Teilsynthetische Herzglykosid-Derivate mit verbesserter enteralen Wirksamkeit. Planta Med. Suppl. 4, 52-60 (1971)

König, E., Ohly, A.: Quantitative Eigenschaften eines neuen Herzglykosids. Med. Klin. 65, 296-299 (1970)

Kongola, G.W.M., Mawer, G.E., Woodcock, B.G.: Steady State Pharmacokinetics of β-Methyl-Digoxin and Digoxin. Br. J. Clin. Pharmacol. 3, 954P-955P (1976)

Kramer, P., Horenkamp, J., Willms, B., Scheler, F.: Das Kumulationsverhalten verschiedener Herzglykoside bei Anurie. Dtsch. Med. Wochenschr. 95, 444-453 (1970)

Kramer, P., Köthe, E., Saul, J., Scheler, F.: Uraemic and Normal Plasma Protein Binding of Various Cardiac Glycosides under "in vivo" Conditions. Eur. J. Clin. Invest. 4, 53-58 (1974)

Kuhlmann, J., Reiche, J., Bruns, J.: Distribution of Digoxin, β-Methyl-Digoxin and Ouabain after Single and Multiple Doses in Dogs. Naunyn-Schmiedeberg's Arch. Pharmacol. 293, R 29 (1976)

Larbig, D.: Herzinsuffizienz: Digitalistherapie. Therapiewoche 25, 48-61 (1975)

Larbig, D., Haasis, R.: Radioimmunchemische Bestimmungen der Konzentration von Digoxin und Digoxin-Derivaten. Digitalistheraphie — Beiträge zur Pharmakologie und Klinik. Berlin-Heidelberg-New York: Springer-Verlag 1975, pp. 62-75

Larbig, D., Haasis, R.: Untersuchungen zur Elimination von Digoxin und β-Methyl-Digoxin. Verh. Dtsch. Ges. Inn. Med. 82, 1717-1719 (1976)

Larbig, D., Haasis, R., Bundschu, H.D., Buckesfeld, R.G., Lankisch, P.G., Ilg, R., Girndt, J.: Radioimmunchemische Bestimmung von Digoxin und Digoxin-Derivaten im Serum und Urin bei normaler und eingeschränkter Nierenfunktion. Verh. Dtsch. Ges. Inn. Med. 80, 1077-1080 (1974)

Larbig, D., Scheler, F., Schmidt, H.-J., Betzien, G., Kaufmann, B.: Untersuchungen zur enteralen Resorption von β-Methyldigoxin. Klin. Wochenschr. 49, 604-607 (1971)

Marinow, J., Olcay, A., Schaumann, W., Weiss, W.: Serum Glycoside Concentrations after Single or Repeated Intravenous Doses of β-Methyl-Digoxin and Digoxin. Eur. J. Clin. Pharmacol. 11, 213-218 (1977)

Rennekamp, H., Rennekamp, Ch., Abshagen, U., Bergmann, K.v., Rietbrock, N.: Pharmacokinetic Behaviour of 4'''-Methyldigoxin in Man. Naunyn-Schmiedeberg's Arch. Pharmacol. 273, 172-174 (1972)

Rietbrock, N., Abshagen, U.: Stoffwechsel und Pharmakokinetik der Lanataglykoside beim Menschen. Dtsch. Med. Wochenschr. 98, 117-122 (1973)

Rietbrock, N., Abshagen, U., Bergmann, K.v., Kewitz, H.: Pharmacokinetics of Digoxin and its 4''' -acetyl- and methyl-derivates in the Rat. Naunyn-Schmiedeberg's Arch. Pharmacol. 274, 171-181 (1972a)

Rietbrock, N., Rennekamp, Ch., Rennekamp, H., Bergmann, K.v., Abshagen, U.: Demethylation and Cleavage of Glycosidic Bonds of 4''' -Methyl-digoxin in Man. Naunyn-Schmiedeberg's Arch. Pharmacol. 272, 450-453 (1972b)

Rietbrock, N., Abshagen, U., Bergmann, K.v., Rennekamp, H.: Disposition of
β-Methyldigoxin in Man. Eur. J. clin. Pharmacol. 9, 106-114 (1975)

Rietbrock, N., Guggenmos, J., Kuhlmann, J., Hess, U.: Bioavailability and Pharmacokinetics of β-Methyldigoxin after Multiple Oral and Intravenous Doses.
Eur. J. Clin. Pharmacol. 9, 373-379 (1976)

Risler, T., Grabensee, B., Grosse-Brockhoff, F.: EKG-Veränderungen und
Digoxin-Serumkonzentration bei Digitalisintoxikationen. Dtsch. Med. Wochenschr. 100, 821-825 (1975)

Schaumann, W., Koch, K.: β-Methyl-Digoxin: VI. Tissue Distribution and Therapeutic Ratio in Guinea Pigs in Comparison with Digoxin. Naunyn-Schmiedeberg's Arch. Pharmacol. 282, 9-14 (1974a)

Schaumann, W., Koch, K.: β-Methyl-Digoxin: VII. Tissue Distribution, Positive
Inotropic and Central Action in Cats in Comparison with Other Digitalis
Glycosides. Naunyn-Schmiedeberg's Arch. Pharmacol. 286, 195-210 (1974b)

Schaumann, W., Wegerle, R.: β-Methyl-Digoxin: I. Cardiotoxizität bei enteraler
und parenteraler Gabe. Arzneim. Forsch. 21, 225-231 (1971)

Schaumann, W., Zielske, F., Kohler, K., Koch, K.: β-Methyl-Digoxin: III. Speed
of Absorption in Guinea Pigs in Comparison to Other Cardiac Glycosides.
Naunyn-Schmiedeberg's Arch. Pharmakol. 272, 32-45 (1972)

Somogyi, G., Gosztonyi, G., Gachalyi, B., Herpai, Z., Szirtes, M., Simonyi, G.:
Changes of Cerebrospinal Fluid Digoxin-Level on Therapeutic Doses. Orvosi
Hetilap (1978a) (in press)

Somogyi, G., Gosztonyi, G., Gachalyi, B., Ibranyi, E.: Serum Digoxin Concentration in Acute Hepatitis. Orvosi Hetilap (1978b) (in press)

Somogyi, G., Kaldor, A., Gachalyi, B., Ibranyi, E.: Verhalten der Plasma-beta-
methyl-Digoxin-Konzentration nach oraler Belastung bei der Leberzirrhose.
Klin. Wochenschr. (1978c) (in press)

Steinorth, G., Schweers, A.: Bericht über die klinische Prüfung von Lanitop. Med.
Welt 24, 1310-1317 (1973)

Storz, H.: Die quantitative Wirksamkeit des Herzglykosids β-Methyldigoxin. Med.
Welt 21, 2066-2070 (1970)

Strobach, H., Greeff, K., Horster, F.A., Wildmeister, W.: Radioimmunologische
Glykosidbestimmungen nach Gabe von Digoxin und Digoxin-Derivaten beim
Menschen. Naunyn-Schmiedeberg's Arch. Pharmacol. 274, R 113 (1972)

Sumner, D.J., Russel, A.J., Whiting, B.: Digoxin Pharmacokinetics: Multicom-
partmental Analysis and its Clinical Implications. Br. J. Clin. Pharmacol. 3,
221-229 (1976)

Tofanetti, O., Siena, M.A., Albiero, L.: Attivitá Farmacologica di un Nuovo
Glucoside Semisintetico, la β-Metildigossina. Annali Dell' Università die Fer-
rara, Sezione XI, Band 3, 225-234 (1971)

Weiss, W., Olcay, A., Teufel, W., Glocke, M.: Vergleichende Untersuchungen der
Glykosid-Konzentration im Serum bei Erhaltungstherapie mit Lanicor®,
Card-Lamuran®, MF 708 d und Lanitop.® Med. Klin. 70, 1367-1374 (1975)

Wirth, K., Bodem, G., Dengler, H.J.: Resorption, Ausscheidung und Stoffwechsel
von Digoxin und Digoxin-verwandten Verbindungen. In: Aktuelle Digitalisprobleme. Pharmakokinetik. Digitalis bei Herzinfarkt. Berliner Arbeitstagung

Dez. 1970. Schröder, R., Greeff, K., (eds) München, Urban & Schwarzenberg: 1972, pp. 51-61

Zilly, W., Richter, E., Rietbrock, N.: Pharmacokinetics and Metabolism of Digoxin and β-Methyl-Digoxin-12α-^{3}H in Patients with Acute Hepatitis. Clin. Pharmacol. Ther. <u>17</u>, 302-309 (1975)

Discussion

Flasch, Hamburg: How did you measure the solubilities shown on your first Figure, and how do you explain the difference between digoxin and the more lipophilic β-methyl-digoxin?

Schaumann: The water solubility in Table 9.1 is the maximum solubility obtained by shaking. The high solubility of β-methyl-digoxin is probably a matter of crystal structure.

Flasch: Are you sure that you reached the physicochemical equilibrium when you made these studies?

Schaumann: Yes.

Flasch: On your last slide, you showed the concentration of β-methyl-digoxin in the brain. We found indeed higher concentrations for this glycoside. Did you determine tritium water in these experiments?

Schaumann: We used material in the 12-α position according to Wartburg and we found no tritium water in cats. The difference between your results and ours is probably due to the difference in the dosing schedule. You gave the glycosides for several days and assayed 5 h after the last dose, and you compared your figures with those obtained by Benthe 5 h after a single dose.

Abshagen, Berlin: You showed that the plasma concentrations after intravenous administration of β-methyl-digoxin were only slightly higher — by about 15% — than after intravenous administration of digoxin; on the other hand, you stressed that the cardiac activities of digoxin and β-methyl-digoxin were almost identical. Presuming the well-known fact that β-methyl-digoxin and digoxin are eliminated to an almost equal degree — with a daily loss of 20%-30% in steady-state conditions — how do you explain that the maintenance dose of β-methyl-digoxin recommended by you is in the range of 0.2 mg per day and that for digoxin is considerably higher? If we assume that the concentrations of β-methyl-digoxin were distinctly higher, as shown previously by us by about 50%, you could explain the above-mentioned discrepancies by the fact that the concentrations in blood with these different doses were then in the same range as a consequence of a lower distribution volume of β-methyl-digoxin. This would also be consistent with your first slide in which the water solubility of β-methyl-digoxin was fairly higher.

Schaumann: The essential factors detemining the average serum concentration $\bar{c}$ which in this presentation I took for a parameter of activity, is the dose D multiplied by absorption R and divided by total clearance Cl_{tot} and dosage interval τ.

$$\bar{c} = \frac{D \circ R}{Cl_{tot} \cdot \tau}$$

Identical doses D of β-methyl-digoxin were injected (R = 1) at τ = 24 h intervals. That means that the difference in serum concentrations $\bar{c}$ of 15% is due to a difference in total clearance. According to our recommendations for oral dosage, 0.2 mg β-methyl-digoxin is equivalent ot 0.33 mg digoxin. Taking into account the difference of 15% in total clearance, 0.2 mg of β-methyl-digoxin give the same serum concentrations as 0.23 mg of digoxin. The ratio of 0.33:0.23 = 1.43 is due to the better absorption of β-methyl-digoxin. I do not think that there is any discrepancy.

Marcus: I have been following the literature with interest on β-methyl-digoxin. We do not have this available in the United States. I have not been convinced of any important clinical advantage of this drug.

Schaumann: There are four studies showing less variation of β-methyl-digoxin plasma levels than of digoxin. One is from Larbig, who routinely assayed the minimum serum concentrations of his patients. He had one group of patients treated with 0.5 mg digoxin daily, and another group with Lanitop®, which is our brand of methyl-digoxin. The variation of the minimum serum concentrations was definitely less for β-methyl-digoxin than for digoxin. We observed the same thing in a single-dose study comparing the areas under the serum concentration time curve in volunteers receiving comparable doses of both compounds (Fig. 9.3). A similar observation was made by Kongola et al. and by Johnson et al.

Grahame-Smith: Could I ask you about the data sheet. One of the things stressed there for β-methyl-digoxin is the speed of onset of action. Could you tell me whether there is really any difference by whatever route between the speed of onset of action of digoxin and β-methyl-digoxin?

Schaumann: I am glad you asked this question for two reasons. One is that in this country a good part especially of elder doctors favor strophanthin for rapid action. The meaning of stressing the rapid onset of action is: if you want to have rapid action you can as well inject β-methyl-digoxin, go on with the same drug orally, and stick to the maintenance dose which you have established intravenously. The second reason is that given orally, the onset of action is more rapid because of the more rapid absorption. I do not know of any intravenous studies comparing the rate of onset of action of digoxin and β-methyl-digoxin.

Benthe: We did experiments about the binding velocity of four radioactively labeled glycosides, strophanthin or ouabain, digoxin, methyl-digoxin, and digitoxin to the heart. First, we studied the absorption of these glycosides in cats by comparing the blood level curves in cats after intraduodenal injection and intravenous infusion. In Figure 1 on the ordinate the blood concentration is plotted. After 30 min there was no further increase of the blood level. At that time the animals were killed and we counted myocardial radioactivity. On the left of Figure 1 the experiment for strophanthin and on the right side for digoxin is shown. There is a much higher ^{3}H activity in the myocard if digoxin is applied by intravenous infusion (fast declining curve). In contrast to digoxin, strophanthin is stored to a higher concentration in the myocard, after intraduodenal injection. That means that strophanthin is extracted quickly from plasma to the heart. This observation is in accordance with the fast therapeutic effect of strophanthin. Also, experiments with methyl-digoxin and digitoxin were done. Figure 2 shows the results for digitoxin (right side). There are higher blood and higher myocardial concentrations after infusion. Surprisingly, methyl-digoxin is stored to a higher amount after

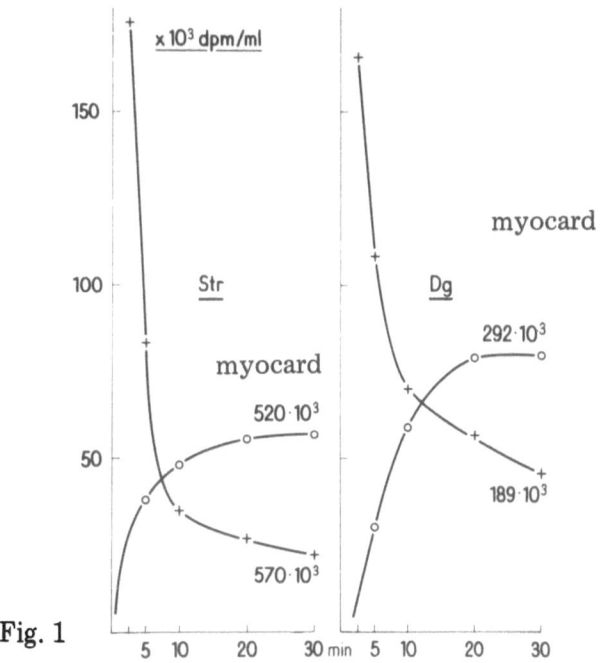

Fig. 1

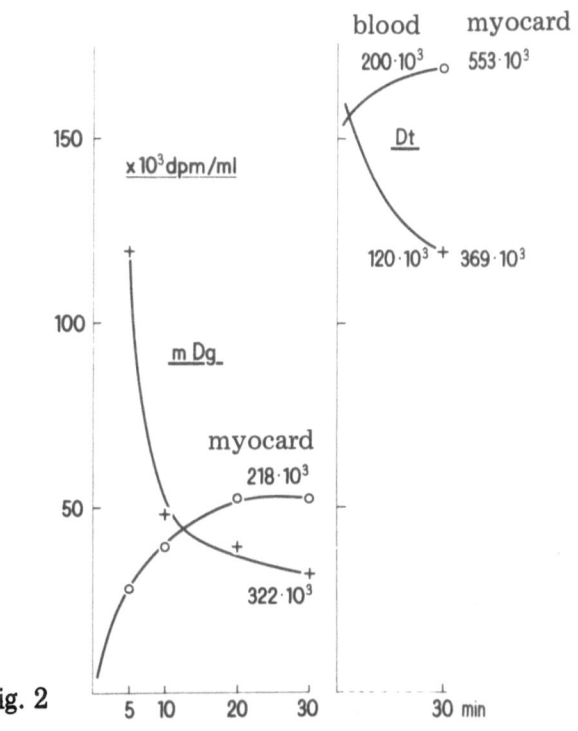

Fig. 2

the intraduodenal injection (left side). That means that the binding velocity of methyl-digoxin is faster than that of digoxin and that might explain the quick therapeutic effect.

Schaumann: Thank you very much for the helpful comment. I am becoming more and more reluctant, however, to draw conclusions from tissue content to the pharmacodynamic activity of a drug.

Lukas: Thank you, Dr. Schaumann.

10 Tissue Distribution of Cardiac Glycosides

J. KUHLMANN, N. RIETBROCK, and B. SCHNIEDERS

The treatment of cardiac failure is complicated by the difficulty in determining the optimal therapeutic response and undesirable side-effects. The side-effects of cardiac glycosides can be categorized into two general classes, those of a neurologic nature including fatigue, loss of appetite, vomiting, color vision, central scotoma, states of confusion and delirium, and those of a cardiac nature, primarily those of alterations in cardiac rate and rhythm (Schwiegk and Jahrmärker, 1960; Lely and van Enter, 1972). Both organ-specific side-effects can occur with varying duration and either simultaneously or independently of each other (Fowler et al., 1964; Bloch, 1964; Lely and van Enter, 1970). The existing dissociation between the duration of cardiac and central effects has been shown in a case study of digitalis delirium by Church and Marriott (1959). This study is of particular interest, since the psychotic state outlasted the cardiac side-effects of digoxin intoxication. Four days after digoxin administration was stopped, a normalization of heart rate and sinus rhythm without extrasystoles in the ECG was observed. In contrast, the central side-effects such as anorexia, dizziness, blurring of vision, and the symptoms of a typical digitalis delirium lasted longer than 2 weeks. The different duration of the cardiac and central effects of digitalis preparations may be caused by different elimination rates of both tissue compartments. This could be confirmed by the following studies in dog and man.

Methods

Distribution and Excretion of Cardiac Glycosides in Dogs

Experimental studies were performed on beagle dogs with an average body weight of 15 kg. Dogs were used since the tissue distribution of digoxin appears to be similar to that observed in humans (Doherty et al., 1961; Doherty and Perkins, 1966). Furthermore, digoxin concentration in plasma and positive inotropy are correlated, and some of the typical symptoms of digitalis intoxication in man such as loss of appetite, vomiting, and weariness can also be seen in dogs (Deutscher et al., 1972). The dog is, therefore, especially suitable for distribution studies on the course of cardiac effects and also central intoxication symptoms as one can draw conclusions from these for man.

Glycosides were administered intravenously as a single or as repeated doses: 0.0125 mg/kg tritium-labeled digoxin, β-methyl-digoxin, ouabain, and MD/D mixtures with a ratio of 60%:40% and vice versa (spec. activity 700-800 μCi/mg). The animals were sacrificed 24 h after a single dose or 24-144 h after discontinuation of multiple doses, and samples weighing 0.5-2.0 g were immediately taken from various tissues in order to determine the total radioactivity. Venous blood samples from each animal were collected 24 h after administration during treatment and for 7 days after cessation of drug administration. Two dogs were placed in metabolism cages and urine and feces were collected during treatment and for 24 days after administration of tritiated digoxin and β-methyl-digoxin had ceased. After measurement of total volume, radioactivity in urine and, after extraction with acetone, also in feces was counted in a liquid scintillation spectrometer. The detailed methods of extraction steps and TLC separation of the total radioactivity have been described previously (Kuhlmann et al., 1975).

Renal Excretion of β-Methyl Digoxin in Man

Two volunteers were given intravenously 0.4 mg β-methyl-digoxin (Lanitop®) once daily for 14 days (Keller et al., 1977). The urine was collected for 24 days after the intravenous administration of methyl-digoxin had ceased and the urinary glycoside concentrations were measured by a H^3 radioimmunoassay.

Results

Elimination

The renal excretion over a period of 24 days after cessation of a daily dose of 0.4 mg β-methyl-digoxin in the two volunteers shows two slopes (Fig. 10.1). During the first 14 days, a mean half-life of 48 h was observed followed by a second half-life of 131 h. The linear regression of the daily excretion rates shows close correlations in both phases (r=0.996 and 0.967 for the first regression and 0.912 and 0.940 for the second regression). The same phenomenon was observed for renal and fecal excretion of digoxin and β-methyl-digoxin in dogs. During the first 14 days, renal and fecal half-lives of 29 and 36 h followed by a terminal half-life of 136 h for digoxin (r=0.994 and 0.917 for the first phase and 0.924 and 0.824 for the second phase of renal and fecal excretion). Corresponding half-lives of 42 and 37 h for the first slope and 134 and 216 h for the second with similar correlation coefficients were observed after β-methyl-digoxin administration. This retarded terminal excretion of glycoside reflects a slowly equilibrating tissue pool which could be — in good agreement with the clinical course of central signs of digitalis intoxication — the brain. Considering that the terminal half-life could be determined only from the 14th day after cessation of glycoside injection, when nearly 95% of the total dose is excreted, it could be supposed that the deep compartment is small.

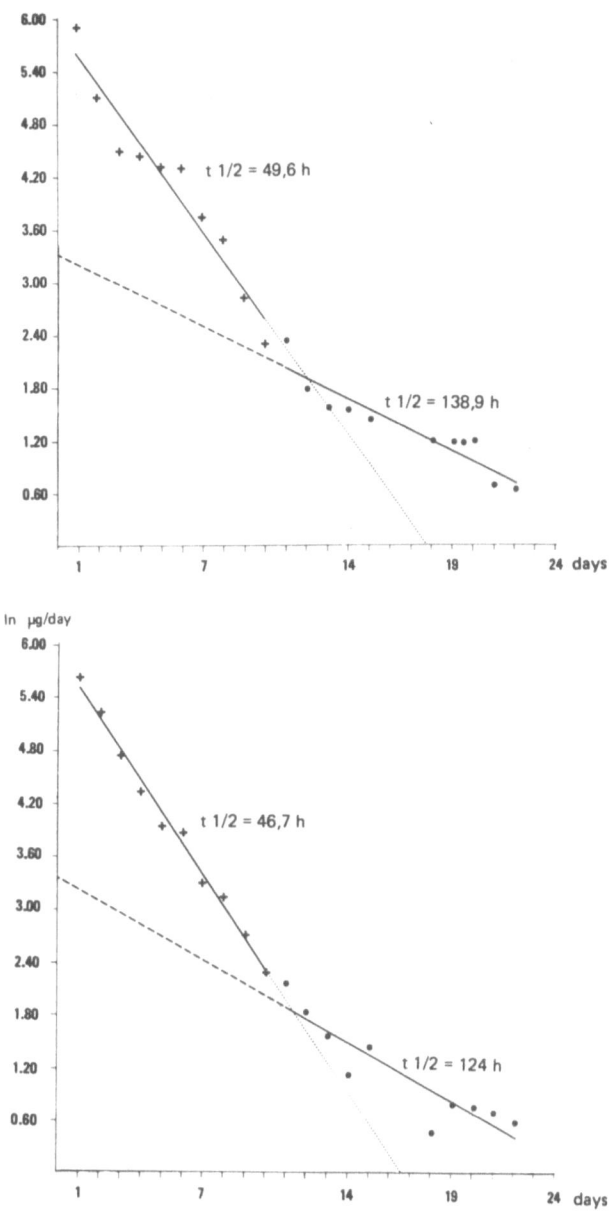

Fig. 10.1. Renal excretion (µg/day) of two volunteers after cessation of multiple dosing of 0.4 mg β-methyl-digoxin daily for 14 days (Keller et al., 1977)

Tissue Distribution in Dogs

The following glycoside concentrations were found in the various tissues 24 h after a single i.v. dose of 0.0125 mg/kg H³ digoxin (Fig. 10.2) : heart atria 12 ng/g

111

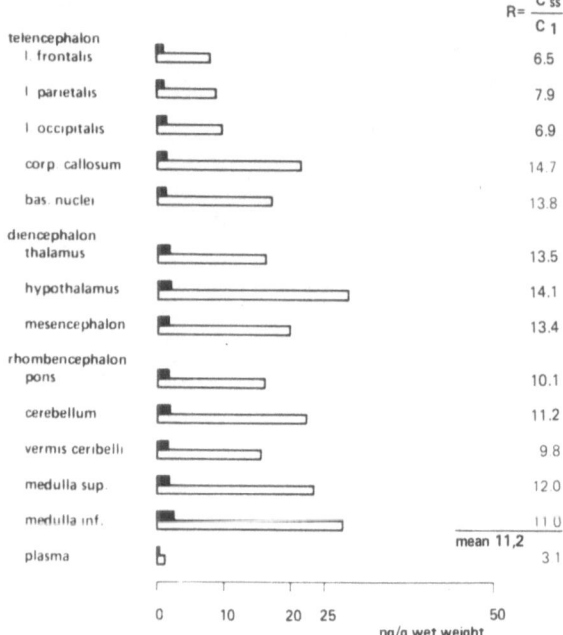

$$R = \frac{C_{ss}}{C_1}$$

telencephalon	
l. frontalis	6.5
l. parietalis	7.9
l. occipitalis	6.9
corp. callosum	14.7
bas. nuclei	13.8
diencephalon	
thalamus	13.5
hypothalamus	14.1
mesencephalon	13.4
rhombencephalon	
pons	10.1
cerebellum	11.2
vermis ceribelli	9.8
medulla sup.	12.0
medulla inf.	11.0
	mean 11,2
plasma	3.1

0   10   20 25   50
ng/g wet weight

in different tissues of beagles

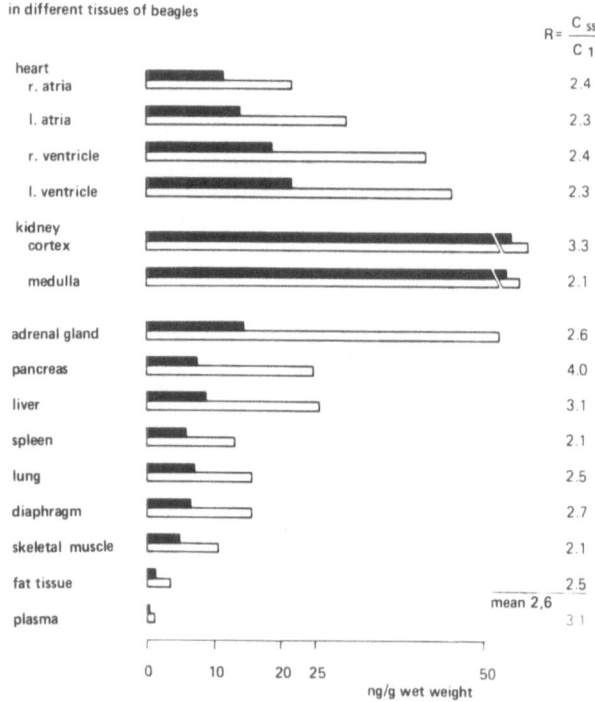

$$R = \frac{C_{ss}}{C_1}$$

heart	
r. atria	2.4
l. atria	2.3
r. ventricle	2.4
l. ventricle	2.3
kidney	
cortex	3.3
medulla	2.1
adrenal gland	2.6
pancreas	4.0
liver	3.1
spleen	2.1
lung	2.5
diaphragm	2.7
skeletal muscle	2.1
fat tissue	2.5
	mean 2,6
plasma	3.1

0   10   20 25   50
ng/g wet weight

■ 24 hours after a single intravenous dose of 0,0125 mg/kg Digoxin
□ 24 hours after a daily intravenous dose of 0,0125 mg/kg Digoxin
   during 10 days

Fig. 10.2. Concentration of H³-Digoxin

112

wet wt and heart ventricle 22 ng/g wet wt, higher in the left than in the right heart; adrenal gland 14 ng/g wet wt; plasma, fat tissue, skeletal muscle, diaphragm, lung, spleen, pancreas, and liver between 0.35 ng/ml and 8.7 ng/g wet wt. In the kidney cortex, the digoxin concentrations are 7-8 times and in the kidney medulla 4 times higher than in the heart ventricle. Compared with other tissues, the concentration in the brain 24 h after a single dose is still relatively low, but the concentrations differed between the various brain areas from 1.1 ng/g in the telencephalon to 2.5 ng/g in the medulla.

The concentration in plasma and in the various tissues except the brain were 2.1-4.0 times higher 24 h after the last daily dose of 0.0125 mg/kg tritiated digoxin, administered over a period of 10 days, than 24 h after a single dose. A much larger enrichment of digoxin was obtained in all brain areas; 7-8 times higher concentrations are measured in the telencephalon and 10-14-fold in the other brain areas.

A similar enrichment after single and multiple doses of 0.0125 mg/kg tritiated β-methyl-digoxin and oubain was observed in the various tissues. In contrast to digoxin, β-methyl-digoxin is similarly distributed between all brain areas with a mean cumulative factor of 12.4, while ouabain showed a lower accumulation with cumulative factors between 4.5-10 in the different brain areas (Kuhlmann et al., 1976a). After daily doses of β-methyl-digoxin and ouabain, 1.5-2.0 times higher concentrations were measured in the renal cortex, heart, liver, adrenal gland, and lung. In skeletal muscle and in brain, the ouabain concentrations amounted only to one-half and one-fourth of the digoxin levels, respectively. In contrast, β-methyl-digoxin concentrations were 13 times higher in the telencephalon and 3-4 times higher in the medulla as compared with digoxin (Fig. 10.3).

Chromatographic analysis showed that the radioactivities were chemically identical with the applied glycoside. Only in the liver could 10%-20% $CHCl_3$-insoluble metabolites be found after digoxin and β-methyl-digoxin application. A demethylation of methyl-digoxin to digoxin, which was revealed as a main metabolic degradation step in man (Rietbrock et al., 1975), could not be established in the dog. The variable ratio of MD/D after MD administration in man may influence the distribution of β-methyl-digoxin or digoxin in the tissues. The enrichment after single and multiple doses of such MD/D mixtures (60%-40% and vice versa) were comparable to those observed after separate digoxin or β-methyl-digoxin administration. The mean cumulative factors were 2.2 in the various tissues and 12-15 in the different brain areas.

After multiple doses of these mixtures, the glycoside concentrations in the most tissues are equal to or only slightly higher than those achieved with digoxin alone (Fig. 10.3), but 4-6 times higher accumulation could be seen in the telencephalon and 2-4 times higher in the other brain areas. Therefore, it is possible that a higher portion of methyl-digoxin may be accumulated in the brain than in other tissues. This could be proved by thin layer chromatographic analysis (Fig. 10.4). In heart, liver, and kidney, equal portions of digoxin and β-methyl-digoxin could be detected after a MD/D mixture of 40%-60% while in all brain areas 90% β-methyl-digoxin and only 10% digoxin could be recovered. Also, inversion of the

MD/D ratio led to a reduced portion of digoxin of up to 20% in the tissues, while in brain only traces of digoxin could be discovered.

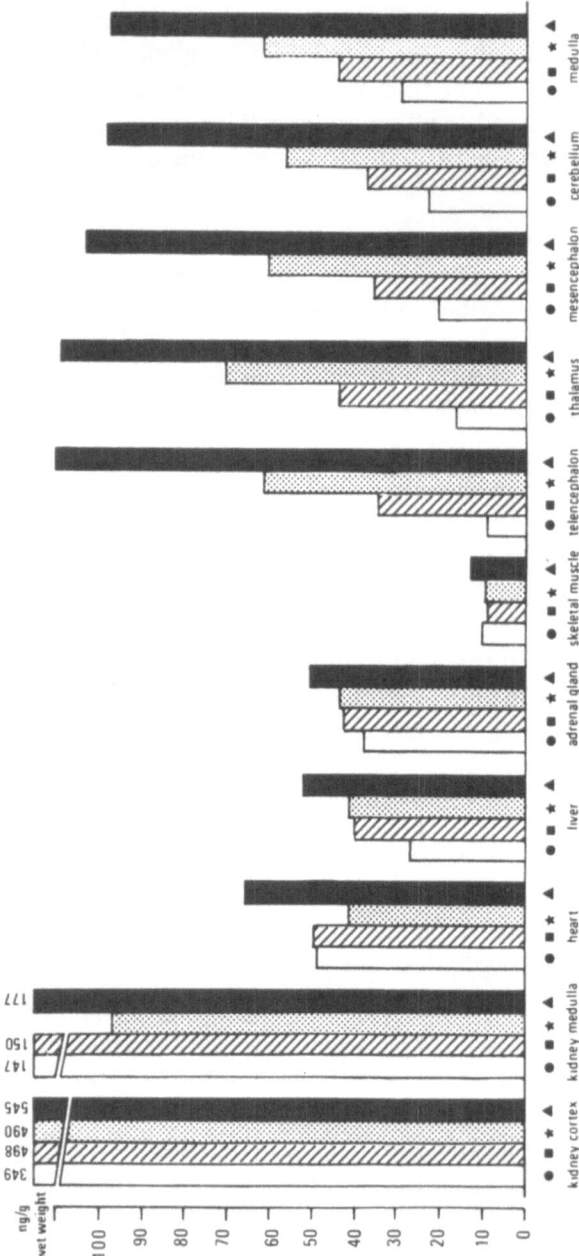

Fig. 10.3. Total radioactivity in different brain areas and tissues of beagle dogs 24 h after the last daily dose of 0.0125 mg/kg tritium-labeled digoxin (●), digoxin/methyl-digoxin 60%:40% (■), digoxin/methyl-digoxin 40%:60% (*), and methyl-digoxin (▲) over a period of 10 days

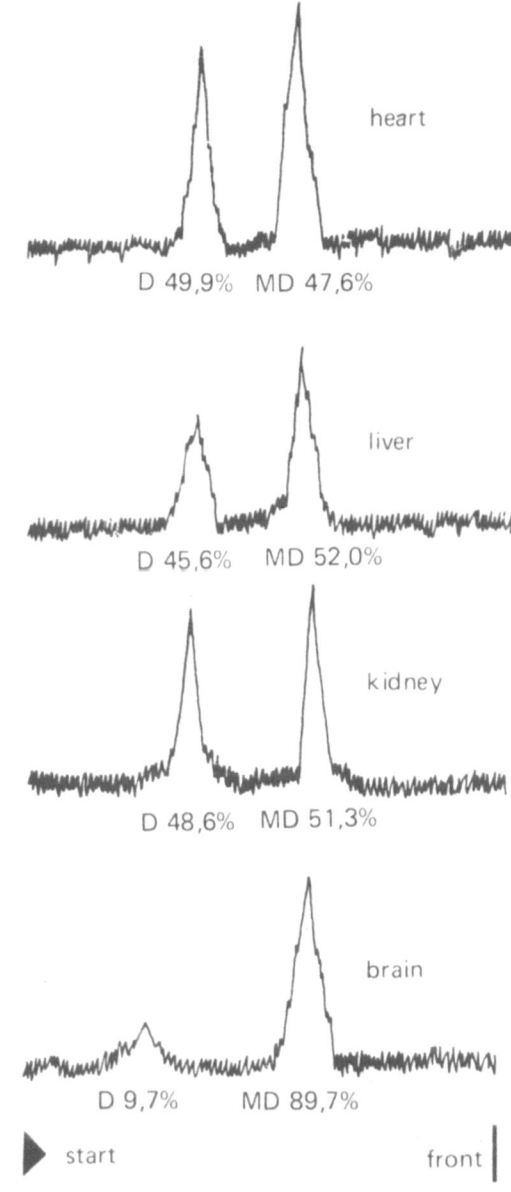

heart

D 49,9% MD 47,6%

liver

D 45,6% MD 52,0%

kidney

D 48,6% MD 51,3%

brain

D 9,7% MD 89,7%

▶ start front |

Fig. 10.4. TLC separation of the CHCl₃-soluble fraction in various tissues of beagle dogs 24 h after the last daily dose of 0.0125 mg/kg tritium-labeled digoxin/methyl-digoxin 60%:40% over a period of 10 days

After discontinuation of multiple digoxin injections, the glycoside concentration in the different tissues, including heart, decline with a mean half-life of 31 h (Fig. 10.5). In contrast, the digoxin elimination from the brain occurs markedly slower with a half-life of 72-96 h for the various brain areas (Kuhlmann and Rietbrock, 1976b). As a consequence of the slower diminuation of digoxin in brain, the concentration was about 2-3 times higher than that obtained in other tissues, except the kidney, 144 h after cessation of digoxin administration. A similar elimination half-life in the tissues could be found after β-methyl-digoxin administration compared with digoxin, while in all brain areas the β-methyl-digoxin concentration declined with a longer half-life of 120-150 h (Fig. 10.5). In accordance with the different elimination half-lives from these compartments, there were also great differences in the cumulative velocity. While in the easily equilibrating tissues the steady-state concentrations of digoxin and β-methyl-digoxin were reached after 6-8 days, in the brain a much more extensive accumulation took place over a longer period of time.

Twenty-four hours after cessation of the repetitive doses of digoxin, 5-6 times higher concentrations could be measured in the heart than in the brain. In contrast, the amount of β-methyl-digoxin after multiple doses was 2 times greater in the brain than in the heart. The percentage distribution of both glycosides increases from 1.5% digoxin and 16% β-methyl-digoxin after 24 h to 16% digoxin and 48% β-methyl-digoxin after 144 h.

Conclusions

1. After single or multiple doses of ouabain, digoxin, and β-methyl-digoxin, ouabain shows the highest concentrations in the heart, while in the brain methyl-digoxin attains the highest and ouabain the lowest concentrations. A similar distribution pattern of these glycosides has been described by Flasch and Heinz (1976) after repetitive doses in cats. According to Benthe (1975), there exists a close correlation between the distribution coefficient brain: plasma water and the lipoid solubility of the glycoside.
2. The distribution velocity of β-methyl-digoxin from plasma to brain seems to be so much higher than that of digoxin that the receptor sites in the brain are occupied by methyl-digoxin before a considerable amount of digoxin can enter the brain.
3. The elimination half-lives of digoxin and β-methyl-digoxin in the brain are 3-5 times longer than in the other tissues. This pharmacokinetic evaluation gives insight into the properties of the brain as a deep compartment for cardiac glycosides influencing the terminal elimination rate. In contrast to urine and feces, it is often difficult to obtain this terminal slope in plasma as it often occurs in a concentration range near to or just below the sensitivity limit of the methods (Rietbrock et al., 1976).
4. The slow penetration in the brain and the higher accumulation after multiple doses compared with other tissues may help to explain why cardiac glycosides produce central side-effects only with a latent period after a single dose (Bine

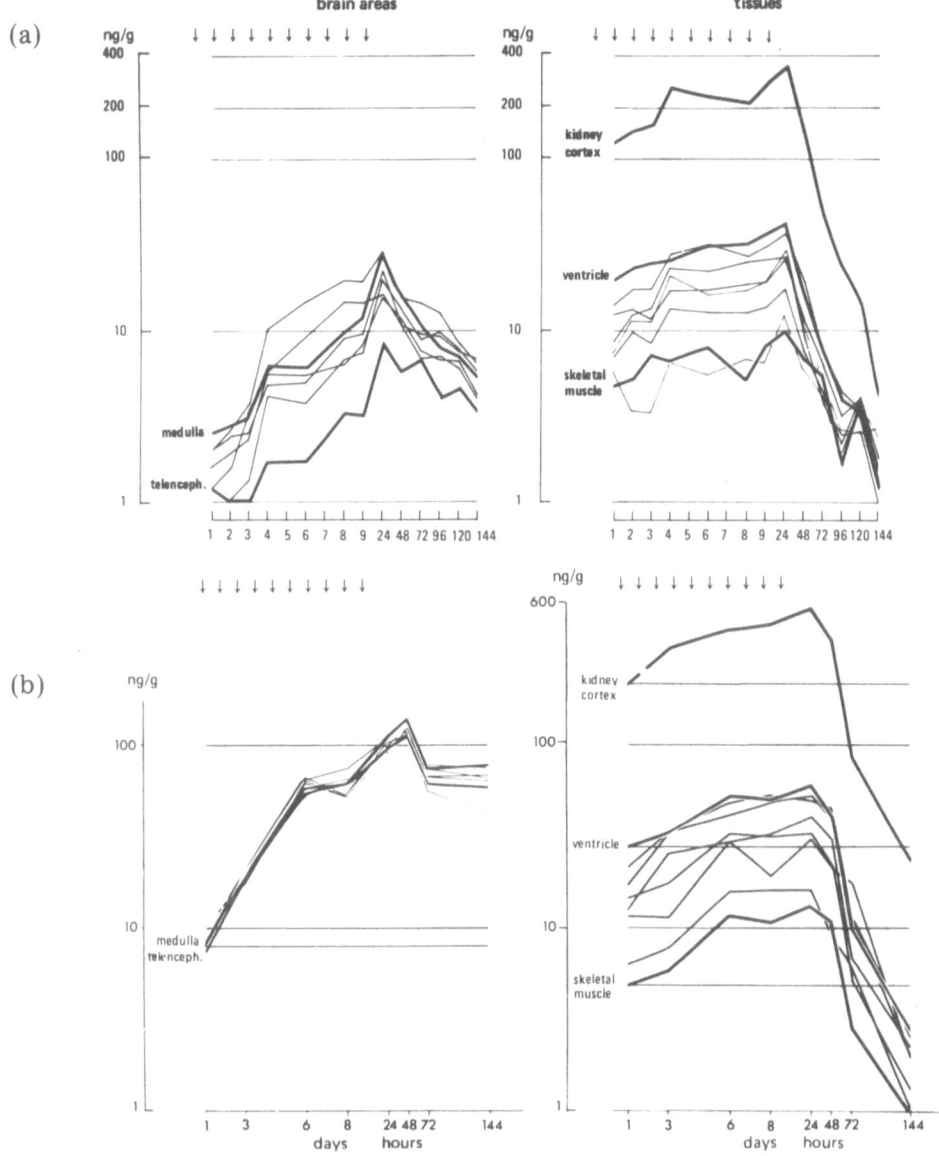

Fig. 10.5. Concentrations of digoxin (a) and methyl-digoxin (b) in different tissues and brain areas of beagle dogs 24 h after 1-10 x 0.0125 mg/kg tritium-labeled digoxin or methyl-digoxin i.v. and 24-144 h after the last daily dose of 0.0125 mg/kg tritium-labeled digoxin or methyl-digoxin over a period of 10 days (↓ : glycoside application)

117

et al., 1951; Fischer et al., 1952) and more often after chronic administration (Gold et al., 1947; Rietbrock and Kuhlmann, 1977).

5. In practice, the clinical use of glycosides is made more difficult by the presence of slowly equilibrating tissues. Since the brain is a small deep compartment, there may be only a poor relationship between glycoside concentration in plasma and the slowly equilibrating brain tissue, and plasma concentration alone cannot indicate with certainty the development of central toxicity.

References

Benthe, H.F.: Organverteilung verschiedener Herzglykoside. In: Digitalistherapie, Beiträge zur Pharmakologie. Jahrmärker, H. (ed.)Berlin-Heidelberg-New York: Springer-Verlag 1975, pp. 25-34

Bine, R., Friedman, M., Byers, S.O., Bland, C.: The deposition of digitoxin in the tissues of the rat after parenteral injection. Circulation 4, 105-107 (1951)

Bloch, K.: Nil nocere!: Digitalisnebenwirkungen. Münch. Med. Wochenschr. 106, 942-952 (1964)

Church, G., Marriott, H.J.L.: Digitalis Delirium. A report on three cases. Circulation 20, 549-553 (1959)

Deutscher, R.N., Harrison, D.C.. Goldman, R.H.: The relation between myocardial ^{3}H-digoxin concentration and its hemodynamic effects. Am. J. Cardiol. 29, 47-55 (1972)

Doherty, J.E., Perkins, W.H., Mitchell, G.K.: Tritiated digoxin studies in human subjects. Arch. Intern. Med. 108, 531-539 (1961)

Doherty, J.E., Perkins, W.H.: Tissue concentration and turnover of tritiated digoxin in dogs. Am. J. Cardiol. 17, 47-52 (1966)

Fischer, C.S., Sjoerdsma, A., Johnson, R.: The tissue distribution and excretion of radioactive digitoxin. Circulation 5, 496-503 (1952)

Flasch, H., Heinz, N.: Konzentration von Herzglykosiden im Myokard und im Gehirn. Arzneim. Forsch. 26, 1213-1216 (1976)

Fowler, R.S., Rathi, L., Keith, J.D.: Accidental digitalis intoxication in children. J. Pediatr. 64, 188-200 (1964)

Gold, H., Modell, W., Cattell, McKeen, Benton, J.G., Cotlove, E.W.: Action of digitalis glycoside on the central nervous system with special reference to the convulsant action of red squill. J. Pharmacol. Exp. Ther. 91, 15-30 (1947)

Keller, F., Blumenthal, H.P., Maertin, K., Rietbrock, W.: Pharmacokinetics of digoxin and β-methyldigoxin after multiple dosing: a one compartment model fit. Clin. Pharmocokinetics in press (1977)

Kuhlmann, J., Kötter, V., Leitner, V.E., Arbeiter, G., Schröder, R., Rietbrock, N.: Concentration of digoxin, methyldigoxin, digitoxin and ouabain in the myocardium of the dog following coronary occlusion. Naunyn Schmiedebergs Arch. Pharmakol. 287, 399-411 (1975)

Kuhlmann, J., Reiche, J., Bruns, J.: Distribution of digoxin, β-methyldigoxin and ouabain after single and multiple doses in dogs. Naunyn Schmiedebergs Arch. Pharmakol. Suppl. 293, R29 (1976a)

Kuhlmann, J., Rietbrock, N.: Glykosidplasmaspiegel unter einer Erhaltungstherapie — Streuung der Konzentrationen und deren Ursachen. Verh. Dtsch.
Ges. Inn. Med. 82 (in press) (1976b)

Lely, A.H., Enter, C.H.J. van: Large-scale digitoxin intoxication. Br. Med. J.
1970/III, 737-740

Lely, A.H., Enter, C.H.J. van: Non-cardiac symptoms of digitalis intoxication.
Am. Heart J. 83, 149-152 (1972)

Rietbrock, N., Kuhlmann, J.: Clinical significance of distribution and elimination of cardiac glycosides. Internal symposium on clinical pharmacokinetics
at Salzgitter-Ringelheim, June 20th to 21st, 1975. In: Practical Experience
in Clinical Pharmacokinetics. Ritschel, W.A. (ed.) Gustav Fischer Verlag
(in press) (1977)

Rietbrock, N., Abshagen, U., v. Bergmann, K., Rennekamp, H.: Disposition of
β-Methyldigoxin in Man. Eur. J. Clin. Pharmacol. 9, 105-114 (1975)

Rietbrock, N., Guggenmos, J., Kuhlmann, J., Hess, U.: Bioavailability and pharmacokinetics of β-methyldigoxin after multiple oral and intravenous doses.
Eur. J. Clin. Pharmacol. 9, 373-379 (1976)

Schwiegk, H., Jahrmärker, H.: Therapie der Herzinsuffizienz VII. Digitalis Into-
xikation. In: Handbuch der Inneren Medizin. Vol.IX: Herz und Kreislauf.
Springer-Verlag 1960, pp. 487-500

Discussion

Greenblatt: When you show the biexponential decay curve for digoxin following
termination of therapy, have you assessed whether the sum of two exponentials
is statistically more stable than a single exponential? It looked like there was a
lot of scatter of the data points around the lines that you drew. I am concerned
about this concept of the "slowly equilibrating deep compartment".
This may be an artefact of measurement — you may be projecting this concept
onto the data when it's not there.

Kuhlmann: We have compared the mono- and biexponential function statistically and the data could be fitted better to a biexponential function. The correlation coefficients for the linear regression of the daily renal excretion rates in
the two volunteers were 0.996 and 0.967, respectively, for the first, and 0.912
and 0.938, respectively, for the second phase. It is very difficult to determine
this second phase in plasma since the plasma level drops fast below measureable
values. The glycoside concentrations in urine, however, are much higher. We
could measure the concentrations exactly over a long period of time.
Similar biexponential decay curves for renal and fecal excretion of digoxin and
methyl-digoxin could be observed in dogs after cessation of multiple dosing of
^{3}H-digoxin and ^{3}H-methyl-digoxin as shown on Figure 1. The correlation coefficients for the linear regression of the daily renal and fecal excretion rates were

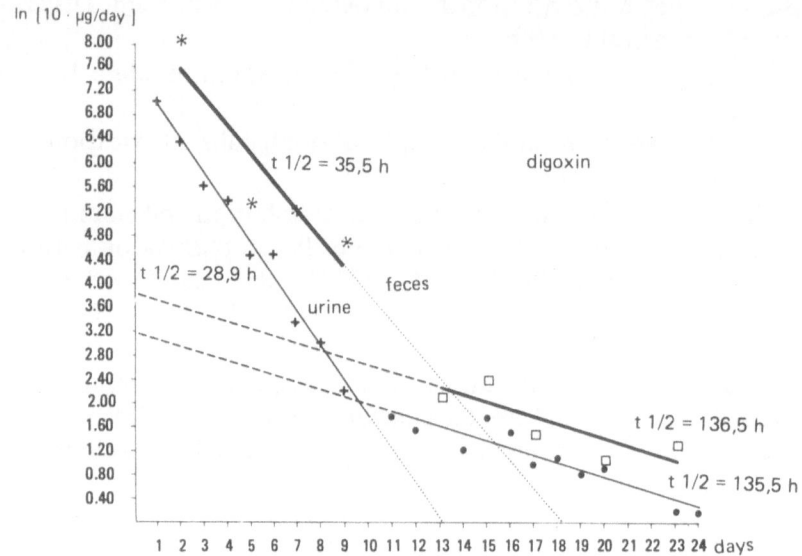

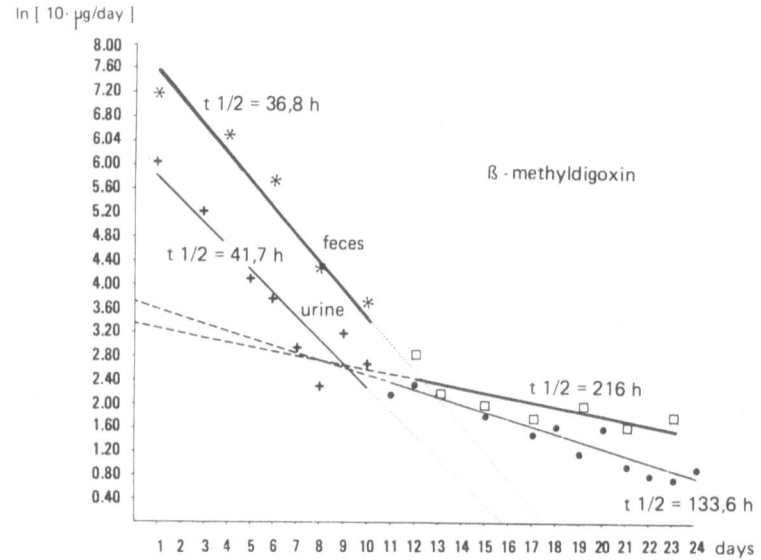

Fig. 1. Renal and fecal excretion (μg/day) of one beagle dog after cessation of multiple dosing of 0.0125 mg/kg H³-digoxin and β-methyldigoxin daily for 10 days. renal + ● fecal * □

similar to those in man. The specific activity of the tritium-labeled glycosides was high enough (800 μCi/mg) to determine the half-life in different organs, and the digoxin half-life in the brain was longer than it could be calculated from the second slope of the renal and fecal excretion. This means that the brain is a deep compartment for cardiac glycosides. This conclusion is in good accordance with clinical observations that central intoxication symptoms occur only with a latent period after a single dose, and these symptoms are much more often diagnosed during chronic administration.

Smith, Boston: There is a great deal of interest now in the effects of cardiac glycosides within the CNS. Some of the central effects are quite rapid in onset, for example the studies of Garan et al. on vasoconstrictor effects on the coronary circulation of digoxin, showing that the CSF levels of digoxin very closely correlate with the vasoconstrictor effect in the coronary bed. These were acute studies, with effects maximal about 15 min after i.v. injection. Your data are very interesting with regard to some of these kinetically slow compartments, but some of the CNS effects may have quite a rapid onset, and in the case of vasoconstrictor effects a relatively rapid offset as well. There may be subcompartments even within the CNS for the different effects of cardiac glycosides.

Erdmann, München: I would like to make a short comment. The tissue distribution alone doesn't necessarily correlate with the effects. In fact, really important is the concentration at the receptor sites. For β-methyl-digoxin and for digoxin we have measured the affinity to the receptor in isolated human cardiac cell membranes, and there we found that the affinity of β-methyl-digoxin to the receptors is about 15%-20% higher than that of digoxin. So I should think that β-methyl-digoxin has a slightly higher affinity, but that does not necessarily influence the tissue distribution, which expresses the drug concentration at mostly unspecific binding sites.

Schaumann, Mannheim: You did not mention that your dogs tolerated about the same doses of the examined glycosides, although you had much higher concentrations of β-methyl-digoxin than of digoxin and ouabain in the brain. The same is true for β-methyl-digoxin and digoxin in cats. Digitoxin penetrates even more into the brain than β-methyl-digoxin, and again there is no difference between the therapeutic margins of digitoxin and digoxin as far as cardiac or cerebral side-effects are concerned. The time course for the increase in cerebral glycoside concentrations and the onset of cerebral side-effects is also different. When you inject a threshold dose intravenously into cats, emesis occurs within 4 h at the latest, whereas the cerebral glycoside concentration increases step by step for several days. All the evidence shows that — at least as far as cerebral glycoside concentrations are concerned — there is absolutely no correlation between the concentration in a tissue homogenate and the concentration at the receptor site.
In a patient treated with digoxin, you showed that the cerebral side-effects persisted longer than the cardiac side-effects. I would like to add that in patients with atrial fibrillation, the decrease in heart rate persisted after withdrawal of the glycosides although the serum concentration had decreased to very low levels.

Kuhlmann: It is not true that dogs tolerate the same doses of digoxin and β-methyl-digoxin. I discussed these results with you several times. After constant daily i.v. doses of digoxin and β-methyl-digoxin over 10 days, the plasma levels of β-methyl-digoxin were 1.6-1.8 times higher in comparison to those of digoxin. The dogs treated with β-methyl-digoxin showed central intoxication symptoms, e.g., fatigue, loss of appetite, and a loss in weight of 10%-20% (Kuhlmann and Rietbrock, 1976). In addition, I don't agree with you that digitoxin penetrates even more into the brain than β-methyl-digoxin. Figure 2 shows lower concentrations in the various tissues after digitoxin than after identical doses of digoxin. Especially in the brain, the digitoxin levels are higher than those of digoxin but reached only one-fifth of the β-methyl-digoxin concentrations. According to Benthe (1975), there exists a close correlation between the distribution coefficient brain: plasma water and the lipid solubility of the glycoside. So the lower digitoxin concentrations in the brain may be caused by the high protein bond of digitoxin. Central side-effects can only take place when the cardiac glycoside accumulates in the brain and so differences in the neurotoxic activity of the glycosides can be

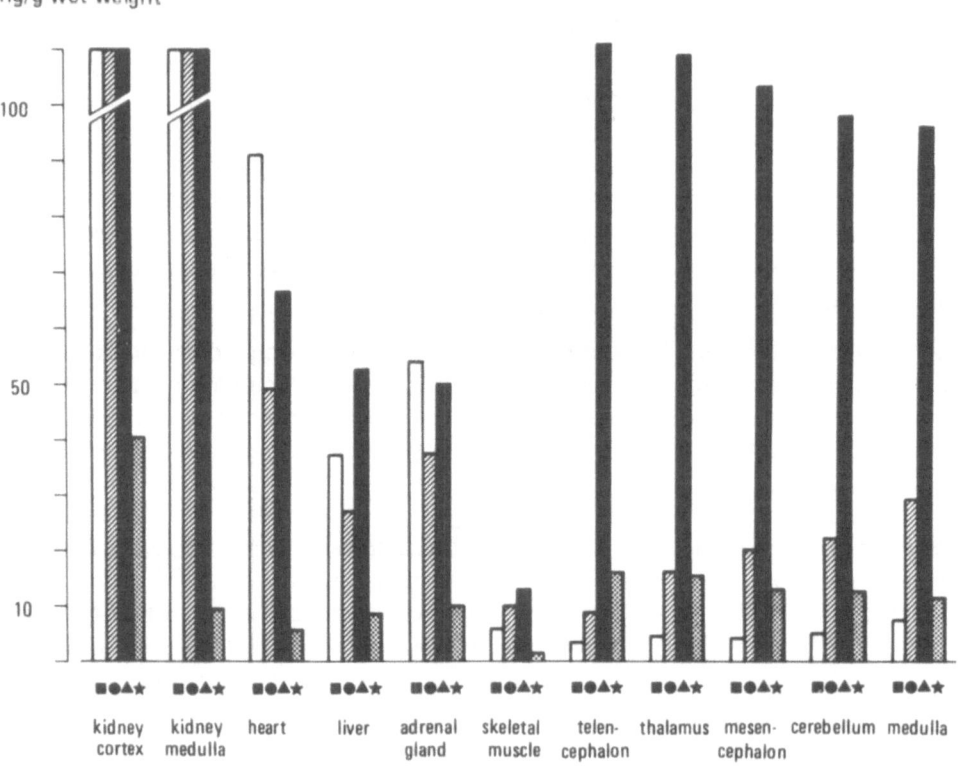

Fig. 2. Concentration of ouabain (■) digoxin (●) β-methyldigoxin (▲) and digitoxin (★) in different tissues of beagles after a daily intravenous dose of 0.0125 mg/kg tritium labeled ouabain, digoxin, β-methyldigoxin and digoxin during 10 days

observed better after repeated administration than after a single dose. There may be a correlation between the glycoside concentration in the brain and the central effects, but perhaps with differences in the threshold dose. Furthermore, it has to be considered that the demethylation of methyl-digoxin to digoxin, which revealed to be a metabolic degradation step in man, could not be observed in dogs. Concerning the other remark you made, it could be shown by many authors, especially recently by Gillis and co-workers, that most of the central effects are the results of the direct action of digitalis on the brain cells. But also some of the cardiac side-effects are of neurologic nature. Your statement that in patients with atrial fibrillation the decrease in heart rate persisted after withdrawal of the glycoside shows that there exists rather a correlation between the pharmacodynamic effect and the glycoside concentration in the tissue than with the plasma level. Moreover, Pace et al. (1974) have shown qualitative differences between digitoxin and digoxin in their effect on the vagus nerve. The slowing of the heart rate after digitoxin seems to be a vagal effect whereas after the administration of digoxin there is an inhibition of the sympathetic nervous tone. The authors supposed that the penetration of digoxin into the CNS may be less resulting in less interaction with the vagal center. These findings are in good agreement with our results that the lipid-soluble glycosides digitoxin and β-methyl-digoxin are equally distributed in all brain areas whereas the more polar digoxin and ouabain show high concentrations only in the brain stem.

P. Reissell, Helsinki: Symptoms of CNS in digitalis intoxication are well-known. The actual concentration of digitalis in the spinal fluid, however, has not been clearly established. This problem was studied in four patients with digoxin intoxication and in seven nontoxic cardiac patients (Table 1). I investigated also the penetration of digoxin into the cerebrospinal fluid by studying two patients during the operation. A catheter was installed in the spinal canal (Table 2), 0.5 mg digoxin was administered intravenously and corresponding serum and cerebrospinal fluid were determined using radioimmunoassay.

Table 1 shows that the concentration of digoxin in the cerebrospinal fluid is low. A correlation with the symptoms of the digitalis intoxication could not be found. This is in accordance with the results by Somogyi et al. though the ratio cerebrospinal fluid digoxin/serum digoxin was higher in their patients. The penetration of digoxin into the cerebrospinal fluid parallels the serum concentration curve (Table 2). Again the amount detected is very low.

Table 1

	Patients	Dose of digoxin (mg)	Digoxin serum level (ng/ml) (24 h after the last dose)	Digoxin concentration in the spinal fluid (ng/ml)	Ratio spinal/fluid serum
Toxic	1. H.T.	0.500	5.10	0.60	0.1
	2. A.G.	0.375	2.30	0	0
	3. A.O.	0.250	2.25	0.50	0.2
	4. A.N.	0.250	1.70	0	0
Control	5. A.M.	0.250	1.60	0	0
	6. K.L.	0.250	1.60	0	0
	7. Y.K.	0.250	1.00	0	0.4
	8. J.T.	0.250	0.80	0.30	0.2
	9. T.P.	0.250	0.45	0.10	0
	10. O.H.	0.250	0.35	0	0
	11. J.O.	0.250	0.25	0.15	0.60

Table 2

Single injection test	Digoxin serum level (ng/ml)	Digoxin concentration in the spinal fluid (ng/ml)	Ratio spinal fluid/ serum
	(mean)	(mean)	(mean)
5 min	16.75	0.15	0
15 min	9.40	0.25	0.02
30 min	8.40	0.05	0.06
60 min	4.55	0.05	0.01
120 min	2.85	0.05	0.02
240 min	1.10	0	0

References

Benthe, H.F.: In: Digitalistherapie. Jahrmärker, H. (ed.) Berlin-Heidelberg-New York: Springer-Verlag 1975, p. 25

Garan, H., Smith, T.W., Powell, W.J. Jr.: J. Clin. Invest. 54, 1365-1372 (1977)

Kuhlmann, J., Rietbrock, N.: Med. Tribune 11 (47), 38 (1976)

Pace, D.G., Quest, J.A., Gillis, R.A.: Eur. J. Pharmacol. 28, 288-293 (1974)

Rietbrock, N., Kuhlmann, J.: Med. Klin. 72, 11, 435-449 (1977)

Somogyi, G., Káldor, A., Jankovich, A.: Int. Z. Klin. Pharmakol. Ther. Toxicol. 4, 421 (1971)

11 Plasma-Tissue Distribution of Different Cardiac Glycosides

D. Larbig and R. Haasis

As shown by other investigators with different methods (Binnion, 1973; Chamberlain, 1973a; Coltart et al., 1972; Doherty et al., 1961, 1967; Güllner et al., 1974; Redfors et al., 1973), tissue glycoside concentrations of patients on digoxin maintenance therapy are usually markedly higher than "steady-state" serum concentrations. Since the relationship between steady-state serum glycoside concentration and cardiac effect is still controversial, glycoside concentrations were determined in various human tissues in order to analyze the correlation between serum concentration and tissue concentration.

Methods and Material

Glycoside concentrations in serum and tissue were determined by radioimmunoassay as previously described (Haasis et al., 1977; Larbig and Kochsiek, 1971). Studies carried out in patients on maintenance therapy with digoxin and digoxin derivatives (β-acetyl digoxin and β-methyl digoxin). Patients treated with digoxin and β-acetyl digoxin were both considered to be on digoxin, because the acetyl group of β-acetyl digoxin is almost completely split of during enteral absorption (Benthe and Chempanich, 1965). Since metabolites of digoxin are also measured using the radioimmunoassay procedure (Larbig and Kochsiek, 1972; Stoll et al., 1972) and β-methyl-digoxin is partially metabolized to digoxin (Rennekamp et al., 1972), the term "glycoside concentration" in patients on therapy with digoxin or digoxin derivatives is preferred. Steady-state serum glycoside concentrations in biopsy studies were determined no earlier than 12-24 h, in autopsy studies 12-36 h after the last dose was administered. Left ventricular papillary muscle biopsies were obtained from patients at cardiac surgery for mitral valve replacement; blood samples for serum glycoside level determinations were drawn just before onset of surgery in order to avoid dilution effects (Chamberlain, 1973b, Coltart et al., 1971; Stunkat et al., 1975). Skeletal muscle biopsies were taken from m. pectoralis major at surgery for implantation of cardiac pacemakers.

Results

Skeletal Muscle

In 19 patients on maintenance therapy with digoxin (n = 5) and β-methyl digoxin (n = 14), the average glycoside concentration of biopsy skeletal muscle was 15 ± 10.4 ng/g with a corresponding serum concentration of 1.5 ± 0.69 ng/ml and a tissue to serum ratio of 10 ± 3.0:1 (Fig. 11.1). There was a highly significant linear correlation between serum glycoside concentration and tissue glycoside concentration (r = 0.8377, p < 0.001). Determinations of glycoside concentrations of autopsy skeletal muscle gave similar results (n = 7, tissue to serum ratio 11 ± 2.6:1) without any statistically significant difference.

Ventricular Myocardium

Glycoside concentrations of left ventricular papillary muscle from biopsy and autopsy specimens in 64 patients in relation to serum concentrations are shown in Figure 11.2. There is a highly significant linear correlation between serum and papillary muscle glycoside concentration (r = 0.7430, p < 0.001), however, associated with marked individual scatter. The tissue to serum ratio for biopsy specimens was 48 ± 10.4:1 and 50 ± 14.1:1 for autopsy specimens, respectively,

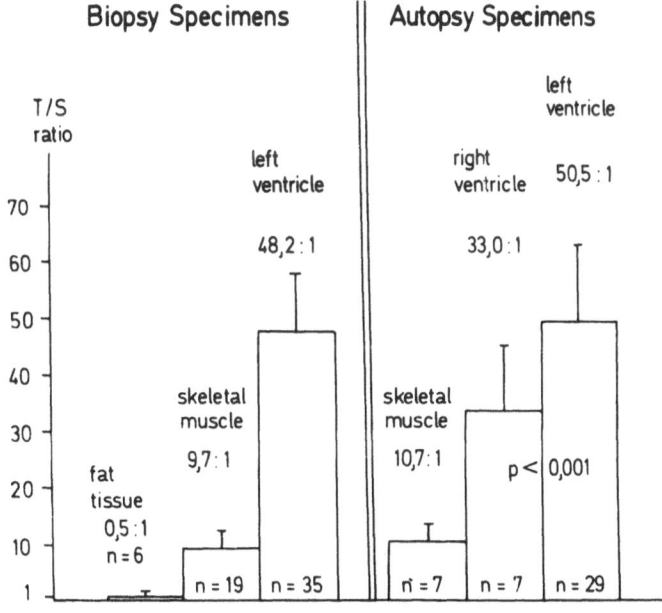

Fig. 11.1. Tissue to serum ratio of glycoside concentrations of biopsy and autopsy specimens of various human tissues from patients on maintenance therapy with digoxin and digoxin derivatives (mean ± SD)

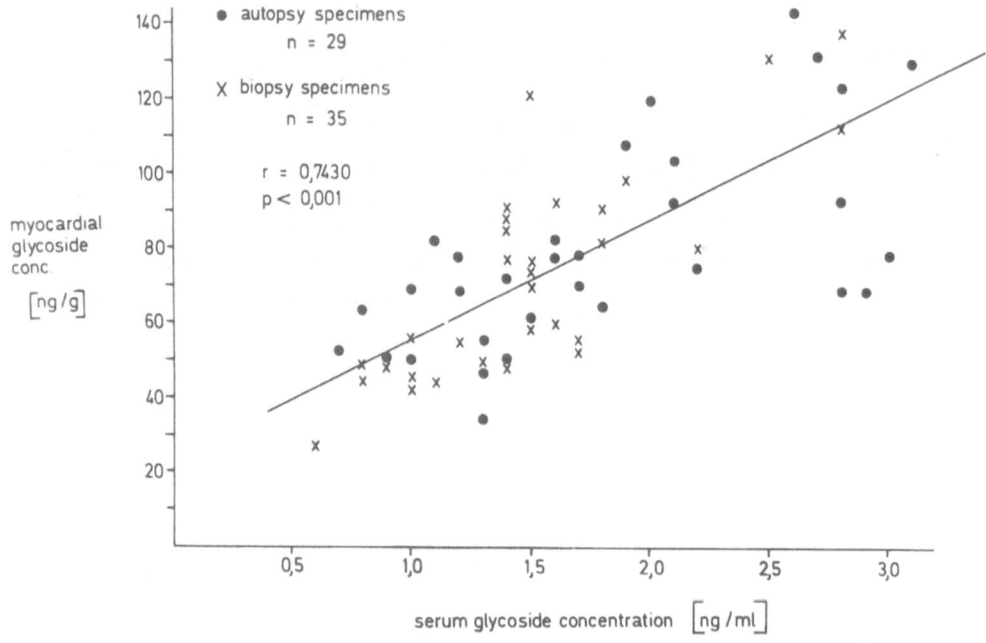

Fig. 11.2. Correlation between steady-state serum glycoside concentrations and left ventricular papillary muscle glycoside concentrations from biopsy and autopsy specimens of patients on maintenance therapy with digoxin and digoxin derivatives (digoxin group n = 26, β-methyl digoxin group n = 38)

without any statistically significant difference. In seven right ventricular papillary muscle specimens, the tissue to serum glycoside ratio was significantly lower (33 ± 7.4:1, p < 0.001). The correlation between serum glycoside concentration and left ventricular papillary muscle glycoside concentration from biopsy specimens of 35 patients on digoxin and β-methyl digoxin was r = 0.8141, p < 0.001; (Fig. 11.3). Out of the total of 64 patients, the tissue to serum ratio of the glycoside concentration in 42 patients with a normal serum creatinine (0.9 ± 0.25 mg%) was significantly higher than the ratio of the remaining 22 patients with an elevated serum creatinine of 3.6 ± 3.30 mg% (51 ± 11.8:1 versus 43 ± 11.1:1; p < 0.01).

Brain Tissue

The results from autopsy analyses of different areas of the human brain of 27 cases in comparison to myocardial determinations are shown in Figure 11.4. Tissue to serum ratios are highest in the gray matter both for the digoxin and β-methyl digoxin group. The tissue to serum ratio of glycoside concentrations of 15 patients on β-methyl digoxin (31 ± 5.0:1) was significantly two to threefold higher than that of 12 patients on digoxin (8.0 ± 1.2:1) (p< 0.01-p< 0.001).

128

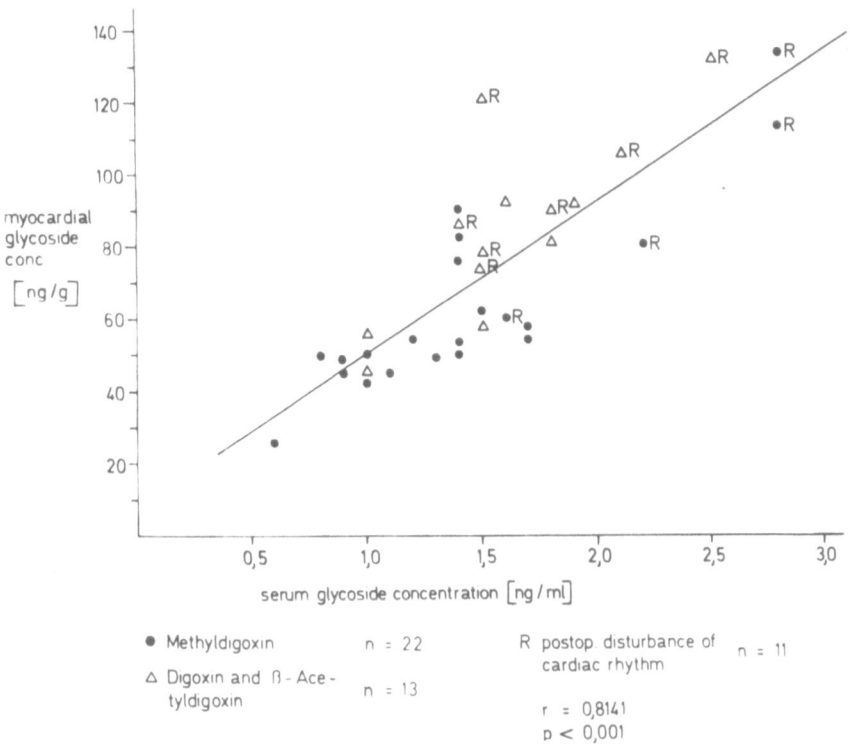

• Methyldigoxin   n = 22   R postop disturbance of   n = 11
cardiac rhythm

△ Digoxin and ß-Ace-   n = 13
tyldigoxin

r = 0,8141
p < 0,001

Fig. 11.3. Correlation between steady-state serum glycoside concentrations and left ventricular papillary muscle glycoside concentrations of biopsy specimens obtained at cardiac surgery from 35 patients on maintenance therapy with digoxin and digoxin derivatives

Discussion

Our results concerning glycoside determinations of skeletal muscle show a highly significant correlation between steady-state serum glycoside concentration and the concentration in skeletal muscle, in close agreement with findings of Coltart et al. (Coltart et al., 1972). Thus, steady-state serum concentrations of patients on maintenance therapy with digoxin and digoxin derivatives mirror glycoside concentrations of a large body pool, since according to Grant (Grant, 1958) skeletal muscle amounts up to 43% of body weight.

As evidenced by our results from left ventricular papillary muscle extractions in 64 cases, steady-state serum glycoside concentrations of patients on digoxin and digoxin derivatives are only about 1/50th of the corresponding concentrations of left ventricular myocardium. However, correlation between serum and myocardial concentration is amazingly good, thus furnishing experimental evidence for the correlation between steady-state serum glycoside concentration and cardiac effect

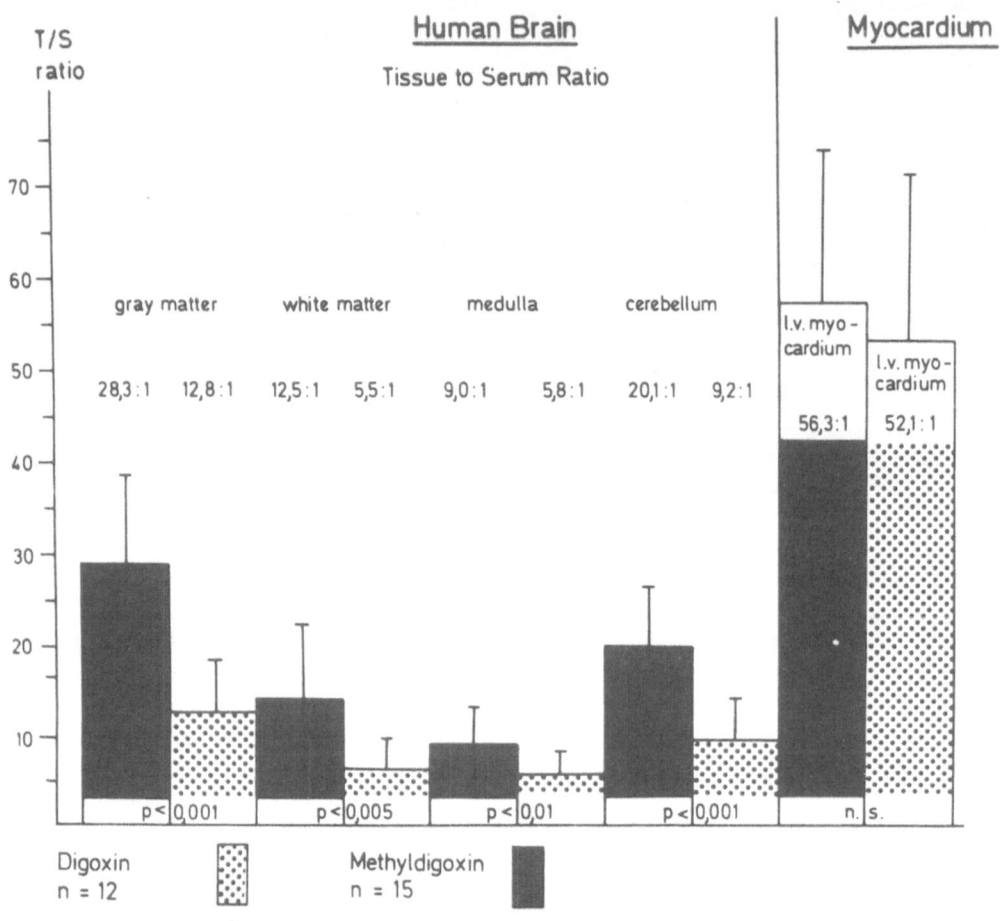

Fig. 11.4. Tissue to serum ratio of glycoside concentrations of different areas of the human brain in comparison to left ventricular papillary muscle to serum ratio from autopsy specimens of 27 cases on previous maintenance therapy with digoxin and digoxin derivatives (mean ± SD)

reasonably well-established from clinical observations (Chamberlain et al., 1970; Haasis et al., 1975; Smith and Haber, 1974). In this respect, it is interesting to notice that in left ventricular papillary muscle biopsy studies of 35 patients at surgery for prosthetic mitral valve replacement both steady-state serum glycoside concentrations and myocardial concentrations were significantly higher (p < 0.001) in 11 patients who developed disturbancies of cardiac rhythm suggestive of digitalis intoxication in the early postoperative period. When 42 patients with a normal serum creatinine out of the total of 64 patients were analyzed separately, the correlation between serum glycoside concentration and myocardial concentration improved from r = 0.7430 to r = 0.8221, whereas the correlation in the remaining 22 patients with an elevated serum creatinine deteriorated to r = 0.5791 (p < 0.01), indicating that the latter group of patients obviously is not a uniform one. In agreement with findings of Jusko et al. (Jusko and Weintraub, 1975), the myocardium to serum ratio of glycoside concentrations in patients with an elevated serum creatinine was significantly lower than that in patients with a normal serum creatinine, possibly decreasing with the degree of impaired renal function. However, in the 22 patients with an elevated serum creatinine, serum potassium was also significantly elevated (p < 0.001), which might also account for the decreased tissue to serum ratio (Marcus et al., 1969).

Autopsy studies of the human brain in 27 cases revealed the highest tissue to serum glycoside concentration ratio in the gray matter and cerebellum both for digoxin and β-methyl-digoxin. The ratio of the cases on β-methyl digoxin was significantly two to threefold higher in all areas of the human brain examined. However, as published earlier (Haasis and Larbig, 1976), we were unable to demonstrate a higher percentage of cerebral side-effects in intoxicated patients on β-methyl digoxin in comparison to intoxicated patients on digoxin.

Summary

Glycoside concentrations of human biopsy and autopsy specimens from various tissues in patients on maintenance therapy with digoxin and digoxin derivatives were analyzed by radioimmunoassay. A highly significant linear correlation was found between steady-state serum glycoside concentration and skeletal muscle glycoside concentration (r = 0.8377), with an average tissue to serum ratio of 10 ± 3.0:1. Left ventricular papillary muscle glycoside concentrations were analyzed in 35 patients from biopsy material obtained at cardiac surgery and 29 autopsy specimens, resulting in a similar highly significant linear correlation (r = 0.7430) and an average myocardium to serum ratio of 49 ± 12.0:1. The correlation between serum glycoside concentration and myocardial glycoside concentration improved, when patients with an elevated serum creatinine were excluded (r = 0.8221), due to the significantly lower myocardium to serum ratio in patients with impairment of renal function (p < 0.01). In autopsy specimens of the human brain, the highest tissue to serum ratio was found in the gray matter and cerebellum both for digoxin and β-methyl digoxin, the tissue to serum ratio being significantly higher in patients on β-methyl digoxin (p < 0.01-p < 0.001).

References

Benthe, H.F., Chempanich, K.: Vergleich der enteralen Wirksamkeit von Digoxin, Acetyldigoxin und Digitoxin. Arzneim. Forsch. 15, 486 (1965)

Binnion, P.F.: Plasma and Myocardial Digoxin Levels in Dogs and Man. Symposium on Digitalis, Oslo, Norway: Gyldendal Norsk Forlag 1973, p. 254

Chamberlain, D.A., White. R.J., Howard, M.R.: Plasma digoxin concentrations in patients with atrial fibrillation. Br. Med. J. 1970, 427

Chamberlain, D.A.: The Ratio Between Myocardial and Plasma Levels of Digoxin. Symposium on Digitalis. Oslo, Norway: Gyldendal Norsk Forlag, 1973a, p. 262

Chamberlain, D.A.: The Influence of Cardiopulmonary Bypass on Plasma Digoxin Cencentrations. Symposium on Digitalis, Oslo, Norway: Gyldendal Norsk Forlag 1973 b, p. 277

Coltart, D.J., Chamberlain, D.A., Howard, M.R., Kettlewell, M.G., Mecer, J.L., Smith, T.W.: Effect of cardiopulmonary bypass on plasma digoxin concentrations. Br. Heart J. 33, 334 (1971)

Coltart, J., Howard, M., Chamberlain, D.: Myocardial and skeletal muscle concentrations of digoxin in patients on long-term therapy. Br. Med. J. 2, 318 (1972)

Doherty, J.E., Perkins, W.H., Mitchell, G.K.: Tritiated digoxin studies in human subjects. Arch. Intern. Med. 108, 531 (1961)

Doherty, J.E., Perkins, W.H., Flanigan, W.H.: The distribution and concentration of tritiated digoxin in human tissue. Ann. Intern. Med. 66, 116 (1967)

Grant, J.C.B.: A Method of Anatomy, 6th ed. Williams and Wilken, Baltimore, USA: 1958, p. 7

Güllner, H.G., Stinson, E.B., Harrison, D.C., Kalmon, S.H.: Correlation of serum concentrations with heart concentrations of digoxin in human subjects. Circulation 50, 635 (1974)

Haasis, R., Larbig, D., Klenk, H.O.: Glykosidkonzentration im Serum und Urin bei Herzgesunden nach Gabe von β-Methyldigoxin. Klin. Wochenschr. 53, 529 (1975)

Haasis, R., Larbig, D.: Vergleichende Untersuchungen der Serumglykosidkonzentrationen bei Glykosidintoxikationen mit extracardialen Nebenwirkungen nach Einnahme von β-Methyldigoxin, β-Acetyldigoxin und Digoxin. Verh. Dtsch. Ges. Inn. Med. 82 (in press) (1976)

Haasis, R., Larbig, D., Stunkat, R., Bader, H., Seboldt, H.: Radioimmunologische Bestimmung der Glykosidkonzentration im menschlichen Gewebe. Klin. Wochenschr. 1, 23 (1977)

Jusko, W.J., Weintraub, M.: Myocardial distribution of digoxin and renal function Clin. Pharmacol. Ther. 16, 449 (1975)

Larbig, D., Kochsiek, K.: Radioimmunchemische Bestimmungen von Digoxin im menschlichen Serum. Klin. Wochenschr. 49, 1031 (1971)

Larbig, D., Kochsiek, K.: Zur radioimmunchemischen Bestimmung von Digoxin und Digoxinderivaten. Dtsch. Med. Wochenschr. 97, 1310 (1972)

Marcus, F.J., Kapadia, G.G., Goldsmith, C.: Alterations of the body distribution of tritiated digoxin by acute hyperkalemia in the dog. J. Pharmacol. Exp. Ther. 165, 136 (1969)

Redfors, A., Bertler, A., Schüller, H.: The Ratio Between Myocardial and Plasma Levels of Digoxin in Man. Symposium on Digitalis. Oslo, Norway: Gyldendal Norsk Forlag, 1973, p. 265

Rennekamp, H., Rennekamp, Ch., Abshagen, U., v. Bergmann, K.: Pharmacokinetic behaviour of 4 ''' methyldigoxin in man. Naunyn Schmiedebergs Arch. Pharmakol. 273, 172 (1972)

Smith, T.W., Haber, E.: Digitalis. Boston, USA: Little, Brown and Company 1974 p. 69

Stoll, R.G., Christensen, M.S., Sakmar, E., Wagner, J.G.: The specifity of the digoxin radioimmunoassay procedure. Res. Com. Chem. Pathol. Pharmacol. 4, 503 (1972)

Stunkat, R., Seboldt, H., Hoffmeister, H.E., Haasis, R., Larbig, D., Kochsiek, K.:
Radioimmunologische Bestimmung der Serumglykosidkonzentration bei
Eingriffen mit extrakorporaler Zirkulation. Thoraxchirurgie 23, 350 (1975)

Discussion

Dengler, Bonn: I sometimes wonder why it is so surprising to find higher concentrations of methyl digoxin and even of digitoxin in the tissue. If any concept
in biochemical pharmacology holds true that higher polarity diminishes the
distribution to the brain then we have to expect your findings. It is just a matter
of distribution and there is nothing to wonder about.

Larbig: Indeed, high concentrations of methyl digoxin in the brain could be
expected. We were surprised, however, about the close correlation between
steady-state serum concentrations and myocardial concentrations. This relationship is the chief aim of our investigations.

Jahrmärker, München: Still there remains the question of the biologic significance
of tissue concentration in general. Would you like to comment on that?

Larbig: I mentioned in the introduction of my paper that this is still controversial,
but at least there is a significant correlation between glycoside concentration and
cardiac effect. We wanted to investigate glycoside concentrations in serum and
various tissues, especially myocardium, and were astonished how well they correlated. Since we have been measuring steady-state serum concentrations for
clinical evaluation quite frequently, we rather feel safe in interpreting them.

Kuhlmann, Berlin: What were your blank values in the various tissues, especially
in the brain, and what was the sensitivity of your method? In my opinion, it is
very difficult to get reproducible results without purification of the extracted
samples.

Larbig: We extracted brain and other tissues of patients who were not on digitalis
and detected up to 2.2 ng/g in the brain and up to 1.2 ng/g of glycoside in the
myocardium as a false positive value. The sensitivity of our radioimmunoassay in
serum is 0.2 ng/ml with a variation coefficient of 4%-5% (intra-assay) and around
8.5% (interassay).

Schaumann, Mannheim: You mentioned that you have arrhythmias post opera-
tively in patients with high glycoside serum concentrations. I suppose that no
additional glycoside dose was given to the patients at this time?

Larbig: No. These were all steady-state concentrations, measured at least 12 h
after the last dose; the blood was drawn immediately before operation.

Schaumann: There might be two explanations for the observed arrhythmias. You
might have a decrease in distribution volume due to the operation with more
glycoside coming out of the tissue and an increase in the serum concentrations
in the post operative state. Or the increasing activity of the sympathetic adds to

the arrhythmogenic activity of the glycosides. Did you do any measurements post-operatively?

Larbig: I think one can only speculate about the explanation for this observation. In fact, patients with relatively high steady-state serum concentrations developed cardiac arrhythmias. On the other hand, there was some overlap. The lowest digoxin plasma concentration we found in patients with toxic arrhythmias was 1.4 ng/ml, which is actually lower than the limit above which an intoxication usually occurs. Apparently, there seems to be — for reasons whatsoever — some change of tolerance due to transient hypoxemia or other factors. But still, it is evident that patients with high concentrations have a greater risk to develop an intoxication.

Benthe, Hamburg: You say that the higher digoxin concentrations in papillary muscle during arrhythmia are due to a higher blood concentration. We have done some experiments in cats with a very constant level of blood digoxin concentration, and in one group we caused ventricular extrasystoly and in the other group there was a normal sinus rhythm. The group of animals with cardiac dysrhythmias showed higher glycoside concentrations in the myocardium. The clearance of digoxin from the myocard seemed to be reduced because there was a reduced blood flow in the arrhythmic myocard. This suggests that we have to expect in arrhythmias that the glycoside concentration in the myocard is higher than in the normal working myocard.

Larbig: Actually, we thought it might be that way, that toxic myocardial concentrations might be higher, so that the tissue to serum ratio in these patients would be increased. But according to our results as demonstrated in Figure 11.3 the ratio is not changed.

Jogestrand, Stockholm: What is the recovery with this extraction method and to what extent was the muscle free from adipose tissue when you measured the concentrations?

Larbig: We did experiments on the percentage of digoxin and methyl-digoxin extractable by this method. It was between 87% and 95% for various tissues. The tissue of cardiac muscle was extracted after fat was removed, but only macroscopically.

Erbel, Koblenz: How do you explain the difference between the concentrations of the right and left ventricle?

Larbig: It is probably due to the facts that the left ventricular muscle has a more dense structure and that there is a more loosely arranged connective tissue between the muscle fibers of the right ventricle. This means that right and left ventricular myocardial glycoside concentrations might be identical. I think there has been some additional experimental evidence by Dr. Erdmann, supporting this explanation.

12 Significance of Plasma Concentration of Digoxin in Relation to the Myocardial Concentration of the Drug[1]

J. COLTART[2]

For almost 2 centuries, dating from the original work of William Withering, considerable interest and research has been applied to the mechanism and action of the cardiac glycosides. These drugs are widely used in clinical practice, for the treatment of patients with heart failure and cardiac dysrhythmias. Despite a widespread use of digoxin, relatively little information is available concerning factors which effect the response of the heart to such medication.

Little is known about myocardial digoxin concentrations in digitalized patients. Knowledge of the clinical pharmacology of the cardiac glycosides has expanded greatly since the introduction of assays capable of measuring concentrations in plasma (Lowenstein and Corill, 1966; Lukas and Peterson, 1966; Smith et al., 1969). Data, however, defining the intramyocardial distribution of digoxin and its relationship to serum levels are lacking, primarily due to the limitation of an adequate supply of myocardial tissue for study. The present study will examine this relation in patients on long-term maintenance therapy with digoxin plasma. In addition, skeletal muscle concentrations were compared with those in myocardium and plasma. In another group of patients, by using the recipient heart removed at the time of cardiac transplantation, a supply of myocardial tissue is realized for more difinitive studies of the distribution of digoxin, as reported in this study.

Although the cardiac receptor, or receptors, which mediates the pharmacologic effect of the cardiac glycosides have neither been fully isolated nor fully identified, evidence suggests that the sodium-potassium activated adenosene triphosphatase, $(Na^+ + K^+)$-ATPase, plays a role in the mechanism of action of the cardiac glycosides (Akera et al, 1970; Besch et al, 1970). In this study, we have identified this enzyme in a microsomal fraction of the heart and measured the activity of the enzyme in vivo and to varying concentration of digoxin in vitro. Furthermore, patients undergoing transplantation in this study had end-stage

---

1 This paper embodies the work performed in the department of Cardiology at St. Bartholomew's Hospital, London and St. Thomas' Hospital, London and the Cardiology Division, Stanford University, California.

2 I would like to acknowledge the help of my co-workers, Drs. Douglas Chamberlain, Robert Goldman, Donald Harrison and Mr. Michael Howard. I also wish to thank Mrs. Fiona Baile for expert secretarial service.

135

cardiac disease due either to severe ischemic heart disease of cardiomyopathy. We have correlated, therefore, the effects of cardiac histology with the distribution of digoxin in the various chambers of the heart on a macroscopic,subcellular, and enzymic level. The mechanism by which hyperkalemia modifies the inotropic effects of digoxin is not totally clear. In this study, variation in plasma potassium concentration enables a biochemical, pharmacologic, and hemodynamic correlation of the mechanism of action of digoxin to be undertaken.

It has been suggested that hyperkalemia alters the inotropic properties of digoxin by decreasing or delaying its tissue uptake (Marcus, Kapadia and Goldsmith, 1969; Goldman et al., 1972). In vitro, Allen and Schwartz (1970) have shown that potassium delays ouabain's binding to the enzyme sodium-potassium adenosine triphosphatase [$(Na^+ + K^+)$-ATPase] and that there is a good correlation between ouabain binding to $(Na^+ + K^+)$-ATPase and inhibition of this enzyme. Besch et al. (1970) and Akera et al. (1970) have presented evidence that membrane-bound $(Na^+ + K^+)$-ATPase is a specific receptor site for the cardiac glycosides because of the close temporal relationship between inhibition of this enzyme and inotropy. Further support for this hypothesis would be provided if it could be shown that potassium inhibits the binding of digoxin to $(Na^+ + K^+)$-ATPase in vivo, and at the same time alters both the inotropic effects and inhibition of $(Na^+ + K^+)$-ATPase by digoxin. Accordingly, a study was designed to determine:
1. The relationship between the inotropic effects of digoxin and $(Na^+ + K^+)$-ATPase inhibition in normokalemic and hyperkalemic animals.
2. The relationship between inhibition of $(Na^+ + K^+)$-ATPase activity and microsomal-bound digoxin concentration.
3. Whether the inhibition of inotropic effects by hyperkalemia could be competitively reversed in vivo by larger doses of digoxin.

Patients and Methods — Study 1

Samples were obtained from eight patients undergoing mitral valve replacement. Their ages ranged from 41 to 60 (mean 54) years; they had been treated with digoxin for a minimum of 7 years. All had normal serum electrolyte and blood urea concentrations at the time of surgery. Venous blood was taken into heparin tubes after induction of anesthesia but before intravenous infusions had been set up or cardiopulmonary bypass initiated. The plasma digoxin concentration in these samples was determined by radioimmunoassay as previously described (Chamberlain et al., 1970).

The mitral valve and subvalvar apparatus was excised in the usual manner, and samples of the left ventricular papillary muscle together with samples of latissimus dorsi (to represent skeletal muscle) were obtained at this time, about 20 min after the start of cardiopulmonary bypass. The biopsy tissue was dried and all excess fatty tissue was removed. It was stored at $-4°C$ to await assay.

Digoxin was eluted from a known weight of tissue by homogenization at room temperature for 30 min with 4 ml of chloroform (analar grade), the supernatant was removed, and a further 5 ml of chloroform was added to the homogenized tissue and stirred magnetically for 30 min. This last procedure was repeated at least twice. The residual homogenate was preserved for further extractions if subsequent analysis showed that the third supernatant solution contained digoxin. The chloroform supernatants were evaporated to dryness and the residues redissolved in 6 ml of barbitone buffer. Aliquots of each were pooled, the digoxin concentration was measured by radioimmunoassay, and the total digoxin content of the original muscle was calculated.

Study 2

Patients selected as described by Clark et al. (1973) as appropriate recipient candidates for cardiac allograft transplantation were studied. There were six men and one woman, whose ages ranged from 42 to 54 years. The primary diagnosis was coronary artery disease in five patients and idiopathic cardiomyopathy in two. All patients needed maintenance digoxin therapy as well as large doses of diuretics before surgery. They all had been treated with digoxin for at least 2 years. The last dose of the patient's usual daily maintenance glycoside therapy was given 5-7 h before the removal of the recipient heart at the time of transplantation. In two patients (cases 6 and 7), their last dose of digoxin was given as tritiated digoxin (specific activity 150 μCi/mg) intravenously 4 and 5 h before the surgical removal of the heart. All had normal serum electrolytes, and all but one (case 2) had normal blood urea nitrogen concentrations at the time of surgery. The patient in case 2 had a blood urea nitrogen level of 60 mg/100 ml at the time of surgery and "toxic" plasma concentrations of digoxin (2.6 ng/ml) immediately before surgery. The patient in case 3 also had a plasma digoxin concentration in the toxic range. Venous blood was taken into heparin tubes after induction of anesthesia but before intravenous infusions had been set up or cardiopulmonary bypass initiated.

The heart was removed by the standard surgical procedure used by our group, which has been discussed elsewhere (Stinson et al., 1969). The heart was quickly devided into its respective chambers, wiped dry, and then quick frozen in dry ice to await pharmacologic, biochemical, and histologic analysis.

Pharmacologic Methods

Tissue specimens of 1 g (wet wt) were cleaned from epicardium and endocardium and then minced with scissors. The tissue was transferred into a Kontes Duall glass tissue grinder (No. 23) with glass pestle and homogenized in 3 ml of 0.04 phosphate buffer, pH 6.6. The homogenate was transferred to a separatory funnel, 15 ml of methylene chloride were added, and the mixture was shaken vigorously for 2 min by hand. This extraction step was repeated once. The clear methylene chloride phases were pooled, placed in a round-bottomed flask, and evaporated to dryness in a Buchi Rotavapor evaporator. The residue was redissolved in 2 ml of trometamol (TRIS)-buffered human serum albumin. The 1 ml of the buffered human serum albumin solution containing the tissue extract was assayed for digoxin by radioimmunoassay as described by Smith et al. (1969). Digoxin in blood serum was assayed by the same method.

The percentage recovery from the tissues was estimated by adding known amounts of digoxin to heart tissue homogenates and determining digoxin by radioimmunoassay. Also ^{3}H-digoxin was added to homogenates and the digoxin content measured after extraction. Recoveries always exceeded 90%. Radioactivity was measured in a Nuclear-Chicago liquid scintillation counter. For determination of ^{3}H-digoxin in heart tissue, the methylene chloride phase containing the tissue extract was evaporated in a scintillation phial with nitrogen gas, Bray's solution was added, and the sample then counted. Counting efficiency was 50%. Recovery was 90%.

Histologic Methods

Tissue sections were taken from immediately next to the muscle used for biochemical and pharmacologic assay. The tissue was fixed in 10% buffered formaldehyde embedded in paraffin. Sections were stained with hematoxylin and eosin and Masson's trichrome stain for fibrous tissue. The histologic sections were classified into three grades: grade 1, minimal morphologic change compared to normal (donor atrium and ventricle); grade 2, moderate to severe fibrosis but with the preservation of architecture; grade 3, severe fibrosis — that is, calcification with disruption or obliteration of architecture. We noted whether the abnormalities in the histologic sections were focal and also the degree of involvement of the section.

Study 3

Mongrel dogs weighing 10.9-22.8 kg were premedicated with morphine sulfate, 2 mg/kg, intramuscularly, then anesthetized with chloralose, 85 mg/kg, and urethane 625 mg/kg, given intravenously. The animals were intubated with a cuffed endotracheal tube and ventilated with a Harvard respirator, using room air. Arterial blood samples were analyzed frequently with a model AME-1 Astrup micromanometer, and tidal volume and respiratory rate adjusted to maintain arterial pO_2 above 80 mm Hg and pH between 7.30 and 7.50. Catheters were placed in the ascending aorta via the carotid artery, the jugular vein, and a femoral vein, and the chest was opened via a midline sternotomy. A BT-250 Bio-Tec solid-state pressure transducer was then placed via a stab wound, into the apex of the left ventricle. A PE-260 polyethylene catheter was positioned in the left atrium via a stab wound in the left atrial appendage, then attached to a saline-filled glass manometer for the measurement of mean left atrial pressure. A left thoracotomy was performed, and an adjustable screw clamp positioned around the descending aorta, immediately distal to the origin of the left subclavian artery, in order to provide a means for controlling aortic pressure. Pacing wires were attached to the right atrium and connected to a Grass Model S-4 stimulator.

Recordings were made on a multichannel photographic recorder. The zero for all pressure measurements was taken at midchest level; aortic pressure was recorded using a Statham P23 Db transducer. Left ventricular pressure was recorded with the Bio-Tec BT-250 solid-state transducer. The first derivative of the left ventricular pressure curve (LVdp/dt) was measured with an RC differentiating circuit, which had a frequency response to a calibrated triangular wave, linear and flat to more than 100 Hz. Aortic mean pressure was derived electronically.

After instrumentation, the animals were given atropine, 0.25 mg/kg, and practolol, 2.5 mg/kg, intravenously over 5 min. After 20 min, half the animals received an infusion of KCl, 1.2 mEq/min, the other half received an equal volume of normal saline. After another 30 min, the rate of KCl and saline infusion was decreased to 0.6 mEq/min for 30 min, then adjusted, as estimated from frequent serum potassium measurements, to maintain serum potassium between 5.0 and 7.5 mEq/liter. Normal saline was administered in isovolumic amounts to normokalemic animals. At the time the KCl infusion was started, right atrial pacing was initiated to maintain heart rate 15-20 beats above control. The aortic mean pressure was increased 15-30 mm Hg, using the aortic constrictor, 30 min after beginning the KCl or saline infusion. This was necessary in order to maintain aortic mean pressure constant after digoxin administration. At zero time, which was 60 min after the onset of the KCl or saline infusion, the aortic constrictor was loosened to allow aortic pressure to return to normal. Half the normokalemic and half the hyperkalemic animals were then given normal saline and served as controls; the other half received 0.08 mg/kg H^3-digoxin (specific activity either 136 or 150 μCi/mg), diluted 1:5 with cold digoxin, intravenously. This is the same dose of digoxin we have previously used in non-β-adrenergic receptor blocked animals, and is the maximally tolerated dose in normokalemic animals which will produce physiologic changes without producing toxic arrhythmias. Serial blood samples and physiologic measurements were then obtained at 10, 20, 30, 45, and 60 min, at which time the animals were sacrificed. Two minutes prior to each physiologic measurement, aortic mean pressure was adjusted to that present just prior to digoxin administration (zero time) using the aortic constrictor.

In order to determine whether hyperkalemia inhibited the inotropic effect of other agents besides digoxin, hyperkalemic and normokalemic animals not receiving digoxin were given 1 cc of 10% $CaCl_2$ intravenously just prior to sacrifice. The maximum increase in left ventricular dp/dt to this agent was then measured.

Biochemical Procedures

After the animals were sacrificed, their hearts were removed, blotted dry, then frozen until analysis. Duplicate samples of left ventricle and plasma were analyzed for digoxin concentration as previously described. Samples were counted in a Packard Tri-Carb liquid scintillation spectrometer to accumulate at least 5000 cpm. Efficiency of counting was determined using either tritiated toluene as an internal standard or the automatic external standard channels ratio method. Results were comparable with either method. Standards and recoveries were run with each sample. Recoveries averaged 85% ± 3% for tissue samples and 75% ± 3% for plasma digoxin. Samples were not corrected for recovery.

Serum sodium and potassium were determined by flame photometry using an Instrumentation Laboratory Model 143.

Microsomal-bound digoxin was determined by extracting a 0.5 ml aliquot of the microsomal fraction containing the ATPase activity (see below) with 10 ml of Bray's solution. The microsomal fraction was shaken overnight at 24°C and then counted in a Packard Tri-Carb liquid scintillation spectrometer with correction for quenching. (Similar results were obtained by complete digestion of the microsomal fraction with 0.2 N KOH at 60°C, indicating that our method completely extracts the digoxin).

A modification of the method of Akera et al. was used to measure myocardial $(Na^+ + K^+)$-ATPase. Approximately 10 g of frozen left ventricle was analyzed within 1 week of the time of sacrifice of the animal. All steps were carried out at 4°C. The 10 g portions of left ventricle were allowed to thaw overnight in the refrigerator, then minced and passed through a tissue press. The material was then homogenized with a power tissue grinder using a Teflon pestle and glass grinding vessel in a total of 19 ml of a solution (A) containing 0.25 M sucrose, 5 mM histidine, 5 mM EDTA 0.15% sodium desoxycholate, 10 μM dithiothreitol (DTT), and Tris base to adjust pH to 6.8. The resulting homogenate was centrifuged at 12,000 $\times$ g for 30 min and the supernatant further centrifuged at 100,000 $\times$ g for 60 min. The pellet was resuspended in a total of 17 ml of a solution (B) containing 0.25 M sucrose, 5 mM histidine, 1 mM EDTA, 10 μM DTT, and Tris base to adjust pH to 7.0 and again centrifuged at 100,000 $\times$ g for 60 min. The resulting pellet was resuspended in 8.5 ml of solution B; 8.5 ml of 2.0 M LiBr was added, and the mixture stirred slowly for 30 min. Following centrifugation at 100,000 $\times$ g for 30 min, the final pellet was suspended in 5-7 ml of solution C (solution B without DTT) and stored frozen at -20°C until assayed. This pellet fraction is hereafter referred to as the microsomal fraction. This fraction contains $(Na^+ + K^+)$-ATPase activity.

The final enzyme-assay mixture was 1.0 ml containing 50 mM Tris-HCl buffer (pH 7.4), 100 mM NaCl, 15 mM KCl, 5 mM $MgCl_2$, 50-70 μg enzyme protein, and 5 mM Tris-ATP. Similar tubes lacking NaCl and KCl were assayed for Mg^{2+}-dependent ATPase activity, and tubes lacking enzyme were assayed for nonenzymic hydrolysis of ATP. All assays were performed in duplicate. The reaction was begun by adding the Tris-ATP. After incubation for 15 min at 37°C, the reaction was terminated by addition of 1.5 ml of freshly diluted 8.3% ice-cold trichloracetic acid. The mixture was centrifuged at 5000 $\times$ g for 3 min at 4°C and 2 ml aliquots were then taken for inorganic phosphate (Pi) analysis. Enzyme acivity was expressed as μM Pi-liberated/mg protein/h, corrected for nonenzymic hydrolysis of ATP. $(Na^+ + K^+)$-ATPase acitivity was calculated as the difference between $(Na^+ + K^+)$-ATPase acitivity and (Mg^{2+})-ATPase acitivity. The $(Na^+ + K^+)$-ATPase activity was completely inhibited by $10^{-6}M$ digoxin.

Enzyme was always prepared by the same individual from a single set of four hearts, one from each of the four experimental groups. Likewise, assays were always performed simultaneously on a single set of four enzyme preparations. Inorganic phosphate liberation was determined by a minor modification of the method of Bonting et al. 0.575 N H_2SO_4 was used in the color reagent, and 2.0 ml of colour reagent was added to 2.0 ml of Pi-containing solution. Standard Pi curves were obtained simultaneously with each assay. Percent inhibition of $(Na^+ + K^+)$-ATPase activity was calculated by subtracting $(Na^+ + K^+)$-ATPase enzyme activity in animals given digoxin from that in controls, prepared at the same time, divided by the activity in the control animals.

Statistical Analyses

The experimental data were evaluated for statistical significance using an IBM 360/50 computer, programmed to calculate means and standard errors and to perform t-test analysis. Each hemodynamic measurement after digoxin administration was compared with that in the same animal just prior to digoxin administration, using a paired t-test. The percentage change of left ventricular dp/dt from its control (zero time) was then calculated. The hemodynamic effects of digoxin in normokalemic and hyperkalemic animals were then compared, using an unpaired t-test. The same analyses were performed for animals that received no digoxin and for our biochemical measurements. Correlations between the percentage inhibition of $(Na^+ + K^+)$-ATPase and the positive inotropic effects of digoxin and microsomal bound digoxin and their statistical significiance were evaluated by the method of Goldstein.

Results

Study 1

The plasma digoxin concentration for the eight patients at the time of surgery ranged from 0.4 to 3.3 ng/ml (mean $1.2 \pm$ SD 0.8). The concentrations in papillary muscle ranged from 15.5 to 132 ng/g (mean 77.7 ± 43.3), with a ratio compared with plasma levels in the individual patients ranging from 39:1 to 155:1 (mean 68 ± 38). The concentrations in skeletal muscle were markedly lower than in myocardium in seven of the eight patients, and ranged from 7.5 to 23 ng/g (mean 11.3 ± 4.9) with a ratio ranging from 3:1 to 58:1 (mean 15.9 ± 18.4). A poor correlation was found between myocardial and skeletal concentrations. The individual results are detailed in the Table 12.1.

Table 12.1. Plasma, myocardial, and skeletal muscle digoxin concentrations and ratios

	Concentration			Ratio	
Case No.	Plasma digoxin (ng/ml)	Myocardial (ng/g)	Skeletal muscle (ng/g)	Plasma/ myocardial	Plasma/ skeletal
1	0.6	31	9	52:1	15:1
2	2.5	125	10	50:1	4:1
3	1.0	54	7.5	54:1	7.5:1
4	0.4	62	10	155:1	25:1
5	1.2	103	12	86:1	10:1
6	3.3	132	11	40:1	3:1
7	1.5	99	8	66:1	5:1
8	0.4	15.5	23	39:1	58:1
Mean	1.2	77.7	11.3	67.7	15.9
(± SD)	(0.8)	(43.3)	(4.9)	(38.3)	(18.4)

Study 2

The individual patient plasma concentration, total myocardial concentration of digoxin, microsomal concentration, and sodium-potassium ATPase activity are shown in Table 12.2. In cases 2 and 7 an in vitro inhibition curve to 10^{-8} and 10^{-7} M concentrations of digoxin was measured, and the sodium-potassium ATPase activities are shown in Table 12.3. In cases 6 and 7, the last dose of digoxin was given as tritiated digoxin, either 4 or 5 h before transplantation, and the radioactive counts in the four chambers of the heart, the total myocardial digoxin concentration, and the total myocardial-tritiated concentration are shown in Table 12.4. The histologic grades of all seven patients are shown in Table 12.5.

Study 3

Hemodynamic Changes

No significant change in either left atrial mean pressure or left ventricular systolic pressure was seen, except in normokalemic animals given digoxin. These animals showed a small but statistically significant decrease in left atrial mean pressure at 10, 20, and 30 min after digoxin administration. Although this decrease in left atrial mean pressure is statistically significant, it is probably too small to be of major physiologic importance.

Table 12.2. Plasma concentrations, total myocardial concentrations, and microsomal concentrations of digoxin and sodium potassium ATPase activity in seven patients

Case No.	Diagnosis	Plasma concentration (ng/ml)	Total myocardial concentration (ng/g heart)				Microsomal concentration (ng/mg protein)		$(Na^+ + K^+)$ ATPase acitivity (μmol/phosphate/mg protein/h)	
			R.A.	L.A.	R.V.	L.V.	R.V.	L.V.	R.V.	L.V.
1	Coronary artery disease	1.8	96	—	76.8	19.2	2.2	1.9	2.55	2.46
2	Coronary artery disease	2.6	54.4	59.2	67.2	75.2	2.8	2.51	3.58	2.51
3	Coronary artery disease	3.0	112	105	144	140				
4	Idiopathic congestive cardiomyopathy	1.4	65	42.8	65.8	76				
5	Coronary artery disease	1.0	45	45	80	120	1.5	1.2		
6	Coronary artery disease	2.1	72	70.9	92	80				
7	Idiopathic congestive cardiomyopathy	1.5	70.5	58	57.5	82				

R.A. = Right altrium. L.A. = Left atrium. R.V. = Right ventricle. L.V. = Left ventricle.

Table 12.3. Results of in vitro incubation of digoxin with ATPase at 37°C for 45 min (case 2) and 30 min (case 7)

	Digoxin concentration (M)	% Inhibition of in vivo ATPase activity
	Case 2	
Right ventricle	10^{-8}	3.4
	10^{-7}	73.6
Left ventricle	10^{-8}	6.8
	10^{-7}	55
	Case 7	
Right ventricle	10^{-8}	32
	10^{-7}	85
Left ventricle	10^{-8}	32
	10^{-7}	88

Table 12.4. Radioactive counts, total and tritiated digoxin concentrations, and total tritiated digoxin ratio in two patients

	CPM	Total myocardial digoxin concentration (ng/g heart)	Tritiated digoxin concentration (ng/^{3}H)	Total tritiated digoxin ratio
		Case 6		
Right atrium	4148	72	14.4	5
Left atrium	2302	70.9	8	8.9
Right ventricle	2381	92	8.29	11.1
Left ventricle	3038	80	10.3	7.8
		Case 7		
Right atrium	2302	70.5	8	8.8
Left atrium	1671	58	5.8	10
Right ventricle	1825	57.5	6.4	9.05
Left ventricle	2764	82	9.6	8.5

Table 12.5. Histologic grades in seven patients

Case No.	Right atrium		Left atrium		Right ventricle		Left ventricle	
	Grade	Comments	Grade	Comments	Grade	Comments	Grade	Comments
1	2	Focal	1		1		3	About 100%
2	1		1	Subendocardial fibrosis	1		1	Subendocardial fibrosis
3	1		1	Subendocardial fibrosis	1		3	33%
4	2		2	Subendocardial fibrosis	1		1	
5	1		2	Subendocardial fibrosis	2		3	Focal
6	1		1		2		1	
7	1		1		2	Subendocardial fibrosis	2	

Table 12.6. Hemodynamic measurements in normokalemic and hyperkalemic dogs (M ± SEM)

Group	No. Time:	-30s	-10s	-5s	0s	+10s	+20s	+30s	+45s	+60s
						Left ventricular dp/dt (mm Hg/s)				
Normal K, no dig.	6	3350± 284	3313± 237	3483± 266	3204± 316	3183± 289	3196± 316	3271± 254	3250± 270	3238± 349
Hyper K, no dig.	6	3300± 207	3692± 247	3592± 248	3550± 255	3533± 231	3617± 233	3483± 189	3425± 224	3375± 184
Normal K, dig.	6	3125± 185	3112± 172	3125± 188	3150± 181	4158± 169[b]	4392± 231[c]	4495± 226[c]	4683± 315[c]	4916± 351[c]
Hyper K, dig.	6	3568± 278	3333± 230	3317± 250	3429± 271	3617± 300[c]	3579± 303[b]	3646± 324[b]	3704± 324[b]	3766± 337[b]

Abbreviations: dig. = digitalis.

[a] $P < 0.05$ compared with zero time value.
[b] $P < 0.025$ compared with zero time value.
[c] $P < 0.01$ compared with zero time value.

Aortic mean pressure was essentially unchanged in all groups of animals studied. In hyperkalemic animals, only at 45 min after being given 0.08 mg/kg digoxin was aortic mean pressure increased from 141 ± 4 mm Hg at zero time to 143 ± 5 mm Hg. Using paired data, this increase in aortic mean pressure was statistically significant (p <0.05). At all other time periods studied, there was no significant increase in mean aortic pressure.

Left ventricular dp/dt is shown in Table 12.6. No significant change in left ventricular dp/dt was seen in animals not given digoxin, while in animals administered digoxin, significant increases in left ventricular dp/dt were observed at all time periods studied. The percentage change in left ventricular dp/dt in animals given digoxin is illustrated in Figure 12.1. At 60 min after the administration of 0.08 mg/kg digoxin, left ventricular dp/dt increased 53.1% ± 8.3% in normokalemic animals, but only 9.5% ± 2.5% in hyperkalemic animals. The differences in the left ventricular dp/dt responses of normokalemic and hyperkalemic animals to digoxin were statistically significant at all time periods studied (p <0.01).

In hyperkalemic animals, 1 cc of 10% $CaCl_2$ increased left ventricular dp/dt 87.9% ± 12.7%, while in normokalemic animals, $CaCl_2$ increased left ventricular dp/dt 76.4% ± 2.3%. The difference in the response between normokalemic and hyperkalemic animals is not statistically significant.

Biochemical Results

Figure 12.2 shows left ventricular digoxin concentrations. In normokalemic animals, left ventricular digoxin concentration was 316.7 ± 13.3 ng/g tissue, while in hyperkalemic animals, left ventricular digoxin concentration was 243.0 ± 10.9 ng/g tissue (p <0.01). Microsomal-bound digoxin concentration is shown in Figure 12.3. In hyperkalemic animals, microsomal-bound digoxin concentration was 20.4 ± 2.1 ng/mg protein, while in normokalemic animals, microsomal-bound digoxin was 29.1 ± 3.0 ng/mg protein (p<0.025). Serum digoxin levels are presented in Figure 12.4. Serum digoxin levels were slightly higher in hyperkalemic than normokalemic animals. The differences between the two groups were significant only at 20 and 30 min (p <0.05).

Figure 12.5 shows the $(Na^+ + K^+)$-ATPase and (Mg^{2+})-ATPase activity in normokalemic and hyperkalemic control animals. In normokalemic animals, $(Na^+ + K^+)$-ATPase activity was 26.5 ± 0.9 μM Pi/mg P/h, while in hyperkalemic animals, $(Na^+ + K^+)$-ATPase activity was 27.9 ± 1.9 μM Pi/mgP/h. (Mg^{2+})ATPase activity was 2.9 ± 0.7 μM Pi/mg P/h in normolakemic animals and 3.2 ± 0.6 μM Pi/mg P/h in hyperkalemic animals. The differences in $(Na^+ + K^+)$-ATPase and (Mg^{2+})-ATPase activity between normokalemic and hyperkalemic animals were not statistically significant. In Figure 12.6 the per cent inhibition of $(Na^+ + K^+)$-ATPase in animals given digoxin is shown, compared to their simultaneously prepared and assayed controls. In normokalemic animals, $(Na^+ + K^+)$-ATPase activity was

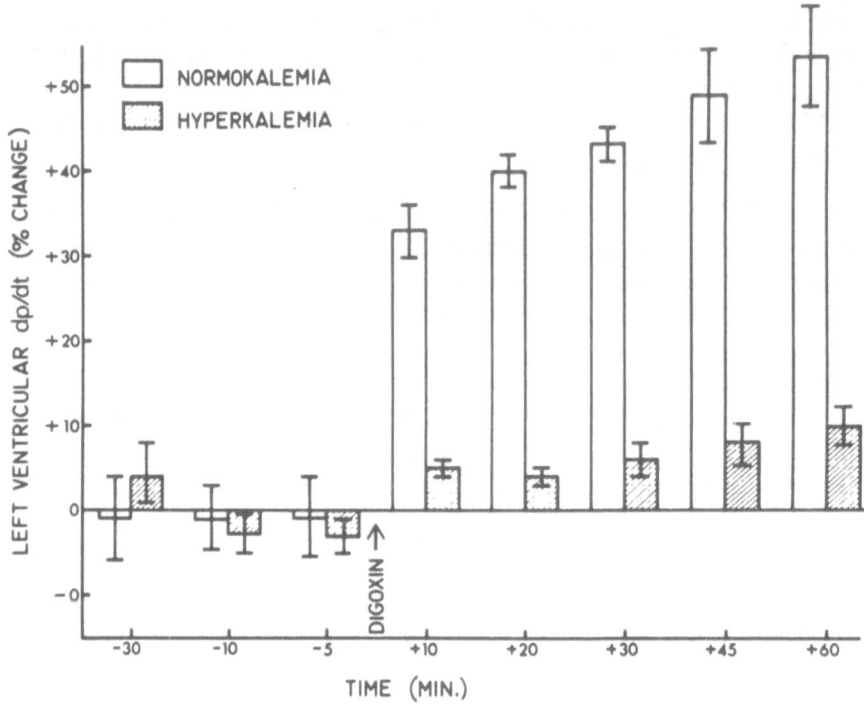

Fig. 12.1. Percentage change in left ventricular dp/dt in normokalemic and hyper-kalemic dogs given 0.08 mg/kg digoxin. Mean ± SEM changes in left ventricular dp/dt are shown for both groups of animals before and after digoxin administration. In this and all other Figures, each mean is from six animals

43.3% ± 2.4 % less than its control, while for hyperkalemic animals, $(Na^+ + K^+)$-ATPase acticity was 27.4% ± 2.5% less than its control. The difference between these two groups is significant ($p < 0.01$). (Mg^{2+})-ATPase levels were similar in normokalemic and hyperkalemic animals given digoxin.

Figure 12.7 shows the correlation between the positive inotropic effects of digoxin and the per cent inhibition of $(Na^+ + K^+)$-ATPase in normokalemic and hyperkalemic animals. There was a significant correlation between the inotropic effects of digoxin and $(Na^+ + K^+)$-ATPase inhibition, $r = 0.73$ ($p < 0.01$). Figure 12.8 shows the correlation between $(Na^+ + K^+)$-ATPase inhibition and microsomal bound digoxin. The correlation coefficient was $r = 0.63$, which is significantly different from zero ($p < 0.05$). In all animals, arterial pH was maintained between 7.30 and 7.50 by varying the respiratory rate or volume. In animals given a KCl infusion, serum potassium was maintained well above 5.0 mEq/liter. Composite data for all experiments filed with the National Library of Medicine, Bethesda, Maryland.

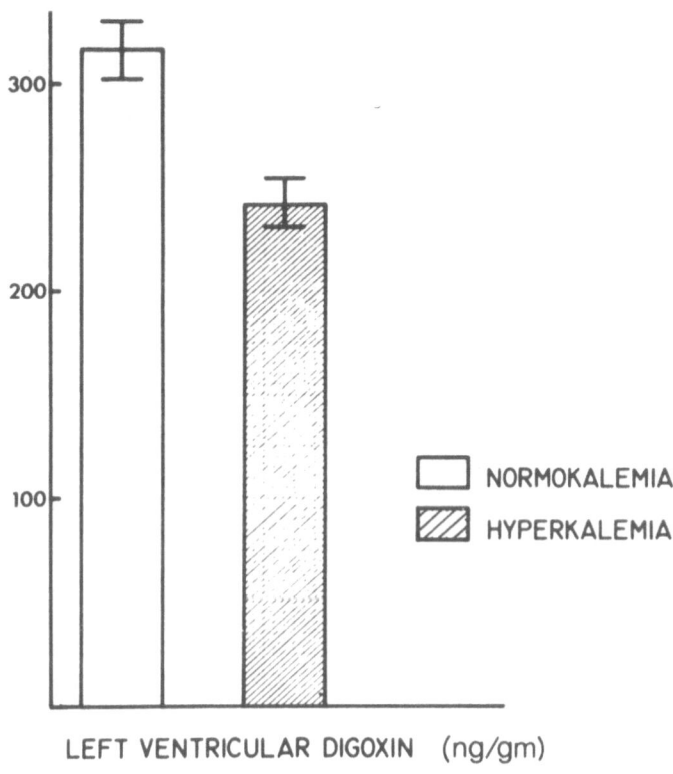

Fig. 12.2. Left ventricular digoxin concentrations in normokalemic and hyperkalemic animals given 0.08 mg/kg digoxin 60 min prior to sacrifice

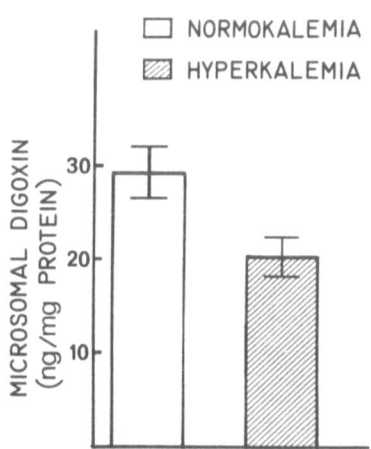

Fig. 12.3. Microsomal-bound digoxin concentration in normokalemic and hyperkalemic animals. Mean ± SEM are shown for normokalemic and hyperkalemic
animals

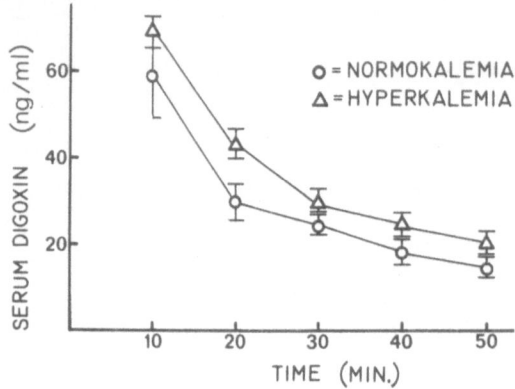

Fig. 12.4. Serum digoxin levels in normokalemic and hyperkalemic animals. Each value represents the mean ± SEM of six animals. At 20 and 30 min hyperkalemic animals had significantly higher serum digoxin levels than normokalemic animals

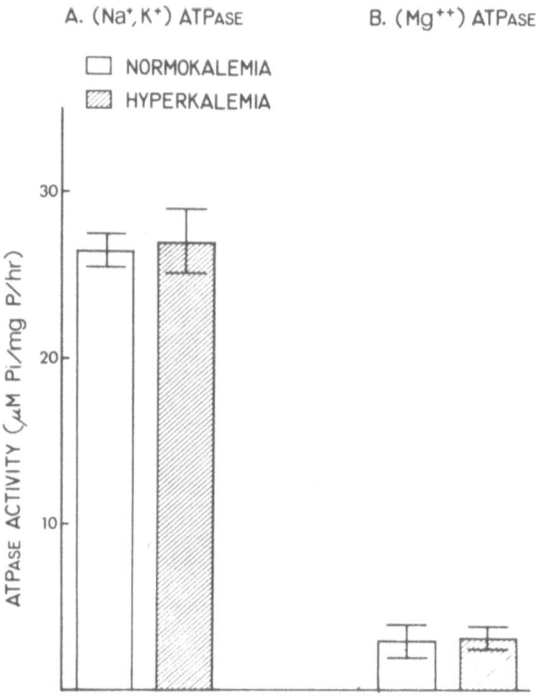

Fig. 12.5. $(Na^+ + K^+)$-ATPase and (Mg^{2+})-ATPase activity in normokalemic and hyperkalemic animals not given digoxin. Mean ± SEM are shown

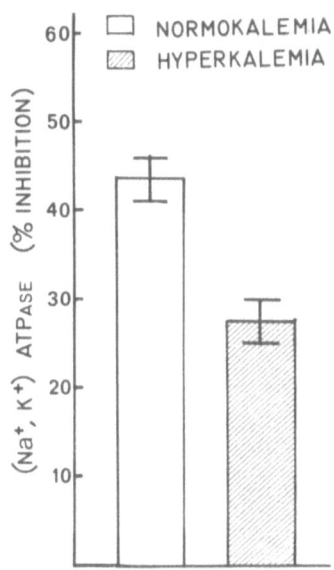

Fig. 12.6. The percentage inhibition of $(Na^+ + K^+)$-ATPase in normokalemic and hyperkalemic animals sacrificed 60 min after digoxin administration is shown. Each bar represents the mean ± SEM of six pairs of animals. There was no change in (Mg^{2+})-ATPase activity (not shown) in animals given digoxin

Discussion

Whereas a vast amount of knowledge has been developed relating to concentration and excretion of the cardiac glycosides, very little is known of their distribution in the tissues and organs of the body. This is particularly true for the damaged heart where tissue fibrosis is common in patients given digitalis. Thus, we directed our studies toward the disposition of digoxin which is related to its distribution within and the elimination from the body. Since digoxin is given in clinical practice for its effect upon the heart, it is particularly pertinent to study its distribution within the various chambers of the diseased human heart. Human cardiac transplantation provides an opportunity to study large amounts of fresh human heart tissue after the administration of drugs. Our results show clearly that when the morphologic architecture of the heart is altered severely owing to a fibrotic process secondary to old myocardial ischemia, there are alterations in the myocardial content of digoxin.

Minimal general fibrosis and milder specific histologic alterations in the structure do not alter the distribution between various chambers. When fibrotic tissue such as occurred in case 1 is present, the content of digoxin is markedly reduced in the scar tissue. Analysis of the microsomal fraction which may represent the location of the active receptor site of digoxin, however, shows that the disparity in drug distribution is decreased even when fibrosis is severe as in case 1 and is relatively

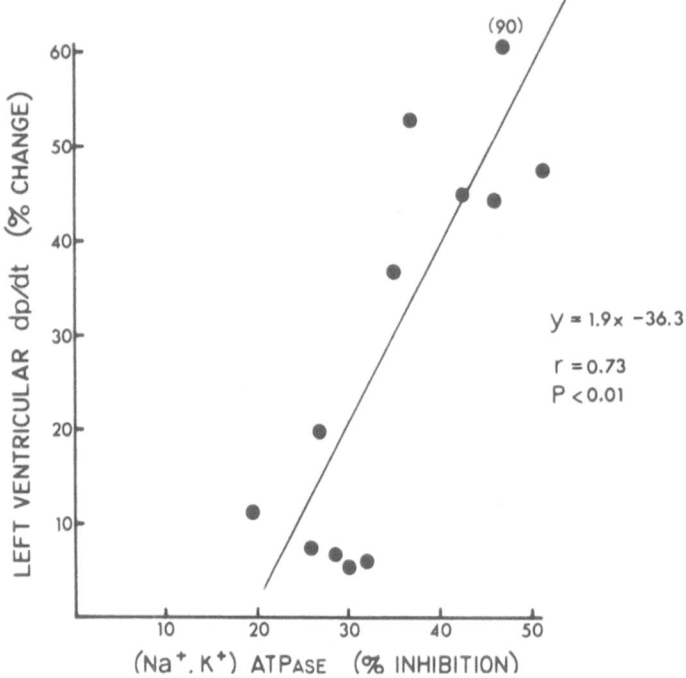

Fig. 12.7. Correlation between the change in left ventricular dp/dt and the percent inhibition of $(Na^+ + K^+)$-ATPase for normokalemic and hyperkalemic animals after digoxin administration. Each point represents the change in left ventricular dp/dt at 60 min after digoxin administration and the per cent inhibition of $(Na^+ + K^+)$-ATPase in normokalemic and hyperkalemic animals sacrificed at this time

normal in other cases with fibrosis (cases 3 and 5). The discrepancy is clearly shown in case 1. In this patient, there was a fourfold difference between the total concentration in the left ventricle and that in the right ventricle whereas the microsomal digoxin concentrations were quantitatively similar to the plasma concentrations. In case 2, the histologic appearances were uniform throughout the four chambers of the heart as was the total myocardial concentration. In case 3, the plasma concentration at the time of transplant was high, and higher total myocardial concentrations were also observed. In case 4, the patient had idiopathic cardiomyopathy and the concentration in the four chambers of the heart was similar. In case 5 where the histologic abnormality was focal in nature, the total myocardial digoxin concentrations was uniformly distributed. In the two patients given labeled digoxin for their last dose, the ratio of labeled to total myocardial concentration was relatively constant for all four chambers. Our results suggest that even 5-7 h after administration there is equilibration between the serum and the myocardium for all four chambers of the heart.

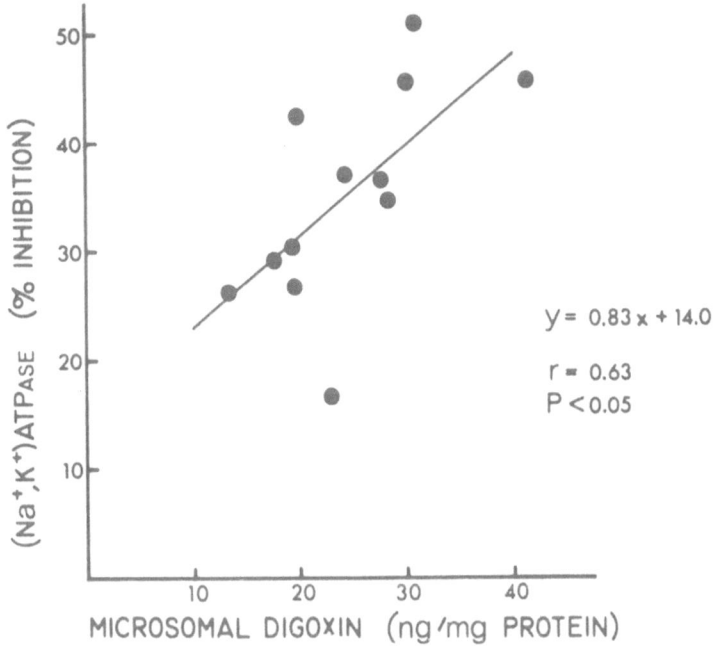

Fig. 12.8. Correlation between $(Na^+ + K^+)$-ATPase inhibition and microsomal-bound digoxin in normokalemic and hyperkalemic animals sacrificed 60 min after digoxin administration

The enzymic estimations of ATPase activity we performed were difficult to interpret owing to the lack of excellent control human tissue. The only control analysis we performed was on the histologic appearances of the donor atria and ventricle. Caution, therefore, must be taken in extrapolating these results, particularly in relationship to previous work of enzymic analysis in a different species. Nevertheless, the results do have significance since they can be compared with the relative information from control animal experiments. It is difficult to differentiate the effects of digoxin on sodium-potassium ATPase activity for those secondary to the underlying myocardial disease process. In the two patients in whom in vitro inhibition to various concentrations of digoxin was assessed, however, the enzyme was inhibited in a dose-responsive fashion. This suggests that there is still further activity of the enzyme in vivo. Gibson and Harris (1970) have reported low values for sodium-potassium ATPase in human heart samples from postmorten myocardium. These workers found that the activity of the cardiac microsomal sodium-potassium ATPase did not differ in patients dying from cardiac disease and those dying from other causes. They interpreted this finding as supporting their previous experimental evidence that myocardial hypertrophy and prolonged administration of digitalis or diuretics had no effect on the activity of this enzyme. Other studies have not agreed with these findings in the failing heart, where decreased ATPase activity per gram of muscle have been noted (Yazaki and Fujii, 1972).

Our results also confirm the previously reported experimental finding of an alteration in digoxin distribution in the experimental, acute, and chronically ischemic left ventricle (Beller et al., 1972). These workers found the pattern of digoxin uptake partly reflected in regional blood flow to infarcted, ischemic, and nonischemic tissue. Furthermore, they speculated that quantitative differences of digoxin in infarcted myocardium combined with ischemic may well contribute to the reported increase in electrophysiologic arrhythmias seen in patients with coronary artery disease treated with cardiac glycosides.

Previous work on plasma and total myocardial digoxin concentrations have suggested that there is a constant relationship between these two, and hence, it might be expected that conclusions regarding a receptor site could be extrapolated from a plasma concentration (Doherty et al., 1967). Our results tend to suggest that such conclusions would be wrong in the presence of severe myocardial fibrosis and necrosis as far as total tissue digoxin levels are concerned but not as far as microsomal-bound digoxin is concerned. There was a direct relationship between plasma and microsomal concentrations of digoxin. This study emphasizes the importance in understanding the active receptor site for the mechanism of action of a drug.

In order to study the inotropic effects of digoxin, we measured changes in left ventricular dp/dt in normokalemic and hyperkalemic animals in which other determinants of myocardial contractility, such as heart rate, left atrial mean pressure (preload), aortic mean pressure (afterload), and sympathetic tone were maintained constant. Since hyperkalemia itself did not alter myocardial contractility in animals not given digoxin, the positive inotropic effects seen after digoxin administration were attributed to the digoxin.

In normokalemic animals, digoxin had a significantly greater inotropic effect than in hyperkalemic animals. This greater inotropic effect was associated with increased microsomal-bound digoxin and a more pronounced inhibition of $(Na^+ + K^+)$-ATPase activity. Since hyperkalemia itself did not alter contractility or $(Na^+ + K^+)$-ATPase activity in control animals (Fig. 12.5), our results suggest that the mechanism by which hyperkalemia alters digoxin-induced inotropy and $(Na^+ + K^+)$-ATPase inhibition must be secondary to hyperkalemia's effect on the interaction between digoxin and its site of action, the microsomal fraction containing $(Na^+ + K^+)$-ATPase. Support for this hypothesis is also provided by the in vitro studies of Allen and Schwartz and by our data showing a good correlation between $(Na^+ + K^+)$-ATPase inhibition and inotropy. Our experiments on the effects of hyperkalemia on the inotropic properties of $CaCl_2$ also indicate that hyperkalemia had a specific effect on digoxin-induced inotropy, rather than a nonspecific effect on other inotropic agents.

Our study also shows a significant correlation between microsomal-bound digoxin and $(Na^+ + K^+)$-ATPase inhibition (Fig. 12.8). This correlation was not as strong as that between the inotropic effects of digoxin and $(Na^+ + K^+)$-ATPase inhibition. Moreover, the correlation between inotropy and microsomal-bound digoxin showed a correlation coefficient of only $r = 0.54$, which is of borderline significance ($t = 2.02$, $p < 0.10 > 0.05$). The reasons for these results are not clear.

154

However, a number of possibilities should be considered. First, Kim et al. have presented evidence that loosely bound digoxin rather than total microsomal-bound digoxin correlates best with inotropy. Their method of preparation of the microsomal fraction differs from ours. In order to increase the specific activity of $(Na^+ + K^+,)$-ATPase, our microsomal fraction is stirred with LiBr, then washed twice with a sucrose media. This procedure may separate loosely bound digoxin from $(Na^+ + K^+)$-ATPase. When we attempted to measure loosely bound digoxin in our microsomal fraction, no radioactivity was detected. Second, the fraction we call "microsomes" is a very impure and heterogeneous fraction which contains the $(Na^+ + K^+)$-ATPase activity within it. We may have large amounts of binding of digoxin to microsomal protein which does not contain $(Na^+ + K^+)$-ATPase activity. This would mask the small amount of specific binding of digoxin to $(Na^+ + K^+)$-ATPase. Although the studies of Matsui and Schwartz, which showed that nonspecific binding in vitro accounts for only 1%-2% of total digoxin bound to $(Na^+ + K^+)$-ATPase when digoxin concentration is less than 10^{-7} M, suggest that this is not the explanation, the amount of nonspecific binding of digoxin $(Na^+ + K^+)$-ATPase in vivo has not been determined. Using isolated guinea pig atria, Kuschinsky et al. estimated that only 10% of tissue digoxin is bound to specific receptor sites. Third, Akera and Brody have shown, in vitro, that there are at least two types of binding of cardiac glycosides to $(Na^+ + K^+)$-ATPase. One type is inhibited by potassium while the second is not. The contribution of each type of binding to total microsomal-bound digoxin is not known nor is it clear whether each type of binding procedures quantitatively similar effects on $(Na^+ + K^+)$-ATPase or inotropy.

Although the present investigation has focused on the interaction of potassium and digoxin with membrane-bound $(Na^+ + K^+)$-ATPase, potassium may be involved at other sites in the myocardial cell and thereby alter the pharmacologic properties of digoxin. However, Schwartz et al. found that H^3-digoxin and H^3-ouabain did not affect or bind to two other cardiac organelles: cardiac relaxing system vesicles and mitochondria. The binding of H^3-ouabain to $(Na^+ + K^+)$-ATPase was, however, related to the inhibitory effect of ouabain on $(Na^+ + K^+)$-ATPase, suggesting that the effect of glycosides on $(Na^+ + K^+)$-ATPase is a specific rather than a nonspecific effect. Repke has also provided important information of the specificity of $(Na^+ + K^+)$-ATPase as a digitalis receptor. He showed that only cardioactive glycosides inhibit $(Na^+ + K^+)$-ATPase, while inactive glycosides had no effect on $(Na^+ + K^+)$-ATPase.

References

Akera, T., Brody, T.M.: J. Pharmacol. Exp. Ther. 176, 545 (1971)
Akera, T., Larsen, F.S., Brody, T.M.: J. Pharmacol. Exp. Ther. 173, 145 (1970)
Allen, J.C., Schwartz, A.: J. Mol. Cell. Cardiol. 1, 39 (1970)
Beller, G.A., Smith, T.W., Hood, W.B.: Circulation 46, 572 (1972)
Besch, H.R., Jr., et al: J. Pharmacol. Exp. Ther. 171, 1 (1970)
Chamberlain, D.A., et al: (1970). Br. Med. J. 1970/III, 429

Clark, D.A., et al: Am. J. Med. <u>54</u>, 563 (1973)

Doherty, J.E., Perkins, W.M., Flanigan, W.J.: Ann. Intern. Med. <u>66</u>, 116 (1967)

Gibson, K., Harris, P.: Cardiovasc. Res. <u>4</u>, 201 (1970)

Goldman, R.H., et al: Circulation <u>48</u>, 830 (1973)

Goldstein, A.: Biostatics. An Introductory Text. New York: Macmillan 1968

Kim, N.K., Bailey, L.E., Dresel, P.E.: J. Pharmacol. Exp. Ther. <u>181</u>, 377 (1972)

Kuschinsky, K., Lahrtz, H., Lullmann, H., Van Zweiten, P.A.: Br. J. Pharmacol. <u>30</u>, 317 (1967)

Lowenstein, J.M., Corrill, E.M.: J. Lab. Clin. Med. <u>67</u>, 1048 (1966)

Lukas, D.S., Peterson, R.E.: J. Clin. Invest. <u>45</u>, 782 (1966)

Marcus, F.I., Kapadia, G.G., Goldsmith, C.: J. Pharmacol. Exp. Ther. <u>165</u>, 136 (1969)

Matsui, H., Schwartz, A.: Biochim. Biophys. Acta <u>151</u>, 655 (1968)

Repke, K.: Proceedings of the Second International Pharmacology Meeting. New York: Pergamon Press 1965 pp. 65-87

Schwartz, A., Allen, J.C., Harigaya, S.: J. Pharmacol. Exp. Ther. <u>168</u>, 31 (1969)

Smith, T.W., Butler, V.P., Haber, E.: N. Engl. J. Med. <u>281</u>, 1212 (1969)

Stinson, E.B., et al: Am. J. Surg. <u>118</u>, 182 (1969)

Yazaki, Y., Fujii, J.: Jap. Heart J. <u>13</u>, 73 (1972)

Discussion

Erdmann, München: I think you demonstrated good results which I would like to confirm with some of our binding studies of labeled glycosides to isolated human cardiac cell membranes (Fig. 1). The lower curve shows the binding of ouabain to the cell membranes without potassium, and the upper experimental line displays ouabain binding in the presence of 5 mM potassium. You see on this double reciprocal plot that there is an apparently competitive type of binding between cardiac glycosides and potassium. This curve implies that potassium actually displaces cardiac glycosides from the receptor site or inhibits the rebinding to the receptor by a conformational change of the enzyme protein.

Smith, Boston: Some investigators, in studies extending back over several years, have suggested that the inhibition of cardiac glycoside binding by K^+ is probably an allosteric interaction. I agree that your curve does appear to be competitive, but this concept cannot go unchallenged from the work of others.

Erdmann: Up to a concentration of 8 mM it follows a competitive type of binding, but beyond that, it doesn't any more.

Smith: The concept that sodium potassium ATPase is in fact the receptor for the inotropic effect of cardiac glycosides continues to arouse controversy. Although my own bias is that there is a great deal of circumstantial evidence that supports this idea, at least three papers have been published within the last year or so that call this into question. One is from Noble's group at Oxford University, who have shown by microelectrode techniques evidence that at concentra-

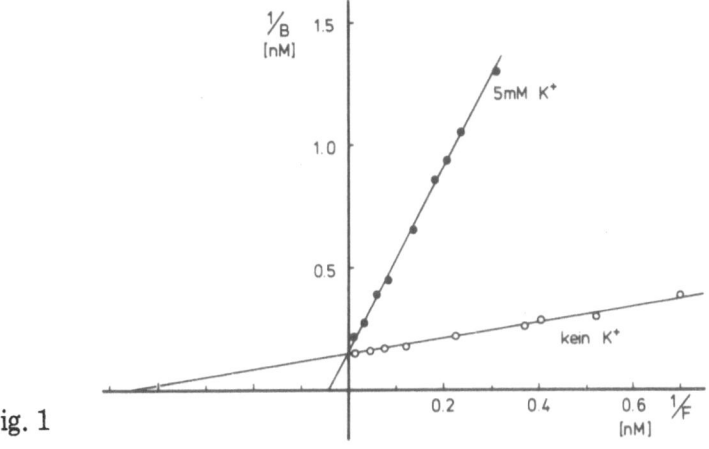

Fig. 1

tions of the order of $10^{-8}M$ there is a stimulation rather than an inhibition of the sodium pump. A second study from Copenhagen by Steiness and colleagues suggests that sodium potassium ATPase inhibition could not be demonstrated, and a third study of Marks and co-workers failed to show significant inhibition of sodium potassium ATPase in animals given a steady-state infusion of ouabain to a positive inotropic end point. I wonder if you would like to comment on that.

Coltart: I'm aware of the controversy, and that's why I've carefully used such words as the "supposed" active receptor site and the "putative", and never to say I was certain. When these studies were designed, there appeared to be nothing better that we could look at — and indeed probably as we stand here today — than to measure $(Na^+ + K^+)$-ATPase enzyme concentration as a receptor site and recognizing the controversy.

Smith, Boston: Dr. Hougen and I now have some evidence using a direct assay of monovalent cation transport that in an infusion regimen which produces low steady-state plasma ouabain concentrations of around 10^{-8} M, with no toxicity even when extended or hours, inhibition of active rubidium uptake in serial myocardial biopsy samples does occur. I agree with you that this is the most likely "receptor" currently under study. It's important, however, to call attention to these other studies which present a different view.

Grahame-Smith, Oxford: These are very nice studies. Assuming for the moment that the sodium potassium ATPase is some sort of receptor, as I have stated before, it is probable that the receptor is not in a stable state because the ATPase has to be in a particular state for digoxin to bind it. In our recent studies on the binding of tritiated digoxin to red cell membranes of red cells removed from patients receiving digoxin, we have found that during the first 5-6 days of treatment there is a decrease in the amount of digoxin that combined to the red cell membrane. After a time, however, the amount of digoxin that will bind to the red cells starts to increase again and may in fact increase above what we presume is the normal level from our control data. It seems to us that perhaps treatment with digoxin may be altering intracellular cation levels and producing an environ-

157

ment in which the ATPase may turn on as far as binding digoxin is concerned. In that case, you may end up with more ATPase available for binding. If in fact various factors can alter the degree of binding of digoxin to the sodium potassium ATPase, it becomes very difficult to know exactly where you are when you are taking postmortem specimens and you only have one instant of time to look at.

Marcus: If you had extended your experiment to maintain hyperkalemia for a longer period of time, may there not have been equilibration of both inotropy and digitalis uptake to the control level? Some time ago, we performed experiments in which we perfused cat papillary muscles with a hyperkalemic solution and then administered tritiated digoxin. At 45 min, there was a decrease in inotropy and a decrease in ^{3}H-digoxin uptake as compared to papillary muscles infused with normokalemic solutions. However, with continued perfusion with the hyperkalemic solution, there was a gradual increase in tritiated digoxin uptake to equal the control level. We concluded that hyperkalemia decreased in rate, but not the total uptake of tritiated digoxin. Also, hyperkalemia decreased the rate of development of digoxin-induced inotropy, but not the ultimate magnitude of the inotropic effect. I wonder if you would comment on these observations.

Coltart: In our experiment, we didn't take any further measurement than the time and the doses I mentioned. Clearly, the variables mentioned are a possible factor which one must take into account. This is why it would be very nice in clinical human experiments to be able to have some type of sampling technique whereby one can look at, more than one instant in time, the digoxin myocardial kinetics.

13 Influence of Thyroid Function on the Pharmacokinetics of Cardiac Glycosides[1]

H. J. GILFRICH and T. MEINERTZ

The clinical observation that larger than usual doses of cardiac glycosides are required to control ventricular rate in hyperthyroid patients with atrial fibrillation (Frye and Braunwald, 1961) has been attributed to an altered intrinsic myocardial function which modifies its response to digitalis (Buccino et al., 1967; Peacock and Moran, 1963). In addition, Doherty and Perkins (Doherty and Perkins, 1965), using single-dose tritiated digoxin showed lower plasma levels in hyperthyroid and higher digoxin serum concentrations in hypothyroid patients. Similar findings were reported by Eickenbusch et al. (Eickenbusch et al., 1969) for ouabain and digitoxin. Doherty and Perkins (Doherty and Perkins, 1965) found no significant differences in either digoxin excretion rate or serum half-life time and proposed the hypothesis that a difference in the volume of distribution of the drug in these conditions may be responsible. Studies in dogs with altered thyroid function, however, failed to demonstrate significant changes in tissue digoxin concentrations. Recently, Croxson and Ibbertson (Croxson and Ibbertson, 1975) studied hyperthyroid patients during the steady state of oral digoxin therapy and found that the lower levels of digoxin in patients suffering from thyrotoxicosis were closely related to changes in renal function. These findings prompted us to reassess the pharmacokinetics of digoxin in hyperthyroidism and to study in which way individual patients alter their handling of digoxin after treatment of their disease.

We studied five hospitalized patients (three women and two men) with marked hyperthyroidism before and after treatment. They were not taking therapeutic digoxin or other drugs known to affect the pharmacokinetics of digoxin. Digoxin was given intravenously as a single dose of 1.0 mg (Lancior®, Boehringer Mannheim GmbH). Blood samples were taken in frequent intervals up to 48 h after administration. Urine was collected every 12 h for 7 days. Completeness of urine collection procedure was controlled by the determination of the total urinary creatinine excretion. After completing this study, the patients were treated with thyrostatic drugs and when they were clinically and biochemically euthyroid the procedure was repeated. Plasma and urine concentrations of digoxin were measured by radioimmunoassay.

1 This study was supported by a grant of Deutsche Forschungsgemeinschaft, Bonn, W.-Germany.
Expert technical assistance was given by Ursula Bohr and Hannelore Heinemann.

The decline of plasma digoxin concentrations of the five hyperthyroid patients before and after treatment with antithyroid agents is shown in Figure 13.1. Plasma digoxin levels from 2 h after injection were significantly lower in the hyperthyroid patients. These findings are in good agreement with that of Doherty and Perkins (Doherty and Perkins, 1956) after a single administration of ^{3}H-digoxin and also with that obtained during maintenance therapy (Croxson and Ibbertson, 1975). Plasma levels of digoxin seemed to decline more rapidly during thyrotoxicosis. Since in some hyperthyroid patients, digoxin levels 24 h after administration were close to the limit of detection, exact calculations of plasma half-life time could not be carried out. Therefore, urinary excretion rates of digoxin were used to calculate the half-life of digoxin since drug concentrations in urine could be measured for at least 7 days. Since digoxin is mainly excreted in urine as a unchanged drug and plasma half-lives and half-lives calculated using urinary excretion rate of digoxin are in close agreement (Dengler et al., 1973), this approach seems to be correct.

Figure 13.2 represents the urinary excretion rate vs. time data for one characteristic patient. In this subject, half-life of digoxin increased from 19.7 h during hyperthyroidism to 30.5 h after thyroid function had returned to mormal. On the average, half-lives of renal digoxin elimination were shortened from 40 h to 24.1 h. This result is different from the findings of Doherty and Perkins (Doherty

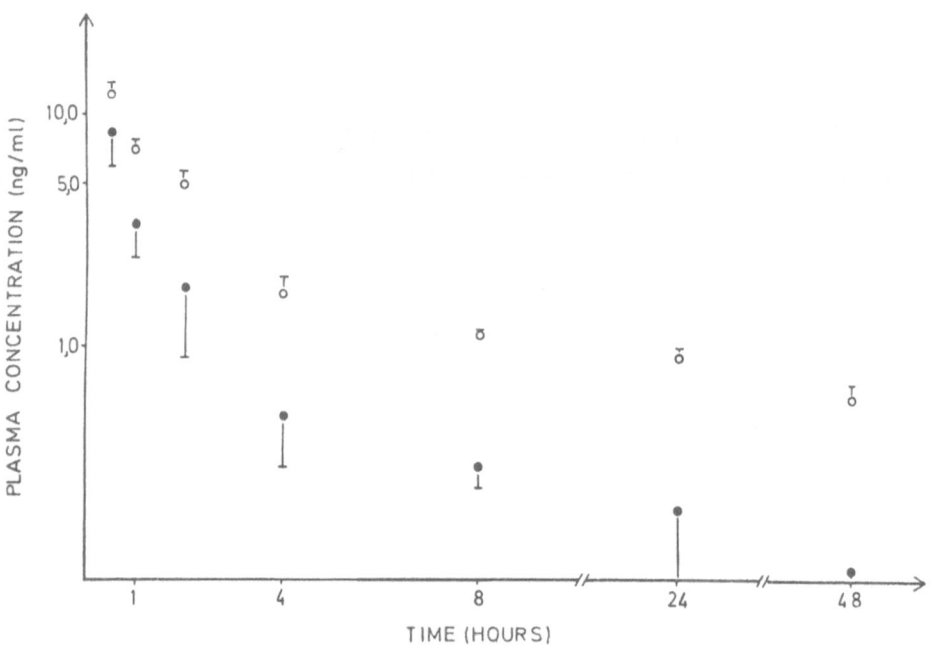

Fig. 13.1. Plasma digoxin concentrations after i.v. injection of 1.0 mg digoxin in five patients ($\overline{x}$ ± SEM) during hyperthyroidism (closed circles) and after thyroid function had returned to normal (open circles)

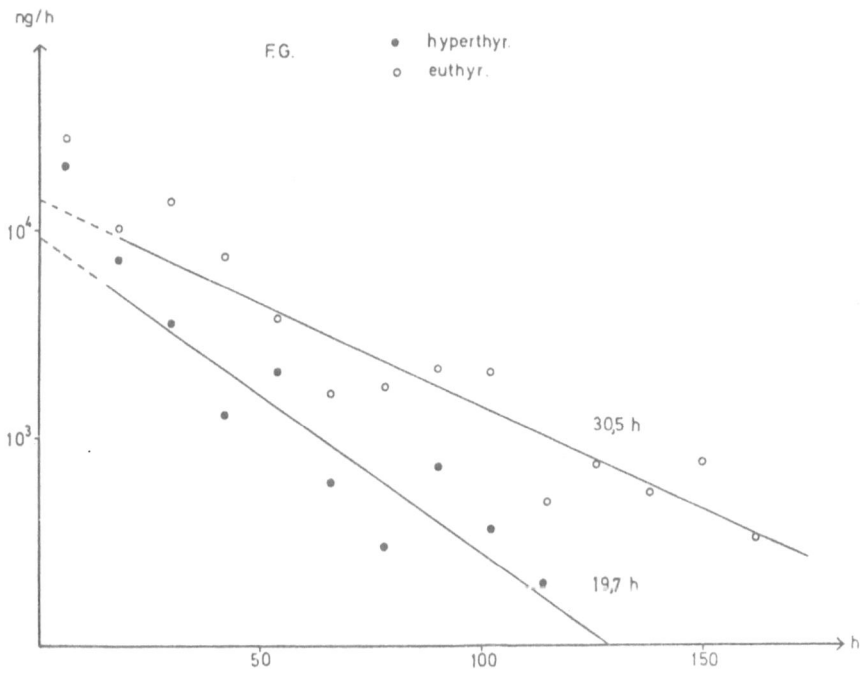

Fig. 13.2. Urinary excretion rate of digoxin in patient F.G. after i.v. injection of
1.0 mg digoxin during hyperthyroidism (closed circles) and after treatment (open
circles). Excretion rates were obtained from urine collection periods of 12 h
for 7 days

and Perkins, 1956) who showed no significant changes of the half-life of urinary
excretion of ^{3}H activity between hyper- and hypothyroid patients. It could be
explained by consistent changes in glomerular filtration rates in patients with
thyroid disease. Inulin clearance was found to be raised in hyperthyroid patients
and decreased in hypothyroidism (Bradley et al., 1974). In agreement with the
findings of Croxson and Ibbertson (Croxson and Ibbertson, 1975), the values of
renal digoxin clearance were markedly higher in our patients during hyperthyroidism, the average renal clearance over the whole collection period being 263 ±
44 ml/min in comparison to 138 ± 20 after treatment. The thyroid state, therefore, influences renal excretion of digoxin. This is one reason for the lower plasma
digoxin concentrations in hyperthyroid patients.

The pharmacokinetic parameters obtained from analysis of plasma concentration
and urinary excretion rate data are summarized in Table 13.1. The apparent
volume of distribution showed large interindividual differences ranging from 709
to 2355 liters (mean 1413 Liters) during hyperthyroidism. Looking at individual
patients, it was found to be significantly larger than that obtained after the thyroid
function had returned to normal. The increase of the volume of distribution might
be explained by an enhanced perfusion of organs which accumulate digoxin or

Table 13.1. Apparent volume of distribution (VD), half-life of renal Elimination of digoxin (T 1/2 $_{urine}$), and cumulative urinary digoxin excretion (A_u ^{7}days) during hyperthyroidism (a) and after thyreostatic treatment (B) ($\bar{x}$ ± SEM, N = 5)

	A	B
VD (L)	1413 ± 373	553 ± 68
T 1/2 Urine (Hours)	24.9 ± 1.6	40 ± 4.0
A_u^7 Days (Fraction of Dose)	0.51 ± 0.08	0.76 ± 0.06

by an increase of binding of digoxin to tissue binding sites. The findings that thyrotoxic animals have higher tissue ($Na^+ + K^+$)-ATPase activities provide a possible explanation for this apparent increase in distribution volume (Ismail-Beigi and Edelman, 1971). The in vitro plasma protein binding was found to be unchanged under the influence of thyroid hormones (Kuschinsky, 1969). When the plasma clearance was compared between both groups, an even more pronounced effect of thyrotoxicosis was observed. Hyperthyroid patients showed a mean digoxin plasma clearance of 724 ml/min, ranging from 1145 to 326 ml/min. The same patients when euthyroid had a digoxin plasma clearance of 174 ml/min. This remarkable difference can partially be explained by the different volume of distribution and renal excretion rate between both groups. However, it further indicates an influence of thyroid function on the metabolic pattern of digoxin. This idea of an increased nonrenal elimination is further supported by comparison of the cumulative urinary excretion data. The total for 7 days urinary excretion of digoxin after intravenous adminstration of 1.0 mg digoxin was appreciably lower during hyperthyroidism (51% of the dose) than after normalization of thyroid function (76% of the dose). The difference in the cumulative urinary excretion of digoxin was observed in all but one patient.

The apparent increase of nonrenal digoxin elimination in patients suffering from thyrotoxicosis could be due to several factors. Marked changes in drug metabolizing activity occur during the hyperthyroid state (Doherty and Perkins, 1956). This may hold true for digoxin also. On the other hand, Hartmann et al. (Hartmann et al., 1975) have demonstrated an increase of the biliary excretion of digoxin and its metabolites in hyperthyroid rats. It has been suggested by Watters and Tomkin (Watters and Tomkin, 1975) that an important factor not adequately investigated yet causing low digoxin plasma levels, may be that of malabsorption due to steatorrhea and disturbances of gastrointestinal motility since the extent of digoxin absorption would be affected by its residence in the upper small intestine. There is only one study on drug absorption during thyroid disorder. Levy et al. (Levy et al., 1972) observed that riboflavin absorption was retarded in hyperthyroidism, whereas in hypothyroid children, absorption of this agent was accelerated. This aspect obviously needs further investigation. To explore this possibility, eight hyperthyroid patients without diarrhea received 1.0 mg of digoxin orally and intravenously in randomized order. The fraction of the dose absorbed was determined by comparison of the areas under the plasma concentration curves during 24 h after administration. In three of the eight patients, there seemed to be a diminished absorption, 38%-51% of the dose administered, whereas five patients demonstrated an absorption of 60%-70% which is in a range obtained in normal subjects with the preparation used (Gilfrich and Clasen, 1976). In all patients, peak levels were seen already 30 min after oral administration, indicating a faster absorption rate than in normal patients.

In conclusion: thyroid status influences digoxin plasma concentrations by a change in the volume of distribution, a change in renal function, in the amount of nonrenal excretion, and in some patients in a different absorption after oral administration.

References

Bradley, S.E., Stephan, F., Coelho, J.B., Reville, P.: The thyroid and the kidney. Kidney International 6, 346 (1974)
Buccino, R.A., Spann, J.F., Pool, P.E., Sonnenblick, E.H., Braunwald, E.: Influence of the thyroid state on the intrinsic contractile properties and energy stores of the myocardium. J. Clin. Invest. 46, 1669 (1967)
Croxson, M.S., Ibbertson, H.K.: Serum digoxin in patients with thyroid disease. Br. Med. J. 1975, 566
Dengler, H.J., Bodem, G., Wirth, K.: Pharmakokinetische Untersuchungen mit ³H-Digoxin und ³H-Lanatosid beim Menschen. Arzneim. Forsch. (Drug-Res.) 23, 64 (1973)
Doherty, J.E., Perkins, W.H.: Digoxin metabolism in hypo- and hyperthyroidism. Studies with tritiated digoxin in thyroid disease. Ann. Intern. Med. 64, 489 (1956)
Eichelbaum, M., Bodem, G., Gugler, R., Schneider-Deters, Ch., Dengler, H.J.: Influence of thyroid status on plasma half-life of antipyrine in man. N. Engl. J. Med. 290, 1040 (1974)
Eickenbusch, W., Lahrtz, H.G., Seppelt, U., Van Zwieten, P.A.: Serum concentration and urinary excretion of ³H-digitoxin in patients suffering from hyperthyroidism or hypothyroidism. Klin. Wochenschr. 48, 270 (1969)
Frye, R.L., Braunwald, E.: Studies on digitalis III. The influence of triodothyronine on digitalis requirements. Circulation 23, 376 (1961)
Gilfrich, H.J., Clasen, R.: Untersuchungen zur biologischen Verfügbarkeit von Digoxin aus Kombinationspräparaten im Langzeitversuch. Inn. Med. 3, 189 (1976)

Hartmann, C.R., Klaassen, C.D., Huffman, D.H.: The biliary excretion of digoxin and metabolites in hyperthyroid rats. Clin. Res. $\underline{23}$, 220 A (1975)

Ismail-Beigi, F., Edelman, I.S.: The mechanism of the calorigenic action of thyroid hormonestimulation of $Na^+ + K^+$ — activated adenosine triphosphatase. J. Gen. Physiol $\underline{57}$, 710 — 722 (1971)

Kuschinsky, K.: über die Bindungseigenschaften von Plasmaproteinen für Herzglykoside. Arch. Exp. Pathol. Pharmakol. $\underline{262}$, 388 (1969)

Levy, G., Macgillivray, M.H., Procknal, J.A.: Riboflavin adsorption in children with thyroid disorders. Pediatrics $\underline{50}$, 896 (1972)

Peacock, W.F., Moran, N.C.: Influence of thyroid state on positive inotropic effect of ouabain on isolated ventricle strips. Proceedings of the Society of Experimental Biology and Medicine $\underline{133}$, 526 (1963)

Watters, K., Tomkin, G.H.: Serum digoxin in patients with thyroid disease. Br. Med. J. 102 (1975)

Discussion

Greenblatt: Although the percent of dose recovered in the urine was small, actually the renal clearance was larger? Did you say that both renal and extrarenal clearances were larger in hyperthyroid patients?

Gilfrich: Yes.

Kramer, Göttingen: Thank you for the permission to present a unique case history (Fig. 1): This was a 51-year-old patient with an intractable iodine-induced hyperthyroidism. He presented all signs of hyperthyroidism except for diarrhea. Because of his tachycardia, we put him on a daily dose of 0.5, later 0.75, and finally 1.0 mg digoxin/day (Lanicor®). The plasma digoxin level rose at last only as high as 1.5 ng/ml and at that time his heart rate decreased. As shown in the Figure, the T_3 and T_4 values had not changed during this time; thus, he was still in a state of hyperthyroidism. I think this case clearly demonstrates that the increase of digitalis tolerance observed in hyperthyroidism is a matter either of low intestinal absorption or high total excretion resulting in a low plasma concentration.

Schaumann, Mannheim: Dr. Gilfrich, you showed a very high volume of distribution and yet a very short half-life, and that usually does not fit together. My question is: how did you calculate the volume of distribution? Under steady-state conditions?

Gilfrich: I can't follow your assumption that an increase of the volume of distribution and shortening of the half-life does not fit together. We calculated the volume of distribution during a single-dose experiment.

Schaumann: How did you calculate V_D?

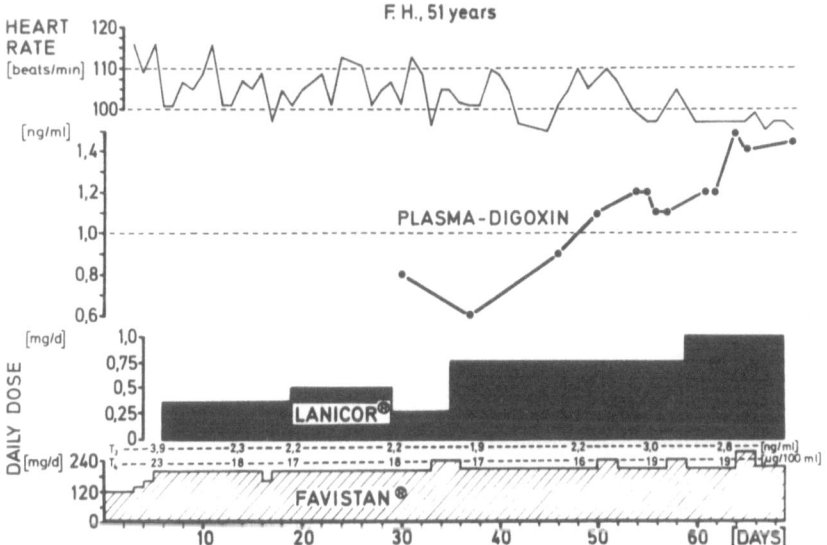

Fig. 1

Gilfrich: We calculated the volume of distribution (V_D) by dividing the dose (D) which was given intravenously by the elimination constant $\beta \times$ the area under the plasma concentration curve from zero to infinity:

$$V_D = \frac{D}{\beta \times \text{area } 0}^{\infty}$$

Klotz: I want to comment on the calculation of the volume of distribution. There are different methods. If you are comparing two different types of patients, you should use the volume of distribution at steady state which is independent from elimination processes. In the study you did, you have two effects. The elimination is changed and by the elimination you alter the volume of distribution. So, for comparing two different patient groups, you should use the volume of distribution at steady state which is defined by the formula:

$$V_1 \frac{(k_{12} + k_{21})}{k_{21}}$$

You have to calculate the rate constants of distribution (k_{12} and k_{21}). Then you can really see if the difference of the volume of distributions is caused by the disease or by some calculation procedure.

Gilfrich: I would like to point out that we studied the same patients during hyperthyroidism and after treatment. That may eliminate your main concern. On the other hand, it is evident that there was not enough time to get the patients in steady state because they suffered from severe hyperthyroidism and they had to be treated.

165

Greenblatt: We should also point out that the steady-state volume of distribution is dependent on the configurations of the compartments, which is ambiguous in a study like this. And secondly, in the vast majority of cases, the difference between $V_{D(ss)}$ and $V_{D(area)}$ is trivial.

Scholz, Hannover: Are you aware of any study on the influence of thyroid hormones on the pharmacodynamic effects of the glycosides?

Gilfrich: In humans, there is the observation of Frye and Braunwald that the administration of triiodothyronine increases the digitalis requirements in patients with chronic atrial fibrillation.

14 Effect of Jejunoileal Bypass on the Bioavailability of Digoxin in Man[1,2]

F. I. MARCUS, D. PERRIER, and M. MAYERSOHN[3]

Seven subjects who underwent jejunoileal bypass surgery for massive obesity participated in a study to examine the relative bioavailability of digoxin before and 1-2 months after surgery. The subjects were given a loading dose of 1 mg digoxin in divided oral doses followed by oral maintenance doses of 0.5 mg daily for 9 days. There were no significant differences in the areas under the digoxin serum concentration time curves, steady-state serum concentrations, or 24 h steady-state urinary excretion of digoxin before and after surgery. We conclude that the bioavailability of digoxin from Lanoxin tablets is not impaired in these patients, although urinary D-xylose and 24-h fecal fat excretion indicated moderate to severe malabsorption after surgery.

Introduction

The effect of various gastrointestinal disease states on the absorption of digoxin continues to be controversial. Heizer and co-workers (Heizer et al., 1971) administered digoxin tablets, 0.25 mg daily, for at least 7 days to 11 patients with different syndromes associated with malabsorption. Four patients had sprue, three had partial resection of the small bowel, two had hypermotility, and two had pancreatic insufficiency. There were ten control subjects who had compensated congestive heart failure but no gastrointestinal disease. A marked decrease in steady-state serum levels was observed in all the patients with malabsorption syndromes except for the two patients with pancreatic insufficiency. It was con-

1 Supported in part by Grant-In-Aid 74-1085 from the American Heart Association, Grants HLI 5265-03 and 1M01RR00714 from the National Heart and Lung Institute and by the Flinn Foundation, Phoenix, Arizona.
2 Results presented in this paper were published previously Marcus, F.I., Quinn, E.J., Horton, H., Jacobs, S., Pippin, S., Stafford, M. and Zukoski, C.: The Effect of Jejunoileal Bypass on Pharmacokinetics of Digoxin in Man. Circulation Vol. 537, March 1977.
3 We gratefully acknowledge the collaboration of Dr. Edward J. Quinn and Dr. Charles Zukowski. We are indebted to the expert assistance of Ms. Herschella Horton, R.N., Ms. Shannon Jacobs, R.N., Susan Pippin, M.S. and Marvin Stafford, M.S.

cluded that digoxin is poorly and erratically absorbed by patients with malabsorption resulting from mucosal defects or hypermotility.

Hall et al. (Hall et al., 1974) studied digoxin absorption in 11 patients with malabsorption due to a variety of causes but none with small bowel resection. The patients and 13 volunteer control subjects were given a single oral dose of ^{3}H-digoxin, either 0.5 or 1.0 mg on a sucrose cube. Radioactivity in serum, urine, and stool was measured for 7 days. They found a decreased serum concentration of ^{3}H-digoxin only during 30-90 min after drug ingestion but not thereafter. There was an increase in stool radioactivity during the 1st day, but the total 7-day fecal excretion of radioactivity was not diminished. It was concluded that digoxin is well absorbed in malabsorption states when soluble forms of digoxin are used. Consistent with the above findings, Beermann et al. (Beermann et al., 1973) observed that partial gastrectomy, vagotomy, and plastic reconstruction of the pylorus and jejunocolostomy had no effect on digoxin absorption when the digoxin was administered as a solution. In another study (Jusko et al., 1974), substitution of digoxin elixir for digoxin tablets in a patient with radiation-induced malabsorption overcame digoxin malabsorption associated with the tablets. Based on the above reports, it would appear that when digoxin is administered in a form from which it is readily available, the various malabsorption syndromes studied do not influence the absorption of digoxin. However, it has not been demonstrated that patients with malabsorption can absorb digoxin well from commercially available tablets which meet the current U.S.P. in vitro requirements.

Very little is known about the influence of jejunoileal bypass surgery on drug absorption kinetics. Removal of large portions of the small intestine will result in substantial reductions of the intestinal surface area available for drug absorption. Similarly, there may be alterations in the structural and functional integrity of the remaining intestinal membrane. Iverson et al. (Iverson et al., 1976) have examined the structural and functional adaptation of the intestine after jejunoileal bypass surgery in man. These investigators have shown increased function per unit length of intestine and increased epithelial surface area 6 months after bypass surgery. The present study was designed to evaluate the effect of jejunoileal bypass, performed for morbid obesity, on the bioavailabilitiy of digoxin in the same patients before and 1-2 months after surgery.

Methods

Subjects and Operative Procedure

Five female and two male patients who were about to have jejunoileal bypass surgery for morbid obesity consented to participate in the study. The patients' ages and weights before surgery, weight loss after surgery, and time from operation to the second study are listed in Table 14.1. Six of the seven patients were restudied within 2½ months after surgery. One patient, C.P., was studied in the reverse sequence. Prior to the operation, he weighed 154 kg. He lost 73 kg after

168

Table 14.1. Patient information

Patient	Age (years)	Weight before (kg)	Weight change (kg)	Time from ileal bypass
K.W.	30	132.3	6.0	Before 1 mo. after
S.R.	37	171.2	12.5	Before 1 mo. after
H.R.	55	127.9	8.5	Before 1 mo. after
B.C.	32	133.7	19.2	Before $2\frac{1}{2}$ mo. after
S.R.	30	173.6	16.9	Before 1 mo. after
G.F.	39	172.5	24.2	Before 6 mo. after
C.P.	50	103.0	22.0	Before $1\frac{1}{2}$ mo. after
Mean values	39	145.0	15.6	

operation, but became weak and had albuminemia, at which time he was first studied. The second investigation was done after reanastamosis when he had gained 22 kg. To avoid confusion, the data relating to this patient are listed in the Tables to conform with the usual sequence of study, i.e., before indicates that his jejunum and ileum have been reanastomosed.

One surgeon performed all the operations which consisted of joining the proximal 12 in. of jejunum, end-to-end, to the ileum 6 in. from the ileocecal valve (Scott et al., 1973). In patient C.P., the jejunum was anastomosed directly to the cecum because the distal stump of the ileum became ischemic after transection. The distal end of the jejunum was closed, and the proximal end of the ileum was anastomosed end-to-side to the ascending colon. The only medications permitted during the studies were sleeping medications (chloral hydrate, flurazepam hydrochloride) and anti-inflammatory drugs (indomethacin, aspirin, acetaminophen). One patient, H.R., took codeine for relief of arthritic pain during her first study.

Protocol

The protocol is outlined in Figure 14.1. The patients received 1.0 mg of digoxin on the 1st day (four tablets of digoxin, 0.25 mg). Thereafter, they took 0.5 mg of digoxin (two tablets in the morning) daily for the next 8 days. Digoxin was given as Burroughs-Wellcome brand Lanoxin tablets (Lot #772B). In vitro tests

Day 1	Digoxin Tablets 0.25 mgm X4
Day 2 - 9	Digoxin Tablets 0.5 mgm once daily
Day 7	Admit to Clinical Study Unit
Day 8	Steady State Digoxin Serum Concentration
	24 - hour urine collection
	24 - hour stool collection
Day 9	Steady State Digoxin Serum Concentration
	Blood Samples for Digoxin ½, 1, 1½, 2, 3,
	6, 8, 12 & 24 hours
	After usual daily dose of 0.5 mgm of Digoxin
	24 - hour urine collection
	24 - hour stool collection
Day 10	D - Xylose Excretion Test
Day 10 - 14	Daily blood samples for determination of Digoxin
	Serum half life

Fig. 14.1. Experimental design of the study. Digoxin given on days 2-9 consisted of two 0.25-mg tablets administered once daily each morning

performed by the Burroughs-Wellcome Company (Research Triangle Park, N.C., United States) demonstrated that 69% of digoxin was in solution within 1 h. The patients were admitted to the hospital the evening of the 7th day of each study. On days 8 and 9, 24-h urine collections were obtained in order to determine total urinary creatinine and digoxin excretion as well as creatinine and digoxin clearance. Blood samples for serum creatinine used in the calculation of creatinine clearance were drawn 8 h after digoxin was given. Blood samples for steady-state serum digoxin levels were drawn 24 h after the previously administered dose on days 7, 8, and 9. On day 9, blood was also drawn at the following times: ½, 1, 1½, 2, 3, 6, 8, 12, and 24 h following administration of the 0.5 mg oral dose. The 24-h area under the serum concentration time curve (AUC) was measured by the trapezoidal rule, and the renal clearance determined by dividing the total amount of digoxin eliminated in the urine during the 24 h by the AUC for the same time interval. The patients were discharged from the hospital on the 10th day. Blood was drawn each morning for 5 consecutive days after the last dose of digoxin was administered in order to calculate the biologic half-life of digoxin.

Tests of malabsorption included serum carotene, total protein, and serum albumin. Two consecutive 24-h collections of stool were analyzed for fecal fat. The dietary intake of fat was not controlled. A D-xylose tolerance test was performed on day 10. Urine was collected and analyzed for D-xylose after administration of 5 g of D-xylose dissolved in 250 ml of water. Serum drawn on day 8 was analyzed for blood urea nitrogen, creatinine, glucose, sodium, potassium, CO_2, chloride, SGOT, thyroxine, and prothrombin time. A complete blood count and urinalysis were also obtained. The same protocol was repeated after surgery.

Analytic Methods

Details of the tritium radioimmunoassay for digoxin in plasma have been described previously (Marcus et al., 1975). The standard solutions were prepared in human pooled plasma in a concentration of 0-4 ng/ml. Digoxin concentration in urine was assayed as follows: 1 ml of urine was diluted with 19 ml of plasma. This solution was assayed in triplicate using 0.5 ml aliquots. An equal amount of blank urine was added to each plasma standard. The digoxin radioimmunoassay involved incubation of the sample with digoxin-specific antiserum and ^{3}H-digoxin. Dextran-coated charcoal was used to separate unbound isotope from that bound to antiserum. The supernatant containing the antibody ^{3}H-digoxin complex was counted in a liquid scintillation spectrometer. The standard curve for each assay was a straight line obtained by plotting the reciprocal of the disintegrations per minute versus digoxin concentration at each standard point. The digoxin concentrations for the patient serum or urine samples were calculated after the slope and the intercept of the standard curve were obtained.

Total serum protein was determined by the biuret method, serum albumin by electrophoresis, serum carotene and urine D-xylose by spectrophotometric analysis. Normal values for serum carotene are 60-200 μg/dl. Normal subjects excrete 1 or more g of D-xylose in urine within 5 h of the oral dose. The normal values for fecal fat are between 5-10 g.

The data were statistically analyzed using the student's paired t-test.

Results

Jejunoileal bypass in our patients caused definite malabsorption as evidenced by a significant decrease in urine D-xylose excretion and by a significant increase in fecal fat (Table 14.2). There was a trend toward a decrease in serum carotene concentration after surgery, but no apparent decrease in the mean concentrations of total serum protein or serum albumin after the jejunal bypass. The digoxin data are summarized in Tables 14.3 to 14.5. Steady-state digoxin serum concentrations are not significantly different before and after surgery (Figure 14.2, Table 14.3). The ratio of these values indicates that the average digoxin bioavailability in these patients after surgery is 87% of that prior to surgery. Another index that may be used to evaluate bioavailability is to compare the AUCs during a dosing interval at steady state. As seen in Table 14.4, the average ratio of the AUCs indicates a 9% decrease in bioavailability after surgery which is similar to the decrease observed in the steady-state digoxin serum concentrations.

The steady-state serum digoxin concentrations and AUCs were adjusted for differences in body weight before and after surgery since there is generally a loss

Table 14.2. Absorption studies

Patient	Time from ileal bypass	Fecal fat (g/24hr)	Serum carotene (μg/100ml)	Urine D-xylose excretion (g/5hr)
K.W.	Before	6.2	168	2.0
	1 mo. after	23.0	35	0.6
S.R.	Before	7.0	62	2.2
	1 mo. after	9.9	96	1.0
H.R.	Before	4.9	93	2.3
	1 mo. after	52.0	20	0.6
B.C.	Before	2.2	110	2.2
	2½ mo. after	8.0	16	0.5
S.R.	Before	22.0	25	1.8
	1 mo. after	33.0	14	0.8
G.F.	Before	12.0	64	2.2
	6 mo. after	56.0	68	0.9
C.P.	Before	19.0	122	1.6
	1½ mo. after	110.0	12	0.4
Mean values				
Before		10.5	92.0	2.0
After		41.7	37.3	0.7
Statistical significance	p	<0.05	<0.1	<0.001

in both muscle and adipose tissue after this operation (Spanier et al., 1976; Brill et al., 1972). If only adipose tissue were lost, this correction may not be warranted since distribution of digoxin into this tissue is negligible (Ewy et al., 1971). When steady-state digoxin serum concentrations and AUCs are adjusted for differences in body weight before and after surgery, the apparent differences in bioavailability are reduced and the average ratio of these respective parameters approaches 1.0. In addition, these adjusted ratios agree closely with the ratios of urinary digoxin recovery before and after surgery (Table 14.5). The urine data is based upon the results in four subjects since there was incomplete urine collection in three patients.

No significant differences were found in the biologic half-lives of digoxin in these patients before and after surgery.

Table 14.3. Digoxin relative bioavailability data

Patient	Time from ileal bypass	Digoxin steady-state concentration			
		ng/ml Mean ± SD		Ratio (after/before) unadjusted[a] adjusted[b]	
K.W.	Before	0.96	0.09		
	1 mo. after	1.04	0.03	1.08	1.14
S.R.	Before	1.13	0.10		
	1 mo. after	0.96	0.08	0.85	0.92
H.R.	Before	1.41	0.05		
	1 mo. after	0.88	0.12	0.62	0.67
B.C.	Before	1.18	0.09		
	$2\frac{1}{2}$ mo. after	1.03	0.12	0.87	1.02
S.R.	Before	0.73	--		
	1 mo. after	0.74	--	1.01	1.12
G.F.	Before	0.84	0.15		
	6 mo. after	0.78	0.11	0.93	1.08
C.P.	Before	0.67	0,65		
	$1\frac{1}{2}$ mo. after	0.48	0.04	0.72	0.91
Mean values ± SD					
Before		0.99	0.27		
After		0.84	0.20		
Ratio after/before				0.87 ± 0.16	0.98 ± 0.16
Statistical significance p		<0.1			

[a] Not corrected for differences in body weight before and after surgery.
[b] Corrected for differences in body weight before and after surgery.

Discussion

These results indicate that there is no apparent impairment of absorption of digoxin from the tablets employed in this study after removal of the distal jejunum
and proximal ileum even though definite evidence of malabsorption was documented in all our patients. When assessing bioavailability from serum concentration data, one usually assumes drug clearance from the body in a given patient
to be constant. However, the influence of jejunoileal bypass surgery on the disposition kinetics of digoxin or drugs in general is not known. As a result, any
changes which surgery of this type may produce in digoxin clearance could influence the interpretation of these data. No apparent change was observed in the
biologic half-life of digoxin in patients after surgery. It is difficult from the data
obtained to determine whether or not there were any changes in the apparent
volume of distribution and hence, any changes in digoxin clearance. Since digoxin is cleared primarily by the kidney, and since no apparent changes in the

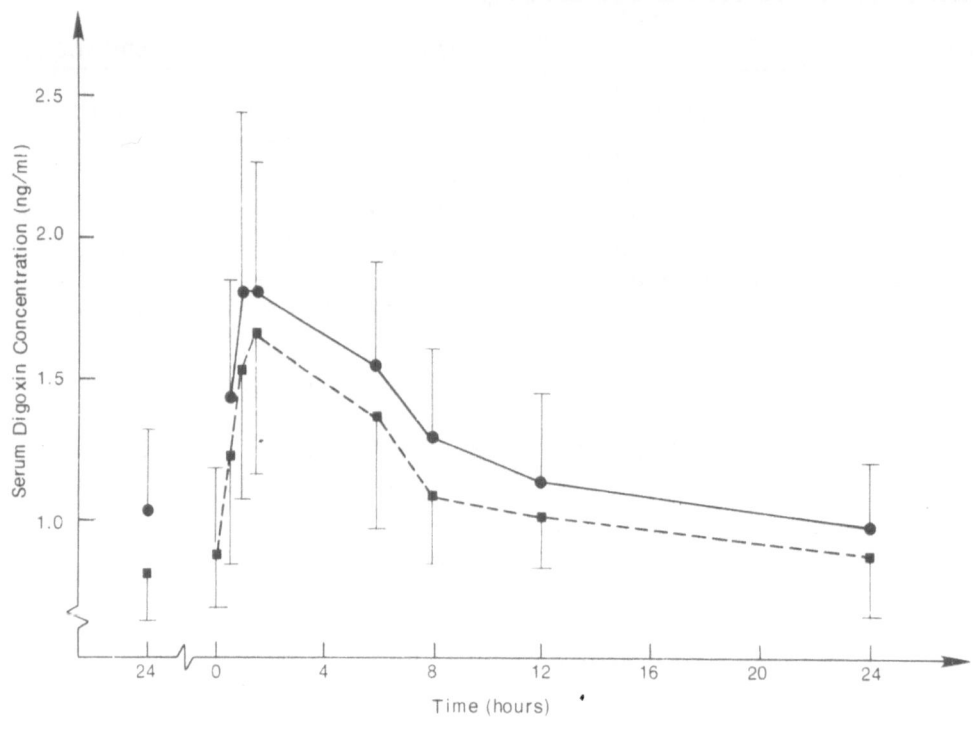

Fig. 14.2. Serum digoxin concentrations during one dosing interval at steady state and after administration of 0.5 mg digoxin in subjects before (solid line) and after (hatched line) the bypass operation. The bars represent mean values ± 1 SD

half-life and renal clearance of digoxin were observed, it would appear that the apparent volume of distribution of digoxin was unchanged. If the loss in weight postsurgery was due to a loss in adipose tissue only, no adjustments in plasma levels and AUCs would be required, since there is no significant distribution of digoxin into adipose tissue (Ewy et al., 1971) and the same dose per kilogram "lean" body weight would have been administered. However, it is possible that the loss in weight after jejunoileal bypass surgery may be a consequence of a loss in both adipose and muscle tissue (Spanier et al., 1976; Brill et al., 1972), and steady-state serum concentrations and AUCs should be normalized for changes in body weight. This has been done (Tables 14.3 and 14.4) and results in a slight but insignificant increase in the ratios of steady-state plasma concentrations and AUCs.

It has been suggested that measurement of urinary excretion of digoxin is less variable and perhaps a more valid measure of digoxin bioavailability than serum concentrations or AUCs (Huffman et al., 1975, 1974). In the present study, urine and serum data agree very well. However, the urine data only represents

174

Table 14.4. Digoxin relative bioavailability data

Patient	Time from ileal bypass	ng/ml x hours	Ratio (after/before) unadjusted[a]	adjusted[b]
		Digoxin steady-state AUC (0-24 h)		
K.W.	Before	24.19		
	1 mo. after	29.04	1.20	1.26
S.R.	Before	29.62		
	1 mo. after	33.31	1.12	1.21
H.R.	Before	37.70		
	1 mo. after	23.93	0.63	0.68
B.C.	Before	36.60		
	2½ mo. after	31.30	0.86	1.00
S.R..	Before	24.67		
	1 mo. after	21.48	0.87	0.97
G.F.	Before	28.42		
	6 mo. after	25.51	0.90	1.04
C.P.	Before	20.04		
	1½ mo. after	15.17	0.76	0.96
Mean values ± SD				
Before		28.75 ± 6.53		
After		25.68 ± 6.22		
Ratio after/before			0.91 ± .10	1.02 ± 0.19
Statistical significance p		< 0.3		

[a] Not corrected for differences in body weight before and after surgery.
[b] Corrected for differences in body weight before and after surgery.

the results of four subjects and hence, this comparison is incomplete. In those subjects where digoxin excretion was determined, approximately 50% of the oral dose was recovered in the urine prior to surgery (range 36%-61%) and 44% after surgery (range 33%-59%). These mean urinary recoveries of digoxin are consistent with the reports of other investigators using digoxin elixir or tablet formulations that had rapid dissolution (Greenblatt et al., 1974a, b,; 1973).

The data in the present study are consistent with the findings of Hall et al. (Hall et al., 1974) and those of Beermann et al. (Beermann et al., 1973) that various malabsorption states do not readily interfere with the absorption of digoxin. Beermann et al. Beermann et al., 1972) found that 40%-60% of the tritiated dig-oxin was absorbed in normal subjects by the time the test solution reached the proximal part of the small intestine (110-200 cm from the nose). Most of the absorption occurred in the duodenum and upper jejunum and only 10% of the

Table 14.5. Digoxin relative bioavailability data

steady-state urinary digoxin excretion (0-24 h)

Patient	Time from ileal bypass	µg	Ratio (after/before)
K.W.	Before	254	
	1 mo. after	294	1.16
S.R.	Before	181	
	1 mo. after	165	0.91
G.F.	Before	259	
	6 mo. after	215	0.83
C.P.	Before	213	
	1½ mo. after	196	0.92
Mean values ± SD			
Before		227 ± 37	
After		218 ± 55	
Ratio after/before			0.96 ± 0.14
Statistical significance p		< 0.7	

tritium label was absorbed in the stomach. These investigators documented that digoxin could also be absorbed in the jejunum since intrajejunal administration resulted in the same 14-day urinary excretion as intragastric drug administration. Absorption of digoxin from the colon has recently been found (Ochs et al., 1975). Anderson et al. (Anderson et al., 1975) also showed digoxin absorption after intrasigmoid administration. It appears, therefore, that the diminished absorption of digoxin in various states of malabsorption reported by Heizer et al. (Heizer et al., 1971) may, in part, reflect the release characteristics of the dosage form used. Evidence to support this hypothesis is provided by Jusko et al. (Jusko et al., 1974) who found that patients with radiation-induced malabsorption had no measurable amounts of digoxin in their serum after being given Lanoxin tablets, but had measurable levels after being given the elixir. Data regarding the dissolution rate of the digoxin tablets used by Jusko et al. (Jusko et al., 1974) were not given. Greenblatt and co-workers (Greenblatt et al., 1973) found that there was a diminished bioavailability of digoxin tablets that have less than 65% dissolution in 1 h compared with the bioavailability of the elixir when given to normal subjects. However, when greater than 65% of the digoxin content of these tablets went into solution within 1 h, they could find no difference in bioavailability between the tablets and the elixir (Greenblatt et al., 1974b). The requirements of the United States Food and Drug Administration promulgated in 1974 specify the dissolution rate requirements for digoxin tablets. Specifically, under standard in vitro conditions specified by the United States Pharmacopeia in 1973, 65% of the digoxin must be a solution within 1 h. If the hypothesis is correct that dimin-

176

ished bioavailability of digoxin was responsible for the malabsorption of digoxin reported by Heizer et al. (Heizer et al., 1971), then malabsorption should no longer be considered a clinical problem with respect to digoxin usage. This does not negate the possibility that isolated cases of decreased absorption of digoxin may occur in patients with malabsorption or if patients receive a digoxin preparation that has a slower rate of dissolution. It should be reemphasized that the digoxin was given in a tablet form from which digoxin appears to be readily released. Serum levels of digoxin will verify diminished absorption of digoxin when this problem is suspected.

References

Andersson, K.E., Nyberg, L., Dencker, H., Gothlin, J.: Absorption of digoxin in man after oral and intrasigmoid administration studied by portal vein catheterization. Eur. J. Clin. Pharmacol. 9, 39 (1975)

Beermann, B., Hellstrom, K., Rosen, A.: The absorption of orally administered (12α-^{3}H) digoxin in man. Clin. Sci. 43, 507 (1972)

Beermann, B., Hellstrom, K., Rosen, A.: The gastrointestinal absorption of digoxin in seven patients with gastric or small intestinal reconstructions. Acta Med. Scand. 193, 293 (1973)

Brill, A.B., Sandstead, H.H., Prive, R., Johnston, R.E., Law, D.H., Scott, H.W.: Changes in body composition after jejunoileal bypass in morbidly obese patients. Am. J. Surg. 123, 49 (1972)

Ewy, G.A., Groves, B.M., Ball, M.F., Nimmo, L., Jackson, B., Marcus, F.I.: Digoxin metabolism in obesity. Circulation 44, 810 (1971)

Greenblatt, D.J., Duhme, D.W., Koch-Weser, J., Smith, T.W.: Evaluation of digoxin bioavailability in single dose studies. N. Engl. J. Med. 289, 651 (1973)

Greenblatt, D.J., Duhme, D.W., Koch-Weser, J., Smith, T.W.: Comparison of one and six day urinary excretion in single dose bioavailability studies. Clin. Pharmacol. Ther. 16, 813 (1974 a)

Greenblatt, D.J., Duhme, D.W., Koch-Weser, J., Smith, T.W.: Equivalent bioavailability from digoxin elixir and rapid-solution tablets. JAMA 229, 1774 (1974 b)

Hall, W.H., Doherty, J.E., Gammill, J., Sherwood, J.: Tritiated digoxin XXII: Absorption and excretion in malabsorption syndromes. Am. J. Med. 56, 437 (1974)

Heizer, W.D., Smith, T.W., Goldfinger, S.E.: Absorption of digoxin in patients with malabsorption syndromes. N. Engl. J. Med. 285, 257 (1971)

Huffman, D.H., Manion, C.V., Azarnoff, D.L.: Absorption of digoxin from different oral preparations in normal subjects during steady-state. Clin. Pharmacol. Ther. 16, 310 (1974)

Huffman, D.H., Manion, C.V., Azarnoff, D.L.: Intrasubject variation in absorption of digoxin in normal volunteers. J. Pharm. Sci. 64, 433 (1975)

Iversen, B.M., Schjonsby, H., Skagen, D.W., Solhaug, J.H.: Intestinal adaptation after jejunoileal bypass operation for massive obesity. Eur. J. Clin. Invest. 6, 355 (1976)

Jusko, W.J., Conti, D.R., Molson, A., Kuritzky, P., Giller, J., Schultz, R.: Digoxin absorption from tablets and elixir: The effect of radiation induced malabsorption. JAMA 230, 1554 (1974)

Marcus, F.I., Ryan, J.N., Stafford, M.G.: The reactivity of derivatives of digoxin and digitoxin as measured by the Na-K-ATPase displacement assay and by radioimmunoassay. J. Lab. Clin. Med. 85, 610 (1975)

Ochs, H., Bodem, G., Schäfer, P.K., Kodrat, G., Dengler, H.J.: Absorption of digoxin from the distal parts of the intestine in man. Eur. J. Clin. Pharmacol. 9, 95 (1975)

Scott, H.W., Jr., Dean, R., Shull, H.J., Abram, H.S., Webb, W., Younger, R.K., Brill, A.B.: New considerations in use of jejunoileal bypass in patients with morbid obesity. Ann. Surg. 177, 723 (1973)

Spanier, A.H., Kurtz, R.S., Shibata, H.R., MacLean, L.D., Shizgal, H.M.: Alterations and body composition following intestinal bypass for morbid obesity. Surgery 80, 170 (1976)

Discussion

Butler, New York: Some years ago, Dr. John Lindenbaum, my colleague at Columbia University, studied about 30 patients with a variety of malabsorptive states giving them two 0.25 mg tablets of good bioavailability and, as you have shown in these single-dose studies, he observed normal areas under serum concentration time curves in 37 of 40 patients. He concluded as you did that, in most of these patients, the absorption seemed to be good but that in an occasional patient with very extensive intestinal resection or bypass it did seem to be significantly impaired.

Lukas, New York: An important issue in the digitoxin study is what happened to the plasma albumin in these patients. If it decreased, I'm sure that would explain the fall in plasma digitoxin concentration.

Marcus: The plasma albumin did not change in this group of patients.

Smith, Boston: I don't remember exactly what the numbers were in all of those patients, but my recollection is that their malabsorption syndromes tended to be worse. Was there any correlation between the severity of the malabsorption by conventional criteria and the change in digoxin excretion?

Marcus: No. We looked at that rather extensively and did not find any correlation between fecal fat excretion, serum D-xylose levels, urinary excretion of D-xylose, and digoxin absorption. The fat intake of these patients was not controlled. Before operation, these patients would eat tremendous amounts of food. We calculated that one patient ate 8000-9000 calories before the operation. Afterward, they had an aversion toward food and especially toward fatty food. Consequently, their intake of fat also decreased. This would affect the fecal fat excretion. Therefore, I think that these patients had rather severe malabsorption that was not reflected by the fecal excretion of fat after, as compared with before operation.

Lukas: I have another question: what happened to the half-life of digoxin in the patients on that drug? Did it change? Steady-state levels of digoxin would very definitely have been affected by such a change.

Marcus: The half-life did not change; it was 1.17 days before operation and 1.36 days after surgery. It was unchanged in the five patients in whom we had adequate data. There was also no change in the renal clearance of digoxin.

Kuhlmann, Berlin: Is there an influence of a severe right heart failure on the absorption of digoxin?

Marcus: I am sorry, but I have no data on which to base an answer to that question.

Dengler, Bonn: I have a short remark on another situation. You investigated the absorption of digoxin after removal of the lower part of the intestine. In our hospital, we have studied digoxin absorption after gastric resection. Here, too, there is no difference between normals and patients with gastric resection.

Marcus: I think one can speculate as to how these patients really absorb digoxin so well. Beermann et al. has shown that digoxin or digitoxin is absorbed well from the duodenum and the proximal portion of the ileum, and this portion of the intestine was intact in our patients. In addition, there have been some recent studies from Dr. Ochs and also by Dr. Andersson in which digoxin was instilled into the colon and there was good absorption of digoxin from this site. So I suspect that the adequate absorption of digoxin in patients with jejunoileal bypass was due to a combination of absorption of this drug from the duodenum, proximal jejunum, and colon.

Greenblatt: What drugs do these people malabsorb, if any?

Marcus: To my knowledge, there has been no other study of other drug malabsorption or absorption in these patients.

Greeff, Düsseldorf: What is your experience with the D-xylose test? Was there a relation between the absorption of D-xylose and digoxin in the individual patient?

Marcus: No, we could not find any such correlation. I think one would have to study much larger numbers to be certain of group correlations.

Hausamen, Dortmund: Patients with jejunoileal bypass have not only malabsorption but also maldigestion. So, perhaps the decreased absorption is mainly due to the increased rapidity of passage of food through the intestine.

Marcus: Before we started this study, we anticipated that there would be a marked decrease in the absorption of digoxin for the reasons that you mentioned, and we were surprised that we did not find it.

Hausamen: You did not give the digoxin as a liquid?

Marcus: No, this was given as tablets.

Bonelli, Wien: Your slide showed that your patients lost weight between the first and second pharmacokinetic studies — is that correct?

Marcus: Yes. The mean weight loss was 15.6 kg.

Bonelli: You must take this weight loss into consideration in your calculations. I think that if you had done so, you would have concluded that there was a significant decrease of absorption.

Marcus: We did correct for the weight loss. The corrected data indicated that the digoxin absorption approximated that obtained before surgery, even to a greater degree than the data uncorrected for loss of weight. We did not study the volume of distribution in these patients, but we think that the volume of distribution was relatively unaltered because the half-life was unchanged and the renal clearance was unchanged , but we did not directly measure the volume of distribution before and after surgery.

15 Bioavailability of Digoxin in Renal Insufficiency and Heart Failure

E. E. OHNHAUS

The absorption of digoxin shows a wide variation in healthy volunteers depending on the different commercial brands and individual conditions (Lindenbaum et. al., 1971). On the other hand, only few studies are available about the absorption of digoxin under pathological conditions. Therefore, in the present study, three different studies were performed. In the first study, different pharmacokinetic parameters after oral administration of digoxin were compared in the same patients in severe right cardiac failure and after clinical remission. In a second study, digoxin was administered intravenously to another group of patients in the same decompensated clinical conditions. From these two studies then an absolute biovailability was calculated. In a third study, the absolute bioavailability was studied in patients with severe renal failure.

Pharmacokinetics of Digoxin in Severe Right Cardiac Failure

Material and Method

Patients

Patients with severe right cardiac failure were included in the study judged by the following clinical criteria: bad clinical condition, cyanosis, jugular venous distension, positive hepatojugular reflux, enlarged liver, extensive edema of the legs, and radiologic signs of right cardiac failure. These signs had to be present in each patient who was included into the study.

First Study

Seven patients in severe right cardiac failure already treated by digoxin before admission were given orally 0.1 mg ^{3}H-digoxin (specific activity 120 μCi) as alcoholic solution after an overnight fasting period. The digoxin was specifically labeled at the 12 α-position. In addition, 0.25 mg digoxin were given as a tablet (Digoxin-Sandoz$^®$) at the same time. Blood samples for the measurement of digoxin in the plasma were taken at the following time intervals: 0, 15, 30, 45, 60, 90, 120, 150, and 180 min. 4, 6, 8, 12, 24, 36, 48, 72, 96, and 120 h. Urine was collected over the following periods: 0-4, 4-8, 8-12, 12-24, 24-48, 48-72, 72-96, 96-120 h. The concentrations in the plasma and urine of the ^{3}H-digoxin was measured in a liquid scintillation counter and the total digoxin concentration by radioimmunoassay ("Digok" Kit from C.I.S./CEA-IRESORIN). The same study was repeated after clinical remission of cardiac failure.

Second Study

Of an additional 12 patients being in severe right cardiac failure, six were given 0.1 mg ^{3}H-digoxin intravenously and the remaining six patients received 0.25 mg unlabeled digoxin as an intravenous injection. Blood samples, urine collections, and measurements were done in the same manner as in the first study.

Pharmacokinetic Calculations

The pharmacokinetic parameters of ^{3}H-digoxin were calculated from the concentrations measured in plasma and urine according to a two-compartment open model assuming first order absorption using a SAAM 25 computer program (Berman and Weiss, 1970). For the radioimmunologic measurements, the "T-interrupt" feature of the SAAM 25 program (Beerman and Weiss, 1970) was used assuming steady-state conditions with a maintenance dose of 0.25 mg/day. An absolute bioavailability was calculated from the ratios of the areas under the plasma curve after oral and intravenous administration and also of the total cumulative urinary excretion after both routes of administration using the values from study 1 and 2.

Statistics

All parameters which are shown in the tables were compared by either the t-test for differences between pairs or the Wilcoxon matched-pairs signed-rank test, in the case of nonhomogeneous variances.

Results

First Study

The ^{3}H-digoxin concentrations measured in the plasma were practically identical under both clinical conditions. The maximal concentration of about 1.1 ng/ml was reached 1 h after administation. In addition, measuring the concentrations of digoxin by the radioimmunassay a similar appearance of the plasma concentration curve was found on the two occasions measured. The baseline values measured were found between 1.5-2.1 ng/ml and the maximal digoxin concentration of 3.2 ng/ml was reached 1.6 h following digoxin administration.

The pharmacokinetic parameters calculated from the concentrations in plasma and urine are seen in Table 15.1. Comparing the pharmacokinetic parameters calculated after oral administration of ^{3}H-digoxin and the digoxin tablet in the same patient in the decompensated and recompensated clinical condition, no significant differences were found. The only significant difference was the invasion rate constant of 3.1 ± 1.5 h^{-1} for the ^{3}H-digoxin solution and 1.1 ± 0.3 h^{-1} for the digoxin tablet representing an absorption half life of 0.3 ± 0.1 or 0.6 ± 0.2 h, respectively (p< 0.05).

Table 15.1. Pharmacokinetic parameters calculated from the measured concentrations in plasma and urine in patients in severe right cardiac failure and after clinical remission of the disease following oral administration of 0.1 mg ^{3}H-digoxin and 0.25 mg digoxin as tablet

	MEAN ±SD	
Plasma values	Before treatment	After treatment
^{3}H-digoxin:		
C_{max} (ng/ml)	1.1 ± 0.3	1.1 ± 0.3
t_{max} (h)	1.0 ± 0.7	0.8 ± 0.3
Invasion rate		
constant (h^{-1})	3.1 ± 1.5	2.8 ± 1.2
α (h^{-1})	0.62 ± 0.25	0.66 ± 0.25
β (h^{-1})	0.017 ± 0.007	0.019 ± 0.004
T α (h)	1.1 ± 0.5	1.1 ± 0.4
T β (h)	46.0 ± 12.7	37.4 ⊥ 8.2
RIA:		
C_{max} (ng/ml)	3.2 ± 1.7	3.2 ± 1.5
t_{max} (h)	1.6 ± 0.7	1.7 ± 1.2
Invasion rate		
constant (h^{-1})	1.1 ± 0.3	1.2 ± 0.5
α (h^{-1})	0.86 ± 0.26	1.19 ± 0.67
β (h^{-1})	0.012 ± 0.02	0.015 ± 0.007
T a (h)	0.8 ± 0.2	0.6 ± 0.3
T β (h)	57 ± 11	47 ± 11
Urine values		
^{3}H-digoxin:		
A_u (120 h) (%)	47 ± 13	46 ± 15
A_u (∞) (%)	62 ± 19	58 ± 15
RIA:		
$A_{u\ ss}$ (%)	44 ± 14	41 ± 19

Second Study

Calculating the pharmacokinetic parameters from plasma and urine concentrations following ^{3}H- and unlabeled digoxin intravenously, nearly the same results were obtained as in healthy volunteers or patients not suffering from severe right cardiac failure (Beveridgy et al., in press; Dengler et al., 1973; Ohnhaus et al.,

1974). Even the volume of distribution for digoxin of 357 ± 141 liters was comparable to other authors.

Calculation of the Absolute Bioavailability

An absolute bioavailability was calculated between the different groups of patients investigated in study 1 and 2 using the urinary excretion of digoxin and the area under the plasma concentration curve for the calculation. These results using the different measurements are presented in Table 15.2. The calculated absolute bioavailability ranged from 75%-99% from the concentrations measured by ^{3}H-digoxin and from 54%-87% for the radioimmunoassay measurement depending on the different calculations used for the estimation of absolute bioavailaibility.

Pharmacokinetics of Digoxin in Renal Impairment

Material and Method

Two groups of patients in chronic renal failure having a mean endogenous creatinine clearance of about 6.9 ml/min were investigated under steady-state clinical conditions. The patients were randomly allocated in a cross over design to an intravenous and oral digoxin administration. ^{3}H-Digoxin was administered in a dose of 0.125 mg to six patients as an intravenous injection and oral solution with an interval of 30 days. In a second group of six patients, 0.5 mg unlabeled digoxin was given intravenously and orally as a tablet (Digoxin-Sandoz[®]). The time interval in this groups was at least 10 days. Blood samples, urine collections, methods for measuring plasma concentrations, and calculating pharmacokinetic parameters were done in the same manner as in the studies of patients in severe right cardiac failure.

Table 15.2. Absolute bioavailability calculated from the area under the plasma concentration curve and the urinary excretion in different groups of patients in severe right cardiac failure after oral or intravenous administration of ^{3}H-digoxin or unlabeled digoxin

	Mean ± SD			
	A_u (120 h)	A_u (∞)	AUC_{TR}	AUC (∞)
[3]H-digoxin	0.99 ± 0.31	0.91 ± 0.33	0.75 ± 0.43	0.80 ± 0.46
RIA	0.55 ± 0.21	0.54 ± 0.26	0.87 ± 0.65	0.86 ± 0.61

Results

The pharmacokinetic parameters of digoxin elimination calculated for both groups were similar to those found by other authors (Doherty et al, 1964; Ohnhaus et al., 1974). In contrast, different results were seen in the parameters concerning digoxin absorption. Comparing the parameters calculated from a study in healthy volunteers given 0.5 mg digoxin (Beveridge et al., in press), significant differences were found in the maximal plasma concentration, the time, in which this maximal plasma concentration was reached, and the invasion rate constant. The maximal plasma concentration in volunteers showed a mean of 2.3 ng/ml reached already after 0.99 h and having an invasion rate constant of 2.8 h^{-1}. The patients in renal impairment reached a maximal plasma concentration of 4.1 ng/ml in about 2 h with a lower invasion rate constant of 0.76 h^{-1}. In contrast, no differences were found in mean absolute bioavailability between volunteers and patients in renal failure, having values of 76% or 71%, respectively. Calculating absolute bioavailability following ^{3}H-digoxin values between 85%-100% were found according to the different methods used for calculation. For the digoxin tablet, an absolute bioavailability was found between 65%-77%.

In conclusion, in all three studies presented, no changes in absolute bioavailability in comparison to normal healthy volunteers were seen after the administration of ^{3}H-digoxin and digoxin as a tablet. However, in patients having renal insufficiency, higher peak plasma levels and a prolonged absorption was observed without influencing absolute bioavailability.

References

Berman, M., Weiss, M.F.: Mathematical Research Branch, Nat. Inst. of Arthritis and Metab. Diseases N.I.H. Bethesda, Maryland 1970

Beveridge, T., Nüesch, E., Ohnhaus, E.E.: Absolute bioavailability of digoxin (Sandoz) tablets. Drug Res. (in Press)

Dengler, H.J., Bodem, G., Wirth, K.: Pharmacokinetic and metabolic studies with lanatoside C, α- and β-acetyldigoxin and digoxin in man. Proc. 5th Int. Congr. Pharmacol. San Francisco 3, 112-126 (1973)

Doherty, J.E., Perkins, W.H., Wilson, M.C.: Studies with tritiated digoxin in renal failure. Am. J. Med. 37, 536-544 (1964)

Lindenbaum, J., Mellow, M.H., Blackstone, M.O., Butler, V.P.: Variation in biologic availability of digoxin from four preparations. N. Engl. J. Med. 285, 1344-1347 (1971)

Ohnhaus, E.E., Spring, P., Dettli, L.: Eliminationskinetik und Dosierung von Digoxin bei Patienten mit Niereninsuffizienz. Dtsch. Med. Wochenschr. 99, 1797-1803 (1974)

Discussion

Greenblatt, Boston: In one of your figures, one can see that in one group of patients the absorption rate constant was almost identical to the a. If those two parameters are close or identical, that causes tremendous problems in getting a reliable and unique fit. Did you consider that?

Ohnhaus: No, we did not consider that, but using our model this problem does not arise.

Vöhringer, Berlin: How can you explain the different values for your absolute bioavailability using different methods? There might be remarkable differences.

Ohnhaus: As you noticed in the first and second study, we had two groups of patients. One got digoxin orally and the second group got it intravenously, and we used these two groups to calculate an absolute bioavailability. There is a different bioavailability of the digoxin solution and the tablet. The only thing that you might criticize is the fact that we did an interindividual comparison. But as you know, it is impossible to do an intraindividual comparison because you cannot use patients with severe cardiac failure as their own controls because they are treated and then are relieved from decompensation. On the other hand, in these two different groups of patients the creatinine clearance was nearly the same. So I think the groups are really comparable mainly judged by the clinical conditions.

Nyberg, Sweden: I want to refer to the remarks of Dr. Greenblatt. We did studies about the absorption rate of digoxin by calculating the absolute absorption rate at different times. We have found that the assumption of a constant absorption rate is a large oversimplification. About 1/2 h after administration, we find a very high absorption rate. About 2 h after administration, this rate has fallen to about 1/10th or 1/20th of the peak rate. Therefore, the absorption rate is not constant but is better discribed by an absorption rate profile. We have confirmed this by means of studies with portal blood and simultaneously sampled peripheral blood and we find virtually the same profile.

May I ask you how you explain the difference in bioavailability found between ^{3}H measurements and radioimmunoassay measurements?

Ohnhaus: The RIA measurements were done properly for the tablets, and there has to be a lower bioavailaibility than for the solution.

Nyberg: Yes, but according to my experience, the digoxin tablets from Sandoz are rapidly dissolved and they should be equal to a solution.

Ohnhaus: According to most of the results of the literature, the solution was found to be nearly totally absorbed in an range of about 80% or 85%. The digoxin Sandoz is the same as the digoxin of Burroughs Wellcome and has a mean of about 68%.

Nyberg: It depends on which studies you refer to. Doherty, for instance, found a bioavailability of about 80%. However, later studies, e.g., by our group, Greenblatt et al., and by Burroughs Wellcome (Johnson et al.) have shown a bioavailability from aqueous solutions, which is slightly less than 70%.

16 Bioavailability Studies: Their Influence on the Clinical Use of Digitalis

T. R. D. SHAW

Introduction

Studies of "bioavailability" inform us about the characteristics of a drug's absorption. They can illustrate not only the typical pattern but also the variations which occur in different circumstances and between different individuals. There has been a recent flood of such studies on digitalis, stimulated by the introduction of assays for the cardiac glycosides. I shall try to outline how this new information has affected the clinical use of the digitalis drugs and will take as a theme the suggestion that we should be working toward greater precision with digitalis therapy since it remains the commonest cause of adverse drug effects. Precision could be increased by several means:
1. By standardizing as many as possible of the factors which influence response
2. By predicting the effect of variations which do occur
3. By measuring events during treatment and using these as feedback to alter the drug regime

Accuracy of Dosage Content

A prime factor for precision is the use of accurate measures of the drug. There have been problems with this aspect. Withering himself (1785) sought to have a standard product by selecting his foxgloves at a particular stage of their growth and by using only the leaves of the plant. Much later, digitalis leaf was assessed by biologic assays. Isolation of the pure cardiac glycosides digitoxin and digoxin allowed standardization by weight alone. However, there have been failures to provide accurate and consistent amounts of digoxin in single tablets. A few years ago, 33 out of 36 digoxin brands in the United States failed to meet the U.S.P. content requirements (F.D.A. Case Studies, 1971). Manninen and Korhonen (1973) found an alarmingly wide range of individual tablet content in European brands of digoxin with some tablets containing nearly twice the stated dose. Only 1/400th of the tablet mass is digoxin, and inadequate mixing with the excipient substances gives irregular distribution. In addition, accurate punch dyes are needed to keep tablet weight constant. Modern manufacturing techniques can overcome these difficulties and the British Pharmacopeia now requires every digoxin batch to be tested and the tablets to be within ± 15% of stated dose.

Bioavailability from digoxin tablets

For a drug to reach the circulation, it must be released into solution at a part of the gut where effective absorption can take place. The application of the digoxin radioimmunoassay to subjects given commercially produced digoxin tablets revealed that different brands could give markedly different rates and extent of absorption. Tablets giving the slowest absorption produced a total absorption at about half that from the fastest absorbed brands.

It became clear that these absorption differences reflected variation in the dissolution rate of the tablets. Some dissolved so slowly that absorption from the small intestine was impaired. In vitro dissolution rate correlated closely with peak digoxin levels during absorption and with steady-state values (Lindenbaum et al., 1973; Johnson et al., 1973) and with clinical effect (Shaw et al., 1973). Digoxin tablets marketed in the United Kingdom were found to have a wide spectrum of dissolution rates, ranging from 19% to 92% in solution at 30 min (Beckett & Cowan, 1973); some brands changed markedly from batch to batch. A similar pattern existed in the United States, Scandinavia, and Australia.

The initial reports of differences in digoxin bioavailability were confirmed by detailed pharmacokinetic studies involving single and multiple doses and a variety of indices of absorption: this bioavailability data has recently been reviewed by Greenblatt et al. (1976). Single-dose experiments have tended to indicate a larger magnitude of difference in bioavailability than that found using steady-state measurements (Preibisz, Butler & Lindenbaum, 1974), but even with the latter, twofold differences in the extent of absorption were found — a variation of major clinical importance. This spectrum of dissolution rates resulted from the effect of manufacturing techniques on the digoxin particle size (Shaw & Carless, 1974).

A change in the brand of digoxin tablet could alter the clinical response and could precipitate toxicity (Redfors et al., 1973; Shaw, 1974). The dissolution rate has been used to bring some standardization to the tablet performance. In the United Kingdom, the Pharmacopeia requires that digoxin tablets have a dissolution rate greater than 75% within 1 h; for the United States, upper and lower limits of 95% and 55% were established, with the latter recently increased to 65%. This international divergence makes interpretation of bioavailability studies more difficult when tablets have been used as a standard. I believe that the dissolution rate limits should be as strict as is technically feasible, since we have consistently found that, although some patients absorb quite well from slow dissolving formulations, others are very sensitive to changes in dissolution rate (Fig. 16.1). The new pharmacopeial criteria have removed one of the factors which make digitalis treatment difficult and the current formulations give slightly less intersubject variation in digoxin levels than did the slow release tablets.

The tablet bioavailability problem also reemphasized two aspects of digoxin absorption known from earlier work — the absorption of digoxin even in solution was incomplete, and there was considerable differences in the extent of absorption between individuals.

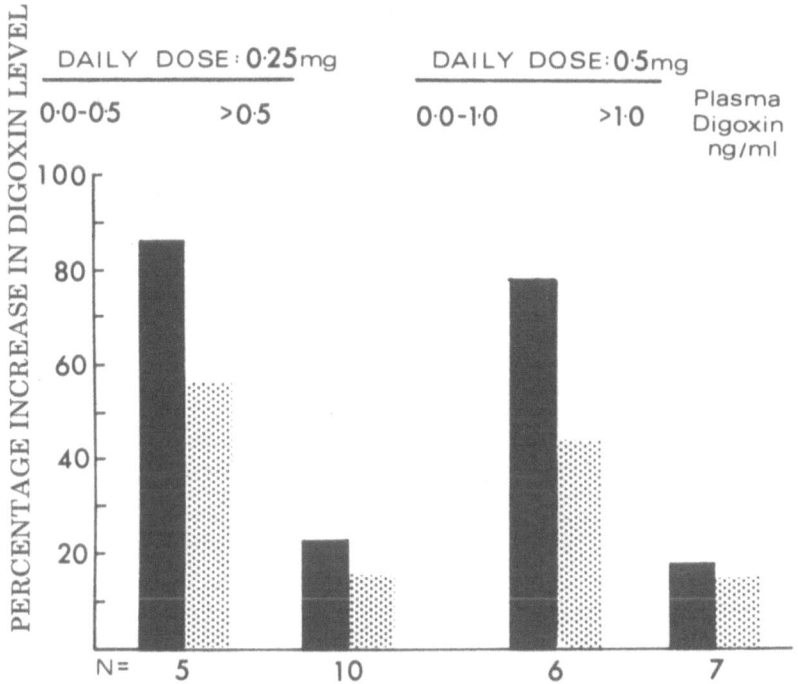

Fig. 16.1. Sensitivity to differences in bioavailability: patients in a randomized cross-over trial of digoxin brands (Shaw et al., 1973) were grouped into those who had "low" or "high" plasma digoxin levels when using the slowest dissolving tablets (0.0-0.5 ng/ml was taken to be "low" for a 0.25 mg/day dose, and 0.0-1.0 ng/ml for 0.5 mg/day). The percentage increase in digoxin level when changed to rapidly dissolving tablets (black columns) was highest in the low level groups: the same trend was seen for use of tablets with intermediate dissolution rate (stippled columns)

Variation between Subjects

The variation between subjects was illustrated by Johnson and Lader (1974) when they gave five digoxin formulations of similar high bioavailability to eight normal subjects (Fig. 16.2). Each person was fairly constant in the percentage of the dose he absorbed but, when assessed by urinary digoxin excretion, there was a threefold difference between subjects. When calculated by the area under the curve method, the highest absorption was 60% greater than the lowest. They later reported that these differences in absorption correlated well with the variation in steady-state levels, suggesting that unpredictable absorption gave a significant contribution to the scatter of digoxin levels found in apparently similar patients. Comparable variation between subjects has been found in most digoxin bioavailability studies.

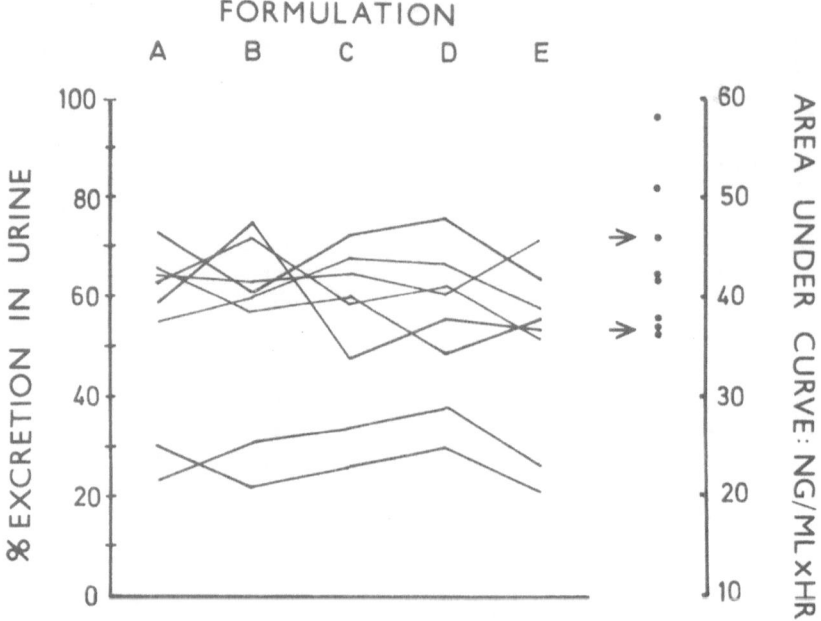

Fig. 16.2. Individual variation in 10-day urinary digoxin excretion in normal subjects following single doses of high bioavailability formulations administered on five separate occasions. Area-under-the-curve values are the means from the five administrations to each subject: the arrows indicate the AUC results for the two patients with the lowest urinary excretion. Adapted from Johnson and Lader (1974)

Absorption of Digoxin Solution and Its Augmentation

The experiments in which oral digoxin solution was compared with intravenous doses confirmed that absorption even of a solution was incomplete. Estimates of the percentage absorbed have varied somewhat, but about three quarters of an oral dose reaches the circulation. A precise figure is now even harder to calculate with recent work showing that a longer infusion time for the same intravenous dose can increase the total urinary digoxin excretion by more than 20% (Greenblatt et al., 1974; Marcus et al., 1976); the reasons for this are unclear.

In general, the closer a drug's absorption approaches 100%, the more consistent is the bioavailability in patients. There would in theory be some benefit to be gained if digoxin absorption could be boosted. Johnson and Bye (1975) suggested that digoxin dissolved in a 10% alcoholic elixir was slightly better absorbed than very rapidly dissolving tablets. A new and more complicated formulation has been developed with digoxin dissolved in polyethylene glycol 400 and encased in a soft gelatin capsule. It gave a more marked improvement in digoxin absorption (Johnson et al., 1976; Marcus et al., 1976). It remains to be seen whether these newer formulations will significantly improve digitalization in patients and whether this will be worth the additional cost of more complex preparations.

Other Glycosides

The awareness of difficulties in digoxin's absorption has stimulated examination of other cardiac glycosides having better absorption characteristics. Digitoxin is more lipophilic than digoxin and is completely absorbed (Beerman, Kellstrom & Rosen, 1971). There are, however, other pharmacokinetic differences which also have to be considered. The half-life of its elimination is four times longer than that of digoxin, and although this is convenient during maintenance therapy, it causes a slow response to a change in dose and makes toxicity last longer. Its high degree of binding to plasma proteins means that changes in albumin concentration have to be considered in interpreting serum level measurements. Its hepatic metabolism is vulnerable to enzyme-inducing drugs (Solomon & Abrams, 1972). On the other hand, its independence from changes in renal function are an advantage (Storstein, 1974). One can now have an even more complex argument as to which is the favorite glycoside.

Methyl-digoxin has appeared as a new rival with some evidence of better absorption. Again one must assess the overall character of the drug; for example, whether the more rapid onset of action might make transient toxicity at peak levels a significant problem.

It would be a disadvantage if too many cardiac glycosides and special formulations came into clinical use since the potential for confusion would be increased. It is perhaps more important to learn how to use better the digitalis preparations we already have.

Impairment of Bioavailability by Other Agents

The quantification of absorption by bioavailability studies has permitted the identification of certain interactions with other drugs and disease states.

Brown and Juhl (1976) followed the in vitro experiments of Khalil (1974) and showed that digoxin absorption is significantly reduced by concomitant doses of antacids, which bind the glycoside. Neomycin, Kaopectate, and cholestyramine also impair absorption. Other drug interactions are likely to be identified. Malabsorption states and thyroid disease may also affect absorption, but their effect is not yet totally clear. Partial gastrectomy had no effect on digoxin absorption (Beerman et al., 1973). When such effects have been documented, then the clinician is in a position to avoid these circumstances or to anticipate the effect.

Bioavailability in Patients

A physician, faced with an individual patient to digitalize, does not of course carry out absorption studies and certainly would not wish the patient to return with 10-days output of urine. The steady-state plasma level is the index normally used to assess how much digitalis is in the body stores. Simple formulas have been developed to help choose the digoxin dose to achieve a satisfactory degree of digitalization (Jelliffe, 1971). These take account of body size and renal function and, in theory, should improve precision. In practice, results have been disappointing. Use of these formulas still gave a wide range of digoxin levels (Christiansen et al., 1973), and computor programs similar to these formulas did not improve the variability of digitalization (Peck et al., 1973; Wagner et al., 1973).

We have measured plasma digoxin concentrations in cardiac patients (Fig. 16.3)
1. When they attended a routine visit to the cardiac follow-up clinic
2. When all were given a standard dose of 0.25 mg digoxin per day
3. When on a daily dose based on a loading dose of 0.015 mg/kg and adjusted for size and serum creatinine

No significant improvement in the wide scatter of digoxin levels has been found, suggesting that body weight and creatinine level may be relatively crude indices and/or that presently unpredictable variation in absorption, metabolism, and tissue binding are of considerable importance.

Conclusions

We are still far from achieving precise digitalization. Bioavailability studies have, however, provided us with better materials to work with. The bioavailability profiles of the various glycosides allow us to make a more informed choice of which digitalis preparation to use. The experiments relating to drug interactions provide some general principles which can be applied to individual cases. At the present time, when assessing an unsatisfactory clinical response to digitalis it is best to use the steady-state level as an overall indication of how much of the drug is being presented to the tissues and to adjust dosage accordingly.

Faced with the presently unpredictable kinetics of digoxin in individuals, we must consider what is the appropriate intensity of digitalization we seek to achieve. Many physicians would agree that the modern diuretics are more important than digitalis in the control of cardiac failure. Even when atrial fibrillation is present, strict control of the ventricular rate is less vital now that unrelieved severe mitral stenosis is seldom seen. This is not to deny the efficacy of digitalis, but in these circumstances it is better to err on the side of safety rather than of toxicity and hence to digitalize gently.

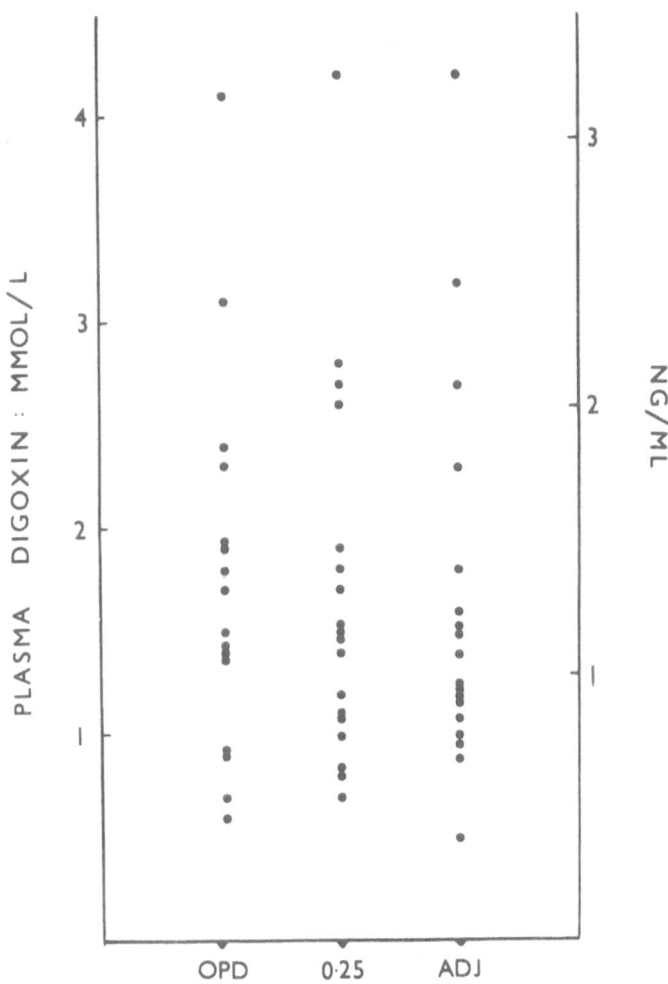

Fig. 16.3. Plasma digoxin levels recorded at steady state in cardiac patients:
1. At a routine visit to the cardiac follow-up clinic (OPD)
2. After each was put on a standard dosage of 0.25 mg/day (0.25)
3. When on a daily digoxin dose based on a loading dose of 0.015 mg/kg and adjusted for renal function (ADJ)

References

Beckett, A.H., Cowan, D.A.: Differences in the dissolution rate of generic digoxin tablets. Pharm. J. 211, 111-113 (1973)
Beerman, B., Hellstrom, K., Rosen, A.: Fate of orally administered ^{3}H digitoxin in man with special reference to the absorption. Circulation 43, 852-861 (1971)

Beerman, B., Hellstrom, K., Rosen, A.: The gastrointestinal absorption of digoxin in seven patients with gastric or small intestinal reconstructions. Acta Med. Scand. 193, 293-297 (1973)

Brown, D.D., Juhl, R.P.: Decreased bioavailability of digoxin due to antacids and kaolin-pectin. N. Engl. J. Med. 295, 1034-1037 (1976)

Christiansen, N.J.B., Kolendorf, K., Steinbaek, K., Hansen, J.M.: Serum digoxin values following a dosage regime based on body weight, sex, age and renal function. Acta Med. Scand. 194, 257-259 (1973)

F.D.A. Case Studies. A composite case study of digoxin tablets. No. 113, 1971

Greenblatt, D.J., Duhme, D.W., Koch-Weser, J., Smith, T.W.: Intravenous digoxin as a bioavailability standard: slow infusion and rapid injection. Clin. Pharmacol. Ther. 15, 510-513 (1974)

Greenblatt, D.J., Smith, T.W., Koch-Weser, J.: Bioavailability of drugs: the digoxin dilemma. Clin. Pharmacokinetics 1, 36-51 (1976)

Jelliffe, R.W.: An improved method of digoxin therapy. Ann. Intern. Med. 69, 703-717 (1971)

Johnson, B.F., Bye, C.: Maximal intestinal absorption of digoxin and its relation to steady-state plasma concentration. Br. Heart J. 37, 203-208 (1975)

Johnson, B.F., Bye, C., Jones, G., Sabey, G.A.: A completely absorbed oral preparation of digoxin. Clin. Pharmacol. Ther. 19, 746-751 (1976)

Johnson, B.F., Greer, H., McCrerie, J., Bye, C., Fowle, A.: Rate of dissolution of digoxin tablets as a predictor of absorption. Lancet 1973/I, 1473-1475

Johnson, B.F., Lader, S.: Bioavailability of digoxin from rapidly dissolving preparations. Br. J. Clin. Pharmacol. 1, 329-333 (1974)

Khalil, S.A.H.: The uptake of digoxin and digitoxin by some antacids. J. Pharm. Pharmacol. 26, 961-967 (1974)

Lindenbaum, J., Butler, V.P., Murphy, J.E., Cresswell, R.M.: Correlation of digoxin − tablet dissolution rate with biological availability. Lancet 1973/I, 1215-1217

Manninen, V., Korhonen, A.: Inequal digoxin tablets. Lancet 1973/II, 1268

Marcus, F.I., Dickerson, J., Pippin, S., Stafford, M., Bressler, R.: Clin. Pharmacol. Ther. 20, 253-259 (1976)

Peck, C.C., Sheiner, L.B., Martin, C.M., Combs, D.T., Melmon, K.L.: Computer-assisted digoxin therapy. N. Engl. J. Med. 289, 441-446 (1973)

Preibisz, J.J., Butler, V.P., Lindenbaum, J.: Digoxin tablet bioavailability. Ann. Intern. Med. 81, 469-474 (1974)

Redfors, A., Bertler, A., Nilsen, R., Wettr, S.: Changing a population from one digoxin preparation to another. In: 'Digitalis'. Storstein, O., Nitter-Hauge, S., Storstein, L. (eds.) Oslo: Gyldendal Norsk Forlag, 1973, pp. 390-395

Shaw, T.R.D.: Non-equivalence of digoxin tablets in the U.K. and its clinical implications. Postgrad. Med. J. 50 (Supp. 6), 24-29 (1974)

Shaw, T.R.D., Carless, J.: The effect of particle size on the absorption of digoxin. Eur. J. Clin. Pharmacol. 7, 269-273 (1974)

Shaw, T.R.D., Raymond, K., Howard, M.R., Hamer, J.: Therapeutic non-equivalence of digoxin tablets in the United Kingdom: correlation with tablet dissolution rate. Br. Med. J. 1973/IV, 763-766

Solomon, H.M., Abrams, W.B.: Interactions between digitoxin and other drugs in man. Am. Heart J. 83, 277-280 (1972)

Storstein, L.: Studies on digitalis I & II. Clin. Pharmacol. Ther. 16, 14-24 & 25-34 (1974)

Wagner, J.G., Yates, J.D., Willis, P.W., Sakmar, E., Stoll, R.G.: Correlation of plasma levels of digoxin in cardiac patients with dose and measures of renal function. Clin. Pharmacol. Ther. 15, 199-204 (1973)

Withering, W.: An Account of the Foxglove, and Some of Its Medicinal Uses: With Practical Remarks on Dropsy and Other Diseases. Reprinted in Classics of Cardiology (1961). Willius, F.A., Keys, T.E., (eds.) New York: Dover, 1785, Vol. I

Discussion

Bodem, Bonn: Is it important whether the tablets were taken before or after a meal?

Shaw: It has been shown that there is some delay in absorption when the tablets are taken after a meal, but the final extent of absorption is not affected.

Johnson, Chapel Hill: I agree that the improvement in the dissolution rate of available digoxin tablets made a big difference in the clinical usage of digoxin. It did lead to reduced variability between subjects. Since then, further improvement is much more difficult to demonstrate. I think it is incumbant upon those of us who are trying to increase the absorption of digitalis products to demonstrate a practical advantage. With one of the oral preparations mentioned by Dr. Shaw, a preparation of digoxin dissolved in polyethylene glycol and encapsulated in soft gelatine, we have been able to produce a further 10%-15% of absorption by comparison with the best available tablets. (Fig. 1) The mechanism for this remains obscure but it has been confirmed. With well-trained, reliable volunteers we were able to show further reduction in the between-subject variability of steady-state plasma concentration in a group of ten volunteers. The reduction was in the order of 40%-50% which could be of clinical importance. This clearly would need to be repeated in a general patient population.

Shaw: We should not only concentrate on the percentage of the dose absorbed. I think the important factor is the variation in the percentage absorbed. If you had a tablet which was only 10% absorbed, but this was always absolutely constant, in everybody and every day, that would be better than one which was 90% absorbed, but with a lot of variation. However, it is usual with drug formulations that the greater the absorption, the less the variation.

Nyberg: Dr. Shaw showed us a slide comparing bioavailability and between-subject variation of digoxin capsules and digoxin tablets. From the literature, I presume that the tablets were Lanoxin[®] made in the United States (Johnson et al., 1976 a, b). The greater variation found with tablets compared with capsules may then have been caused by a moderate dissolution rate from the

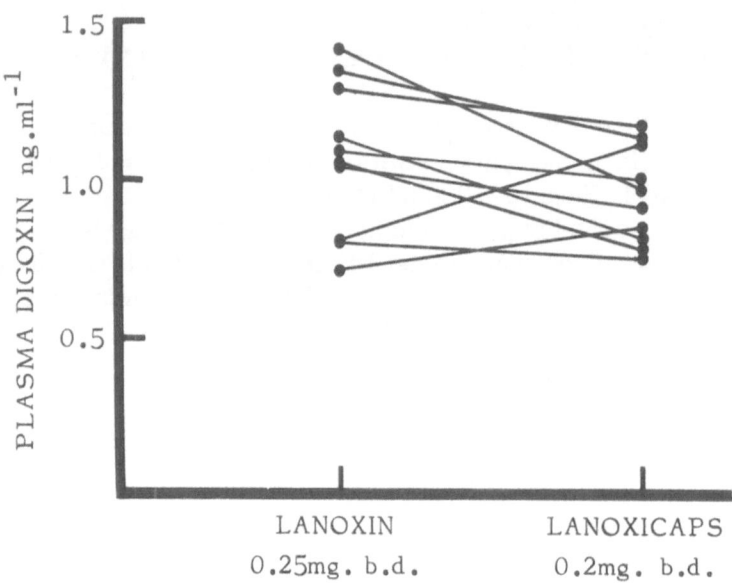

PLASMA DIGOXIN ng.ml⁻¹

LANOXIN
0.25mg. b.d.

LANOXICAPS
0.2mg. b.d.

Fig. 1

investigated tablets. Mallis and colleagues (Mallis et al., 1975) have shown that more readily available digoxin does not give a larger relative standard deviation than digoxin capsules. Therefore, a study with more rapidly releasing tablets would have been interesting, for instance with Lanoxin® tablets made in the United Kingdom.

Johnson: In the study I demonstrated, the Lanoxin tablets were made in England and had a dissolution rate over 95% in 1 h. I agree that in this type of comparison, one should use the digoxin tablets of the highest bioavailability that one can obtain, and that was the case in our study.

Nyberg: But how do you explain the findings by Mallis et al.?

Johnson: All I can say is that in all of our experiments, capsules have been associated with a lower coefficient of variation for measures of extent of absorption by comparison with any other oral preparation including solution.

Nyberg: In addition, I would like to point out that differences in a variability parameter are extremely difficult to evaluate with a statistical significance. In conclusion, I agree with Dr. Shaw that more studies on the actual topic seem to be warranted.

Schaumann, Mannheim: I think we have to keep in mind that bioavailability is not the only source of variation of serum glycoside concentrations. Boerner et al. (Boerner et al., 1976) found a considerable day-to-day variation in the minimum serum concentrations also in patients under intravenous maintenance therapy. If D is the daily injected dose, Cl_{tot} the total body clearance, V_d the

196

volume of distribution, and β the rate constant for elimination at pseudo-equilibrium, the average serum concentration $\bar{c}$ at steady state is

$$\bar{c} \;=\; \frac{D}{Cl_{tot}} \;=\; \frac{D}{V_d \cdot \beta}$$

The serum concentration clearly depends on interindividual differences and intraindividual variations in Cl_{tot}. Short-term variations in V_d will also affect the serum concentration.

Larbig, Tübingen: Dr. Shaw, you showed one slide about experiments in which you adjusted the dosage to body weight and could not find any decrease of the variation of the serum concentration. Is this correct?

Shaw: The dosage was adjusted both for body weight and for renal function as assessed by serum creatinine.

Larbig: And you could not demonstrate any decrease of the scatter?

Shaw: Patients changed places in the order of the scatter, but the overall scatter remained.

Larbig: Would you say that body weight has no influence whatsoever on steady-state serum concentration in patients who do not have any severe decrease of renal function? We were trying to assess this problem analyzing steady-state serum concentrations in a large series of patients on digoxin and methyl-digoxin maintenance therapy. We found that in patients with a low body weight, serum concentrations were significantly higher. But I think you have to have a large group to demonstrate this phenomenon.

Shaw: Weight is a relatively crude index — but we cannot easily measure lean body mass. Multifactorial analysis has shown that there is some influence from body size. The problem is that a patient and his plasma digoxin level are a combination of many different factors, of which body size is only one.

Larbig: Indeed renal clearance of creatinine does correlate with body weight. I do not refer to obese patients but to lean body weight. I personally would give patients with a low body weight a low maintenance dose in order to avoid an intoxication. Would you go along with this?

Shaw: Yes, that would be sensible, particularly since one deals with at least a fourfold range of body weight in the patient population. However, when one tries to quantitate this effect by using these simple formulas to calculate dosage, then no benefit is seen.

Vöhringer, Berlin: I have a question on the interference between digoxin and antacids. Do any kind of antacids interact with digoxin? We have studied the interference of digoxin with magnesium-aluminium-silicate-hydrate and di-magnesium-aluminium-trisilicate (Vöhringer et al., 1976) and we didn't find a alteration of the mean plasma concentrations of digoxin by these antacids. But I don't know about aluminium oxide.

Shaw: Khalil (Khalil 1974) found that magnesium trisilicate was a powerful binder in vitro of digoxin, but other substances used as antacids were not such powerful binders. Brown and Juhl (1976) recorded some reduction in digoxin absorption, not only with trisilicate but with aluminium hydroxyde and magnesium hydroxyde.

Kramer, Göttingen: We have studied the absorption of digoxin and digitoxin by aluminium hydroxyde in the duodenal fluid and there was none. Thus, I don't think that this phosphate binder interferes with the intestinal absorption of cardiac glycosides.

References

Boerner et al.: Eur. J. Clin. Pharmacol. 9, 307 (1976)1976)
Johnson, B.F., Bye, C., Jones, G., Sabey, G.A.: Clin. Pharmacol. Ther. 19, 746-751 (1976)
Idem: Eur. J. Clin. Pharmacol. 10, 231-236 (1976 b)
Khalil: J. Pharm. Sci. 63, 1641-2 (1974)
Mallis, G.I., Schmidt, D.H., Lindenbaum, J.: Clin. Pharmacol. Ther. 18, 761-768 (1975)
Vöhringer et al.: Dtsch. Med. Wochenschr. 101, 106 (1976)

17 Comparative Pharmacokinetics of Various Digoxin Preparations in Man[1]

P. F. BINNION

Introduction

The amount of a drug absorbed from a dosage form and the time course of absorption are covered by the term bioavailability (Lancet, 1975), and this has been investigated more extensively for digoxin than any other drug to my knowledge. Physicians in New York about 6 years ago noted several patients who received large doses of tablet digoxin but still had low serum digoxin concentrations (Lindenbaum et al., 1971). This raised the question as to the intestinal absorption of digoxin and the bioavailability of the digoxin thought to be present in the tablets being used. Using healthy volunteers, marked variation in serum digoxin levels were noted when these preparations were ingested after an overnight fast with one product producing peak levels seven times higher than another preparation (Lindenbaum et al., 1971). At the time this study was published, one of our hospital physicians, under treatment for atrial fibrillation with digoxin in tablet form, had a plasma digoxin level of 0 ng/ml. Changing the brand of tablet digoxin subsequently produced a satisfactory blood level, and this led us to inform the manufacturer that their digoxin tablets could not be absorbed satisfactorily (a statement later proven to be incorrect) (Binnion and McDermott, 1972). However, we did find tablets of digoxin which did not produce a satisfactory blood level. Many others have confirmed that the absorption of digoxin varied widely between different brands of digoxin tablets (Fleckenstein et al., 1974; Preibisz et al., 1974; Bertler et al., 1972; Karjalainen et al., 1974; Shaw et al., 1972). In one dramatic instance, the Burroughs Wellcome and Co. brand of tablet digoxin ("Lanoxin"), which was used in the early American studies as a standard for bioavailability studies (Lindenbaum et al., 1971; Binnion, 1974), was made into the tablet formulation in the United Kingdom by a different technique such that they had a different effective potency. Tablets manufactured after May, 1972 by the same firm had approximately double the potency of the earlier digoxin tablets (Lancet editorial, 1972). Having established that equivalent digoxin tablets do not have equivalent bioavailability, what are the possible and actual reasons for this?

1 Supported by funds from Lederle Division of the American Cyanamid Co., Pearl River, NY, Burroughs Wellcome Co., Research Triangle Park, NC, grant-in-aid (No. 71-1091) from the American Heart Association & with funds contributed by the Pennsylvania Heart Association in 1971 and 1976.

Factors Affecting the Bioavailability of Digoxin — Physical Form

Table 17.1 gives a list of factors which could alter the achievement of a satisfactory blood level of digoxin after the ingestion of digoxin tablets. The amount of digoxin in tablets sold to the public was found to be approximately that stated (Lindenbaum et al., 1971; Binnion, et al., 1973; Sachez et al., 1973), hence this could not be the cause of the marked variation in blood levels seen in volunteers. Although the size of the particles in the digoxin tablets was measured, initially there was discrepancy as to whether this influenced absorption (Jounela & Sothman, 1973; Shaw et al., 1972). However, more recent work has proven conclusively that in general the smaller the digoxin particle size, the greater the amount in solution within an hour (the dissolution rate) and the greater the bioavailability (Shaw et al., 1974; Jounela et al., 1975). Tablets containing the same amount of digoxin made in different ways by the same manufacturer in the United Kingdom (Whiting et al., 1972) produced markedly different blood glycoside levels which suggested that the physical properties of the tablets was of great importance in determining bioavailability. Delayed disintegration of the tablet was initially considered to be the main factor (Shaw et al., 1972; Manninen et al., 1972; Binnion et al., 1973) but further work revealed a better correlation between dissolution rate and biologic availability of the drug (Table 17.2). The solutions used to measure dissolution rates are either a simulated gastric fluid or dilute hydrachloric acid (Bertler et al., 1972; Lindenbaum et al., 1973; Preibisz et al., 1974; Binnion, 1974) or water (Steiness et al., 1973; Wagner, 1974), and there appears to be no significant difference between the methods used (Johnson et al., 1973). Many investigators have proven that the rate of dissolution of digoxin after its ingestion is a major determinant of its absorption, and these references are best summarized in a recent paper (Greenblatt et al., 1976).

Table 17.1. Possible factors affecting bioavailability of tablet digoxin

---

1. Differing amounts of digoxin in the tablets

2. Variable physical characteristics of the tablets
    a) Disintegration
    b) Digoxin in tablets going into solution (dissolution characteristics)

3. Factors interfering with absorption from the gastrointestinal tract
    a) Simultaneous presence of other materials in the gut
    b) Malabsorption syndromes
    c) Alterations in gastrointestinal motility

Table 17.2. Physical characteristics of digoxin tablets

Digoxin in 0.25 mg tablet	Mean = 0.237 mg (Sanchez et al., 1973)		
	92-99% (Binnion, 1973)		
	82.7-96.5% (Lindenbaum et al., 1971)		

Disintegration times	(Manninen et al., 1972)	5 min	Mean serum level	1.7 ng/ml
		9 min	Mean serum level	1.5 ng/ml
	(Binnion, 1974)	1 min	Mean 1 h plasma digoxin level	1.5 ng/ml
		2 min		1.6 ng/ml
		5 min		0.1 ng/ml
		8 min		1.2 ng/ml

Dissolution rate	(Steiness et al., 1973)	60% in solution in 1 h	Area under time-conc. curve	0.50
		95% in solution in 1 h	Area under time-conc. curve	1.22
	(Binnion, 1974)	74% in solution in 1 h	Max. plasma digoxin level	1.7 ng/ml
		70% in solution in 1 h	Max. plasma digoxin level	1.8 ng/ml
		23% in solution in 1 h	Max. plasma digoxin level	0.2 ng/ml

Methods for Assessing Bioavailability

The earlier papers noted reduced blood digoxin levels after the ingestion of tablet digoxin bringing the idea of reduced bioavailability to the notice of investigators (Lindenbaum et al., 1971; Binnion & McDermott, 1972, Fleckenstein et al., 1974). When initial controlled studies were done on the absorption of digoxin, the maximum plasma level reached was first used (Lindenbaum et al., 1971; Binnion & McDermott, 1972; Whiting et al., 1972), but later the area under the absorption (concentration-time) curve was employed (Shaw et al., 1972; Steiness et al., 1973), and the final form of investigation included the previous two methods together with the cumulative excretion of digoxin in the urine over a period of several days (Sanchez et al., 1973). It is probably only necessary to use the urinary excretion technique as a check on digoxin bioavailability now (Greenblatt et al., 1973); however, these various methods of measuring digoxin absorption were being introduced during bioavailability studies and the earlier work did not measure urinary excretion rates. Slow intravenous infusion of digoxin is now used as the standard in bioavailability testing, against which other preparations of digoxin are evaluated (Greenblatt et al., 1974). The gradual introduction of these methods did not invalidate any of the conclusions from earlier work but have given us better standards for evaluating bioavailability.

Factors Interfering With Absorption From the Gastrointestinal tract

Nearly all experimental studies on digoxin absorption were done with subjects in the fasting state which avoided errors in methodology which are exposed when comparison is made between absorption in the fasting or fed state (Sanchez et al., 1973). Digoxin tablets given shortly after eating produce a lower peak serum digoxin concentration and reduced area under the concentration-time curve, but there is no change in the cumulative 5-day urinary excretion of digoxin.

The absorption of digoxin by the rat intestine shows it to be a passive transport process (Caldwell et al., 1969), although the processes regulating digoxin absorption in man are not known (Beermann et al., 1972). The main intake of orally administered digoxin in healthy people occurs in the most proximal part of the small intestine, and it has been demonstrated that drugs which increase gastrointestinal motility will lower serum digoxin concentrations in patients on maintenance digoxin therapy and vice versa (Manninen et al., 1973). It would appear that the initial absorption of a poorly absorbed substance can be altered pharmacologically by substances altering gastrointestinal motility and produce changes in the bioavailability of this material (Ashley & Levy, 1973).

Patients with the malabsorption syndrome have lower circulating digoxin levels after ingesting tablets due either to hypermotility or mucosal defects, whereas pancreatic insufficiency has no deleterious effect (Heizer et al., 1971). It appears that bile salts and pancreatic secretions are not required for digoxin absorption and neither is energy required for this process.

When digoxin is given with neomycin, absorption is decreased (Lindenbaum et al., 1972), and in vitro studies have demonstrated adsorption of digoxin by antacid and antidiarrheal preparations which could also affect bioavailability (Binnion, 1973). This work was done by us to resolve the problem in our physician patient with a zero digoxin level (Binnion, 1974). The tablet digoxin being used (made by Lederle) was proven to be of satisfactory bioavailability (Binnion & McDermott, 1972); therefore, a reason had to be found for the unsatisfactory plasma level in the patient. Other medications being used simultaneously by the patient were large quantities of antacid and antidiarrheal medications. It was considered that adsorption by these medications could be the explanation, and in vitro studies were then performed on ^{3}H-digoxin removal by these agents. Activated charcoal has been demonstrated to reduce the absorption of aspirin in man (Levy & Tsuchiya, 1972) and later proven to be efficacious in the treatment of digoxin overdosage in dogs (Zajtchuk et al., 1975). Activated charcoal interferes with digoxin absorption in adult volunteers taking tablet digoxin (Härtel et al., 1973). Hence, adsorption of digoxin by activated charcoal can certainly be a significant factor in reducing bioavailability. What is the situation regarding more usual therapies in reducing digoxin bioavailability? Our work pointed the way but did not prove the point. In dogs, an antacid did not reduce serum digoxin levels (Loo et al., 1975), but in humans, both antacids and Kaopectate reduced peak serum levels but, more importantly, did reduce the 6-day urinary excretion of digoxin (Brown & Juhl, 1976), i.e., they produced a striking decrease in digoxin bioavailability.

Improving Digoxin Bioavailability

Digoxin in solution as the elixir is better absorbed than tablet digoxin (Johnson & Bye, 1975), and we have recently compared the bioavailability of digoxin in solution in capsules with intravenous and tablet forms of administration (Table 17.3). Capsules containing a solution of digoxin are better absorbed than tablets (Binnion, 1976); the tablets had a dissolution profile consistent with satisfactory bioavailability which has been stated to be 70%-90% of the digoxin in solution in 1 h (Binnion, 1974; Dunning, 1974). The Federal Drug Administration has removed tablets with low dissolution rates from sale to the public (F.D.A. drug bulletin, 1974).

Table 17.3. Improving digoxin bioavailability

Preparation	Max. plasma digoxin conc. (ng/ml)	Area under 6 h conc-time (ng/ml × min)	6-day cumulative excretion (% dose given)
Intravenous	6.0	87.2	69.8
Tablet	1.3	38.5	52.4
Liquid in capsules	2.9-3.3	63-69	64-71

Conclusions

The cause of low blood digoxin levels seen in patients taking tablet digoxin in the beginning of this decade has been shown to be due to the physical characteristics of the tablets, namely the rate at which the digoxin in the tablet goes into solution (the dissolution rate). Other factors can interfere with the satisfactory absorption of digoxin in solid form such as rapid gastrointestinal movements, altered mucosal characteristics, and possibly the presence of powerful adsorbing substances. The large number of investigation on digoxin absorption have given great impetus to studies on the bioavailability of pharmaceutic preparations and culminated in the formulation of an improved oral preparation of digoxin. However, the role bioavailability plays in the actions of digoxin remains to be clarified, for the relationship between plasma digoxin level and cardiac uptake and activity are most complex.

References

Ashley, J.J., Levy, G.: Effect of vehicle viscosity and an anti-cholinergic agent on bioavailability of a poorly absorbed drug (phenolsulfonphthalein) in man. J. Pharm. Sci. 62, 688-690 (1973)

Beermann, B., Hellström, K. Rosén, A.: The absorption of orally administered (12 α-³H) digoxin in man. Clin. Sci. 43, 507-518 (1972)

Bertler, A., Redfors, A., Medin, S., Nyberg, L.: Bioavailability of digoxin. Lancet, 1972/ii, 708

Binnion, P.F.: Absorption of Different Commercial Preparations of Digoxin in the Normal Human Subject, and the Influence of Antacid Antidiarrhaeal and Ion-Exchange Resins. Symposium on digitalis. Oslo, Norway: O. Storstein, (ed.) Gyldendal Norsk Forlag, 1973, pp. 216-224

Binnion, P.F.: The absorption of digoxin tablets. Clin. Pharmacol. Ther. 16, 807-812 (1974)

Binnion, P.F.: Zero plasma digoxin levels in patients on oral digoxin therapy, Ir. J. Med. Sci. 148, 346-349 (1974)

Binnion, P.F.,: A comparison of the bioavailability of digoxin in capsule, tablet, and solution taken orally with intravenous digoxin. J. Clin. Pharmacol. (in press) (1976)

Binnion, P.F., McDermott, M.: Bioavailability of digoxin. Lancet 1972/ii, 592

Binnion, P.F., McDermott, M., LeSher, D.: Bioavailability of digoxin. Lancet 1973/i, 1118

Brown, D.D., Juhl, R.P.: Decreased bioavailability of digoxin produced by antacids and kaopectate. Am J. Cardiol. 37, 123 (1976)

Caldwell, J.H., Martin, J.F., Dutta, S. Greenberger, N.J.: Intestinal absorption of digoxin-³H in the rat. Am. J. Physiol. 217, 1747-1751 (1969)

Dunning, A.J.: The safety of digoxin. Eur. J. Cardiol. 2, 1-2 (1974)

Editorial: The bioavailability of digoxin. Lancet 1972/ii, 311-312.

Editorial: Bioavailability after intramuscular injection. Lancet 1975/i, 261

FDA Drug Bulletin: FDA to correct digoxin problems. 1974

Fleckenstein, L., Kroening, B., Weintraub, M.: Assessment of biologic availability of digoxin in man. Clin. pharmacol.Ther. 16, 435-443 (1974)

Greenblatt, D.J., Duhme, D.W., Koch-Weser, J., Smith, T.W.: Evaluation of digoxin bioavailability in single-dose studies N. Engl. J. Med. 289, 651-654 (1973)

Greenblatt, D.J., Duhme, D.W., Koch-Weser, J., Smith, T.W.: Intravenous digoxin as a bioavailability standard: slow infusion and rapid injection. Clin. Pharmacol. Ther. 15, 510-513 (1974)

Greenblatt, D.J., Smith, T.W., Koch-Weser, J.: Bioavailability of drugs: the digoxin dilemma, Clin. Pharmacokinetics 1, 36-51 (1976)

Härtel, G., Manninen, V., Reissell, P.: Treatment of digoxin intoxication. Lancet, 1973/ii, 158

Heizer, W.D., Smith, T.W., Goldfinger, S.E.: Absorption of digoxin in patients with malabsorption syndromes. N. Engl. J. Med. 285, 257-259 (1971)

Johnson, B.F., Bye, C.: Maximal intestinal absorption of digoxin and its relation to steady state plasma concentration. Br. Heart J. 37, 203-208 (1975)

Johnson, B.F., Greer, H., McCrerie, J., Bye, C., Fowle, A.: Rate of dissolution of digoxin tablets as a predictor of absorption. Lancet 1973/i, 1473-1475

Jounela, A.J., Sothman, A.: Bioavailability of digoxin. Lancet 1973/i, 202-203

Jounela. A.J., Pentikainen, P.J., Sothmann, A.: Effect of particle size on the bioavailability of digoxin. Eur. J. Clin. Pharmacol. 8, 365-370 (1975)

Karjalainen, J., Ojala, K., Reissell, P.: Non-equivalent digoxin tablets. Ann. Clin. Res. 6, 132-136 (1974)

Levy, G., Tsuchiya, T.: Effect of activated charcoal on aspirin absorption in man. Clin. Pharmacol. Ther. 13, 317-322 (1972)

Lindenbaum, J., Mellow, M.H., Blackstone, M.O., Butler, V.P.: Variation in biologic availability of digoxin from four preparations. N. Engl. J. Med. 285, 1344-1347 (1971)

Lindenbaum, J., Maulitz, R.M., Saha, J.R., Shea, N., Butler, V.P.: Impairment of digoxin absorption by neomycin. Clin. Res. 20, 410 (1972)

Lindenbaum, J., Butler, V.P., Murphy, J.E., Cresswell, R.M.: Correlation of digoxin tablet dissolution-rate with biological availability. Lancet 1973/i, 1215-1217

Loo, J.C.K., Rowe, M., McGilveray, I.J.: Effect of an antacid on absorption of digoxin in dogs. J. Pharm. Sci. 64, 1727-1728 (1975)

Manninen, V., Ojala, K., Reisell, P.: New formulation of digoxin. Lancet 1972/ii, 922-923

Manninen, V., Apajalahti, A., Melin, J., Karesoja, M.: Altered absorption of digoxin in patients given propantheline and metoclopramide. Lancet 1973/i, 398-400

Preibisz, J.J., Butler, V.P., Lindenbaum, J.: Digoxin tablet bioavailability: single-dose and steady-state assessment. Ann. Intern. Med. 81, 469-474 (1974)

Sanchez, N., Sheiner, L.B., Halkin, H., Melmon, K.L.: Pharmacokinetics of digoxin: interpreting bioavailability. Br. Med. J. 1973/IV 132-134

Shaw, T.R.D., Howard, M.R., Hamer, J.: Variation in the biological availability of digoxin. Lancet 1972/ii, 303-307

Shaw, T.R.D., Carless, J.E.: The effect of particle size on the absorption of digoxin Eur. J. Clin. Pharmacol. 7, 269-273 (1974)

Steiness, E., Christensen, V., Johansen, H.: Bioavailability of digoxin tablets. Clin. Pharmacol. Ther. 14, 949-954 (1973)

Wagner, J.G.: Appraisal of digoxin bioavailability and pharmacokinetics in relation to cardiac therapy. Am. Heart J. 88, 133-138 (1974)

Whiting, B., Rodger, J.C., Sumner, D.J.: New formulation of digoxin. Lancet 1972/ii, 922

Zajtchuk, R., Corby, D.G., Miller, J.G., O'Barr, T.P.: Treatment of digoxin toxicity with activated charcoal. Am. J. Cardiol. 35, 178 (1975)

Discussion

(General Discussion on Bioavailability of Cardiac Glycosides)

Smith, Boston: I think we can proceed to a general discussion about the bioavailability of cardiac glycosides. The bioavailability problems that are now perceived have come to light under circumstances where there was a very dramatic change in bioavailability. Dr. Binnion's paper provides an example of a thoughtful physician trying to sort out an apparent problem with bioavailability in an individual case and coming up with the recognition that nonabsorbable materials ingested by patients may interfere with absorption. Another example would be the low bioavailability of the preparation Drs. Lindenbaum and Butler recognized in one of the index papers on the bioavailability of different preparations in the United States. When Burroughs Wellcome was changing the digoxin formulation, producing changes in bioavailability, was there any widespread appreciation on the part of the physicians that the incidence of digoxin toxicity changed in the United Kingdom?

Shaw: The time factor was such that the increase in the Burroughs Wellcome Lanoxin® bioavailability occurred a very short time before it was discovered that this had taken place. Physicians were warned and were able to take appropriate action quickly. I think another reason that there weren't more troubles with toxicity was that during the period when slowly dissolving tablets were used most patients continued to be on dosages which were appropriate for well-absorbed preparations — so that really the problems then was underdigitalization rather than overdigitalization. In Scandinavia, Redfors and colleagues changed 91 patients from a slowly dissolving to a rapidly dissolving formulation 6: became toxic and 14 had an improved clinical response.

Smith: I have a question concerning some of the intricacies of these bioavailability studies. If one simplifies matters by specifying patients who do not have gastrointestinal disease, and preparations with dissolution rates that are considered adequate according to current standards, I wonder how many people would accept a figure of 70% ± 10% as a reasonable estimate of the absolute bioavailability of digoxin tablets now marketed? I gather, then, that there is a consensus that formulations now on the market fall somewhere in this range of 70% ± 10%, and now I would submit the following question to the clinicians in the group: do variations within that range matter very much in relation to changes in individual response? We know that changes take place in the individual patient in tolerance to the drug with changes in severity of ischemic disease, with changes in serum potassium levels, with changes in other electrolytes, and with changes in other drugs that are administered. I would like to open this question to discussion and ask the following questions: what percentage variability in steady-state level should we tolerate as physicians, and what kind of standards should we recommend for the pharmaceutic industry? I think that we can waste a lot of their time asking them to come up with a preparation that varies by 2% from day to day if our patients are varying by 20% or by 50% from day to day in their tolerance. I would ask Dr. Marcus first what he thinks is a reasonable variation.

Marcus: I am not sure whether I should thank you for that question and I really do not have an answer. I think that one of the major problems in attempting to answer that question relates to the fact that we do not have an adequate means of measuring the inotropic response in patients on chronic maintenance digitalis therapy. For example, what percentage change in inotropy results from a variation in bioavailability from 60% to a bioavailability of 80%, even assuming that higher blood levels result? We are all familiar with the logarithmic dose-response curve, but where on that dose-response curve is the patient in that particular situation? I have the impression that the factors other than bioavailability that you have mentioned are much more important than the variation in digoxin bioavailability that drug companies are concerned about.

Reissell, Helsinki: In the early 1970s, the problem of bioavailability of the digoxin tablets was very alarming. Later on, a careful standardization of the tablets including studies on bioavailability in humans was required by the Medical Board of Finland. Until it was realized, however, that the bioavailability of some formulations was improved, the lack of communication or of understanding the instructions from the manufacturer to the physicians caused digitalis intoxication in several patients. Information problems have to be taken into consideration when changing the bioavailability of a drug, and all efforts should be made to inform the physicians. In Finland, the uniformity of bioavailability of oral digoxin formulations is probably unique considering that as many as seven preparations are sold in this small country.

Shaw: I've been reflecting on the problem when differences in digoxin bioavailability become of clinical significance. I think as a general principle — no matter how many variables are present — one should always aim to minimize these variables in order to get an easier situation to deal with. The second point is that you've got to bear in mind the "worst possible case."

If there are some patients who are much more sensitive to slight differences in dissolution rate than others, then one must cater to them as much as to the average or best case. We did find that some patients are very sensitive to a change in dissolution rate of their tablets. I agree with you that we are now getting to a stage in digoxin bioavailability where there are very small quantities of difference that we are talking about, and these are overwhelmed by other factors in most patients. In addition, if you plan your treatment by watching carefully the response and by monitoring serum digoxin levels, the slight increases in bioavailability of the newest formulations become less important.

Smith: I think we have a responsibility to try to come up with guidelines. We would probably all agree that variations from day to day of 40% would be intolerable. Even though some patients would tolerate them, others would not. We should have preparations reliable enough that these very sensitive patients are not at risk. I wonder if anyone would like to come up with figures as to what really should be tolerated in day to day steady-state level variability for preparations that are sold to patients. Can I get anyone to express an opinion in numeric terms?

Lukas: That's a very difficult question because what may be varying is not only the preparation but also the patient. I think we are quite well aware of the many factors that can induce enzymes that are capable of degrading drugs, which now apparently include smoking cigarettes and eating charcoal-broiled steaks. It is possible that such induced enzymes will influence steady-state levels of digoxin since the liver may be involved in the net measurement of bioavailability. It is important to know whether the patient himself is intrinsically varying more than the preparation is. However, I know what you are after, and I'd like to hear a figure.

Smith: One problem is that most of the studies that have been quoted and most of the data that have been presented in this session relate to normal volunteers. The variability there is likely to be less than it is in patients.

Schaumann, Mannheim: Dr. Smith, I cannot answer your question; I just would like to point out that in Germany we do not only have on the market several formulations of digoxin with an average absorption of about 70%, but also methyldigoxin and esters of digoxin which are absorbed 80% or 90%. The doctors' acceptance certainly was in favor of these new derivatives, because there is an old experience that a more complete absorption means a more reliable absorption.

Smith: I think most would subscribe to the notion that the higher the bioavailability, the less the variation is likely to be within or among patients. I would like now to open the floor to any other questions or comments that anyone would like to make on the bioavailability problem in cardiac glycosides.

Greenblatt: One issue that came up about drug absorption and absorption rates: we don't assume that drug absorption occurs at a constant rate, even though we assign it a "rate constant".

The rate constant is just a proportionality factor between a continuously changing rate of absorption and the concentration left at the absorption site. Initially, when the drug is "dumped" into the gastrointestinal tract, the rate of removal is rapid; as the drug is removed, so the rate of removal slows. It is a first-order, exponential process, and the iterative computer programs that try to assess absorption rate constants actually try to fit the drug removal process to a first-order function.

Lukas: At lunch, we were discussing the availability of a new method for sampling portal venous blood in man. A catheter is inserted into the portal vein via the umbilical vein at the time of an abdominal surgical procedure and left in place. Do you know of any data on bioavailability and absorption of digoxin in man using this technique?

Greenblatt: I don't know of any such data. I do think that probably too much has been made of first-pass metabolism; it applies only to drugs with very high hepatic clearances and certainly not to most digitalis glycosides. But I think assessment of portal vein concentrations of durgs — particularly of those with high hepatic clearance — is a good way to assess the absolute bioavailability.

Nyberg, Lund, Sweden: I would like to return to the oversimplification involved in assuming a constant absorption rate of digoxin. To avoid misunderstandings, I think I should mention that we calculated the amount of digoxin remaining in the alimentary canal at different times after administration. By fitting these data to a logarithmic decline, we found no overall first-order rate constant. Instead, the absorption rate differed strongly between sampling intervals, thus giving the mentioned profile of rate versus time.

Smith: Are there any other general comments or questions?

Marcus: One of the unsolved questions relating to bioavailability studies is whether or not there is an increased incidence of arrhythmias if you have a drug which has a very rapid dissolution rate and very rapid absorption. I wonder whether anyone here has an opinion or data relating to this problem.

Smith: That is a very important question, with very rapidly absorbed preparations now undergoing clinical testing. Is there anyone who would like to respond?

Grahame-Smith, Oxford: Could I follow up what you said about the absorption profile of the compounds. I have a very simple question that I would like to have your opinions about and that always puzzles me. We always tend to measure steady-state plasma levels. Now, most of the cardiac glycosides, particularly digoxin and digitoxin land up on a receptor at some point and I believe stay there for some time. Presumably, the concentration gradient between the receptor and the blood or the particular compartment that the digoxin is coming from is highest at the peak of the plasma level and at that time you would expect most of the molecules to go on to the receptor. So when you are studying bioavailability by looking at plasma levels, what is the really important function of the plasma level time curve in determining the therapeutic pharmacologic effect?

Shaw: Several studies, including the early clinical work of Wayne and of Gold, have shown that the peak response to digoxin occurs several hours after the time of the peak blood levels and in magnitude is very dampened compared to the shape of the blood level curve, so I think that we should not be too frightened by the size of the peak blood levels.

Dr. Barry Grimaldi and I looked at a few patients who were given 0.5 mg oral doses of liquid digoxin while on maintenance treatment and recorded the ECG over 6 h. We did not record any transient toxicity although some of these patients had previously been shown to have digitalis toxicity when they had steady-state plasma digoxin levels over 2 ng/ml.

18 Digoxin Pharmacokinetics and Their Relation to Clinical Dosage Parameters

H. J. DENGLER, G. BODEM, and H. J. GILFRICH

Introduction

The availability of isotope-labeled cardiac glycosides and the development of the radioimmunoassay made possible for the first time extensive studies on the pharmacokinetics of those cardioactive substances. In the meantime many data have been collected and have contributed to our basic knowledge of the metabolism and the disposition of these very important drugs. There is no doubt, however, that even before these data were available, cardiac glycosides were used very successfully in therapeutics and were handled by rather strict dosage schedules. Historically, they represented the first group of medicines for which — due to their long-lasting action and the need for continuous treatment — therapeutic regimes were established on a mathematical basis (Augsberger, 1951, 1954). It is particularly noteworthy that these calculations were performed without any knowledge of drug concentrations but by the use of analysis of clinical data on drug effects only; this is a rather modern approach.

In the mathematical derivations used by Augsberger in 1951 (which incidentally were intentionally presented in the form of footnotes in order "not to deter physicians") three main variables were used:

1. Absorption rate (Resorptionsquote)
2. Decay rate (Abklingquote)
3. "Vollwirkdosis," a term that is difficult to translate, defined as the body load of a cardiac glycoside at optimal therapeutic effect

It is the aim of this presentation to evaluate the relationship between these terms, which are widely used in therapeutics in European, and other countries, and the pharmacokinetic parameters emanating from modern studies with labeled glycosides or RIA-determinations.

It seems inappropriate to discuss again the absorption rate since it has been dealt with during this symposium under the heading of "Bioavailability." However, a word of reminder is in order: The fact that orally administered cardiac glycosides, or better, pharmaceutical preparations of cardiac glycosides are not too well "absorbed" or not fully "available" was widely recognized. The solutions, to the problem however, were different: in Germany the desire to create better available semi-synthetic glycosides led to the development of a number of new compounds (penta-acetyl digoxin, α-acetyldigoxin, β-acetyldigoxin, β-methyldigoxin); whereas in most other areas the improvement of the bioavailability of digoxin preparations by pharmaceutical means was attempted. The outcome was rather similar in regard to bioavailability and its relative consistency, with the exception that β-methyldigoxin is the digoxin derivative or preparation with the highest bioavailability (Dengler et al., 1970).

Experiments

The following experiments or considerations are aimed at the assessment of the parameters "decay rate" and "body load," in particular "body load at optimal effect" (Vollwirkdosis).

Single dose studies

The pharmacokinetic analysis of single i.v. dose experiments should ideally yield sufficient information to predict the multiple dose situation, provided that inductive and/or nonlinear processes are absent. Doherty (1968) reported in his early studies digoxin half-lives of ~33 h. Data from our own experiments, in which $12\alpha H^3$-digoxin was administered i.v., were described best (least square regression analysis) by a sum of three exponential terms (Dengler et al., 1973):

$$c\,(t) = 44200 \times e^{-6.8t} + 13900 \times e^{0.566t} + 2326 \times e^{-0.0125t}$$

(Eq.1)

The results of i.v. experiments by some authors using digoxin are listed below. The $T_{1/2}$ of the terminal slope, the number of subjects, days of sampling, and model used are given.

The first four studies were performed using tritium-labeled digoxin; in the two last, digoxin was analyzed by radioimmunoassay.

The results of both types of experiments agree sufficiently to indicate mean $T_{1/2}$ of the terminal slope following i.v. administration of digoxin of 40-50 h. Incidentally, this agreement of both methods makes it difficult to believe that such a large percentage of digoxin as reported by Lukas (1977) during this symposium should be present in form of metabolites.

Nonlinear processes can be operating at various stages of drug disposition. The following reports on two sets of data that present some evidence against nonlinear processes in the pharmacokinetics of digoxin.

a) Digoxin was given i.v. in three different dosages in a randomized order. As both the area under the curve and the cumulative urinary excretion are strictly linear to the doses it is likely that in the clinically used dosage range the kinetic behavior is not dose-dependent (Otten et al., 1976).

Table 18.1. Half-life ($T_{1/2}$), number of examined individuals (N), sampling time, kinetic model

	$T_{1/2}$ (h)	N	Sampling days	Model
Blankart & Preisig (1970)	43	10	10	3 Cpt.
Dengler et al., (1973)	53.3	7	4	3 Cpt.
Abshagen (1973)	42	4	6	—
Ohnhaus et al. (1975)	36-54	7	5	3 Cpt.
Koup et al. (1975)	44	8	2 (6)	2 Cpt.
Kramer et al. (1976)	45	5	3	3 Cpt.

b) We observed a number of mostly suicidal cases of digoxin intoxication, with blood levels as high as 20 ng/ml. Depending on the intoxicating dosage, digoxin blood levels were monitored using the radioimmunoassay up to 8 days. There was neither a tendency towards an altered half-life at high levels nor a break in the slope of the individual decay curves, again pointing to linear pharmacokinetics (Bodem et al., 1977).

Multiple-dose studies

a) A study was performed on eight patients 41-66 years old, who were digitalized for medical reasons (I° heart failure). They were on 0.25 mg digoxin daily for at least half a year and spent at least 3 days under controlled intake in the hospital. During this time predose-plasma levels and urinary collections were analysed daily by radioimmunoassay. On the last day of this regimen they received, together with the regular oral dose of nonlabeled digoxin, 50 µCi of tritium-labeled digoxin i.v. Then digoxin therapy was discontinued and plasma samples were drawn for as long as possible. Urine was collected for 12 days.

The results are summarized in Table 18.2. The overall recovery of immunore-active digoxin in the urine after discontinuation of digoxin treatment was 348 μg, i.e., 46% of the daily administered oral dose was excreted in the urine. Extrapolation of the cumulative urinary digoxin excretion to infinity had little influence on the final value. The T½ of urinary excretion was 51.2 h, this is in the same range as reported in single-dose experiments. The cumulative recovery of tritium label in urine was 75%. The average digoxin plasma level before discontiuation of the drug and before the last digoxin dose was 0.62 ng/ml.

Table 18.2. Long term Digoxin Study (N = 8, $\overline{x}$, s $\overline{x}$)

Digoxin urine % of dose/24 hrs	A urine $_o^{10d}$	$T_{0.5}$ in hours (urine)	H^3-recovery urine in % of dose 0-10 d
46.4 ± 3.3	348 μg ± 59	51.2 ± 2.1	75 ± 4.5

Dosage : 0.25 mg orally

Mean digoxin level (c_{ss}) before discontinuation 0.62 ng/ml

Table 18.3. Long-term Digoxin Study

Daily dosage	250 μg
Bioavailability factor	0.60
Available	150 μg
Recovered in urine (RIA digoxin) $_o^{10d}$	348 μg
Recovered in urine (H^3-activity)	75%
Present in body	465 μg
$D*/D_{avail}$	3.04

Calculated bioavailability data and body burden.

The patients received an oral dose of 250 μg per day. The bioavailibility factor for this particular pharmaceutical preparation was 0.6 (Table 18.3). Therefore, 150 μg of digoxin were available daily. Following discontinuation of digoxin intake

214

348 μg of digoxin were recovered in the urine during the next 12 days, representing practically the cumulative urinary excretion extrapolated to infinity.
Corrected for a 75% recovery of a tracer dose of H^3-digoxin, the total amount
of digoxin present in the body during equilibrium was calculated at 456 μg.
The ratio of the body stores of digoxin (D^*) to the daily available dose (D_{avail})
D^*/D_{avail} was 3.04 after, or 2.7 before the last oral dose.

There is no doubt that this calculation depends on a number of assumptions.
First of all it postulates that the recovery of the H^3-digoxin added to the regular
dose on the last day of intake equals that of digoxin already present in the body
and its different compartments. This may not be true, and there are indications
that the observed 75% recovery overestimates the true recovery in steady state.
Unfortunately, our calculation is particularly sensitive with respect to this value.
Assuming that the "true" recovery is 70% and 65%, the corresponding values for
the post-dose ratio D^*/D_{avail} will increase to 3.3 and 3.5, respectively.

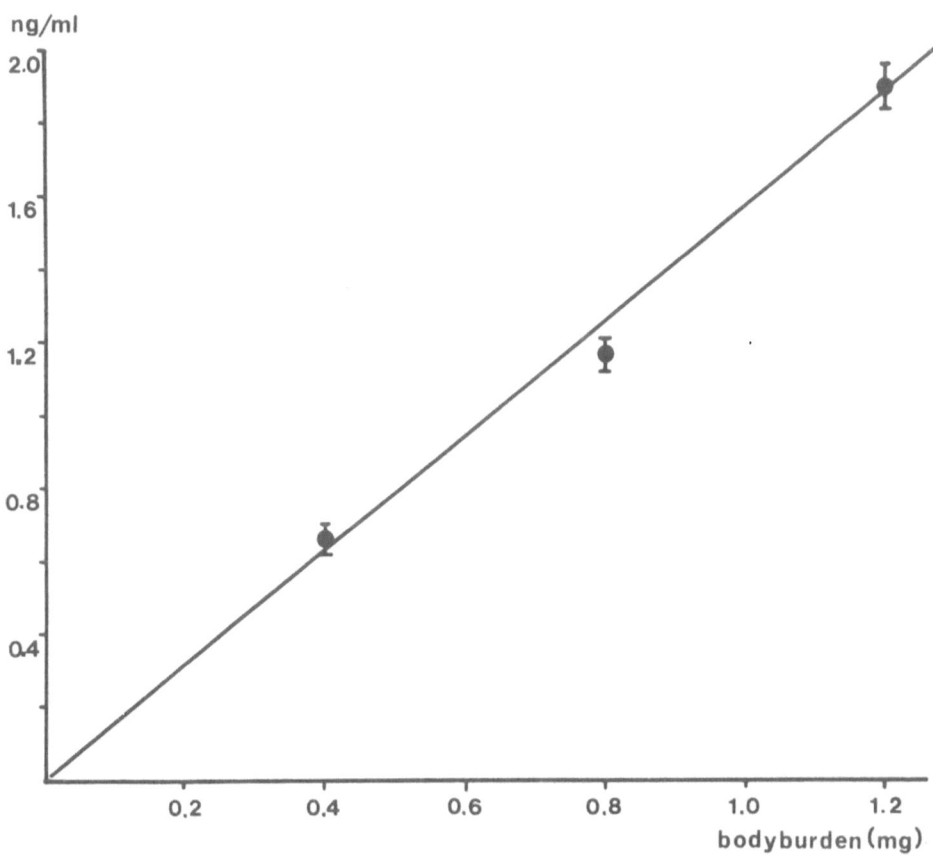

Fig. 18.1. Correlation of digoxin blood level and body burden of digoxin

The second part of this multiple-dose experiment consisted of the achievement of a given body load of digoxin and the correlation of this body load with the digoxin blood levels during steady state in the same individuals 3 weeks after the last dose of digoxin. Experimentally, the following protocol was used: The patients were given 0.4 mg digoxin i.v.. The body burden was increased up to 0.8 mg, 24 h later. Then after another 24 h the body burden was again increased up to 1.2 mg. The blood level of digoxin was determined 9 h after each dose. The adequate dosage for completing the body burden up to 0.8 and 1.2 mg was calculated by assuming identical elimination conditions, as shown after discontinuing the maintenance therapy in the first part of the study (cf. page 213).

A good correlation was established between the amount of digoxin present in the body and the pre-dose digoxin blood level, as shown in Figure 18.1. This diagram can be used as a sort of calibration curve connecting the digoxin blood level and digoxin body load.

b) At this stage the logical consequence was a study on a larger number of patients in which digoxin levels were monitored during digoxin maintenance therapy. In our experiment we emphasized strictly controlled digoxin administration. A daily oral maintenance dose of 0.5 mg digoxin (Lanicor) was given to 46 patients. The intake of the two tablets was checked daily by a doctor. Under this treatment at the 10th, 11th, and 12th day blood was drawn for determining digoxin by radioimmunoassay.

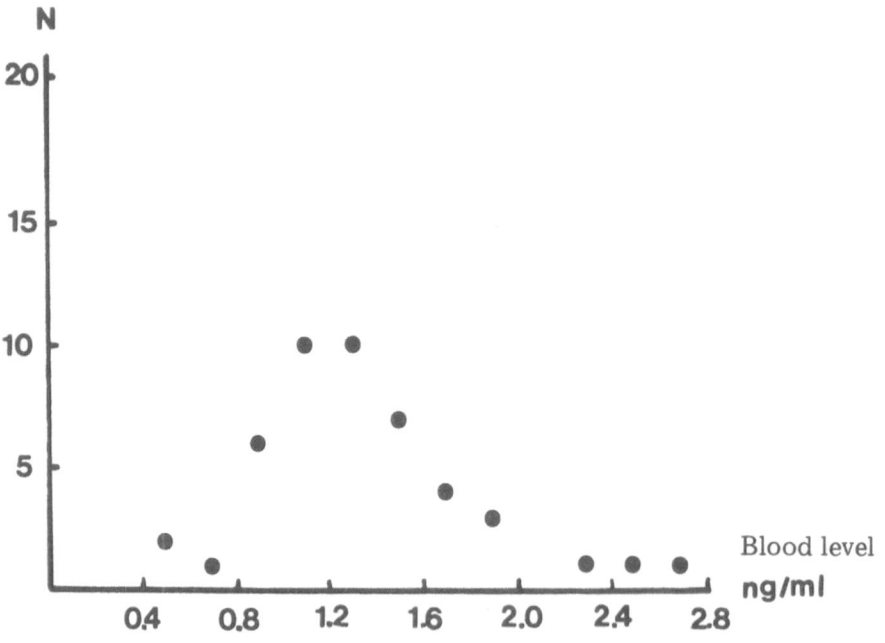

Fig. 18.2. Predose digoxin blood levels of 47 patients during treatment with 0.5 mg digoxin daily (controlled intake); N, number of patients

Figure 18.2 shows the predose serum digoxin levels in a histogram. A more refined analysis of these data is achieved in Figure 18.3, where the blood-level values of the 47 patients are plotted on a probability scale vs a log scale. It is evident that the blood-level values are not normal, but rather log-normal distributed like many other biologic parameters. The mean predose digoxin

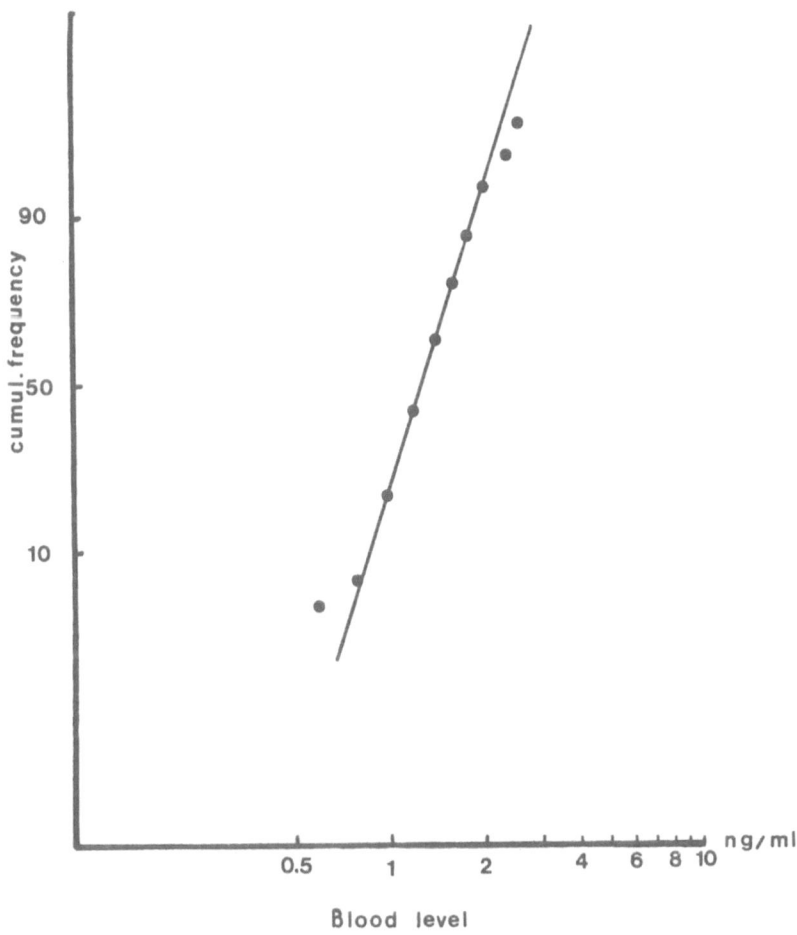

Fig. 18.3. Data of Figure 2 rearranged on a probability-v.-log scale

level (which is not identical with but close to the steady-state level of digoxin) was 1.25 ng/ml in this group of 47 hospitalized patients. According to the diagram shown in Figure 18.1 this blood level corresponds to a mean body load of 0.83 mg. Taking into account the bioavailability factor of 0.7 of this particular digoxin tablet (Lancior) the ratio D^*/D_{avail} equals 2.37 before and 2.72 after the last oral digoxin dose.

217

Theoretical interpretations

In the foregoing studies we attempted to calculate the amount of digoxin present in the body by a balance type of experiment. It should be possible, however, to predict the body load at steady state from pharmacokinetic parameters of single-dose experiments.

One of the methods of doing this is the "Eigenvector Decomposition Principle" (Müller-Schauenburg, 1973). This method is particularly useful when the experimental data are fitted by a polyexponential sum (Nüesch, 1973) as used in our digoxin experiments (Dengler et al., 1973) and recently recommended by J. Wagner (1976) not only for the fitting but also for the calculation of derived parameters, e.g., multiple-dose blood levels. The calculation of the body load D^* after the last dose (D^*_{max}) with the parameters of the digoxin single i.v. injection case is shown in Equation 2.

$$\text{Body load}$$

$$D^* = \frac{\text{max.}}{\text{body load}} = D \times \left[\frac{s_1/s}{1 - e^{-\gamma_1 t}} + \frac{s_2/s}{1 - e^{-\gamma_2 t}} + \frac{s_3/s}{1 - e^{-\gamma_3 t}} \right]$$

$$\text{f.i.} \quad D \times \left[0.03 + 0.12 + \frac{0.85}{0.26} \right] = 3.44\ D$$

$$\begin{array}{lll} \text{Decay rate} & = & \dfrac{D}{D^*} \quad \sim \quad 0.30 \quad \sim \quad 30\% \\ \text{(Abklingquote)} & & \end{array}$$

(Eq. 2) $S_{1,2,i} = \text{area of a } \gamma\text{-process}$ $s = AUC_0^\infty$

In this calculation D^*_{max} is identical with D^*_{max}/D_{avail}, as D_{avail} was assumed to be 1.0. Consequently D^*/D_{avail} before the last dose equals 2.44. When we compare the ratios of D^*/D_{avail} obtained either experimentally in multiple-dose experiments (predose: 2.7 and 2.4, respectively) or calculated by means of data of single-dose experiments (predose: 2.44) we notice a fair agreement between these values, which allow the estimation of the body load by multiplying the available dose with that factor. Furthermore, single dose experiments yield useful data, provided that curves are fitted with appropriate methods.

To study the so-called deep compartment, as postulated by Rietbrock et al., (1977) for digoxin kinetics, we performed the following calculation: to the 3-exponential sum describing the time course of H^3-digoxin blood level (cf. page 212) a fourth exponential term with a $T_{1/2}$ of 72 h and discernible at day 6 from the foregoing slope was added. In this case the total body load changes by only

218

about 10%, due to the fact that this final γ-process contains so little of the dosage. Notwithstanding the accumulation of digoxin in certain tissues, the amount stored there will not essentially influence the predominant half-life and will therefore not alter the body load to any relevant extent.

From Equation 2 the contribution of the single γ-terms to the final value of D^*/D_{avail} can be seen. Practically, the slow term (γ_3) only determines the value of D^*/D_{avail} and therefore the body load. Since s_3/s (area below the process with the rate constant of γ_3 /total AUC) approaches unity, the ratio D^*/D_{avail} can be approximated with $D^*/D_{avail} = 1/1 - e^{-\gamma_3 t}$, the well-known equation for the one-compartment model. In other words: the cumulative behavior of digoxin in the body can be predicted within certain limits of error with the rate constant γ_3 of the main segment of the plasma decay curve, provided this parameter is calculated with high precision.

In the first section (cf. page 213) predominant half-lives were determined in single i.v. dose experiments and after cessation of maintenance therapy and were found to be ~50 h. Equation 3 permits the estimation of the "predominant $T_{1/2}$" using the experimentally assessed body load or the ratio D^*/D_{avail}.

The reported value of the ratio D^*/D_{avail} 2.7 (cf. page 218) corresponds to a predominant $T_{1/2}$ of 53 h which agrees with experimental data measured by the analysis of plasma decay curves.

The decay rate (Abklingquote), which can be calculated as the ratio D_{avail}/D^* was about 30% day.

We also calculated the distribution volumes of digoxin, again by means of the γ-Process Decay Principle (Müller-Schauenburg, 1973). The data are summarized below, the value of total clearance was taken from Dengler et al. (1973).

Distribution volumes:

(1) Steady-state

$$V_{d(ss)} = Cl \left(\frac{S_1}{S} \times \frac{1}{\gamma_1} + \frac{S_2}{S} \times \frac{1}{\gamma_2} + \frac{S_3}{S} \times \frac{1}{\gamma_3} \right)$$

assuming Cl = Clearance = 102.5 ml/min

$V_{d(ss)}$ = 421 liters

S_i = areas of the γ-processes

(2) Pseudodistribution equilibrium

$$V_{d\gamma} = \frac{Cl}{\gamma_3} = 492 \text{ liters} \qquad f = 0.85$$

(3) Central volume = 22 liters

The distribution volume at steady-state — 421 liters — is smaller than the distribution volume at pseudodistribution equilibrium by a factor of 0.85. The central volume was 22 liters, thus being half of the value found by Kramer et al. (1976). This may be due to less frequent sampling early in our experiments.

Conclusions

Finally, we have to assess the validity of the pharmacokinetic data and to compare them with clinically used dosage parameters. We exclude the discussion of "absorption rates," as this is dealt with elsewhere during this symposium.

1. The predominant plasma $T_{1/2}$ of digoxin in the age group of 50-70 years is 50-55 h.

2. This value was obtained both in acute experiments with single-dose i.v. injection of digoxin as well as in the post-maintenance period, as reported here on page 215. Calculation of $T_{1/2}$ by means of the experimentally determined body load points again to a $T_{1/2}$ of 50 h.

3. The ratio D^*/D_{avail} is about 2.5 with good agreement between the experimentally determined values of 2.4 and 2.7 and the one calculated from single dose experiments, 2.44.

4. The decay rate (Abklingquote) is about 30% per day and, therefore, moderately higher than assumed by clinical investigations and quoted widely in the literature (20%).

5. The body load at optimal therapeutic effect (Vollwirkdosis) is definitely lower than almost generally assumend in the past. (about 2.0 mg). There is no doubt that many patients with heart failure are well controlled with a daily oral dose of 0.5 mg. Assuming a bioavailability factor of 0.7, the resulting body load is 0.5 x 0.7 x 2.5, which equals 0.88 mg. The corresponding figures for 0.25 and 1.0 mg are 0.44 and 1.75, respectively.

6. The relationship between digoxin blood levels and pharmacodynamic effects depends on the particular digitalis effect under observation. This is illustrated by Figures 18.4 and 18.5 which depict different experimental situations. The first study (Gilfrich, 1974) relates the velocity of posteriorwall movement assessed by echocardiography with digoxin levels. It demonstrates a very good correlation. The second study (Otten et al., 1976) shows the decay of the digoxin body burden after a single dose of 1.5 mg, and the disappearance of digoxin-induced ECG parameters. Undoubtedly, the disappearance of the digoxin effect on the ST segment and the T-wave follows a different time curve from that of plasma (and heart muscle) levels of digoxin.

7. During maintenance therapy, the day-to-day variation of predose digoxin blood levels and of urinary digoxin excretion (Bodem et al., 1977) show fluctuation to an extent that cannot be explained by analytic or other experimental errors. These are not yet convincingly explained and need further investigation.

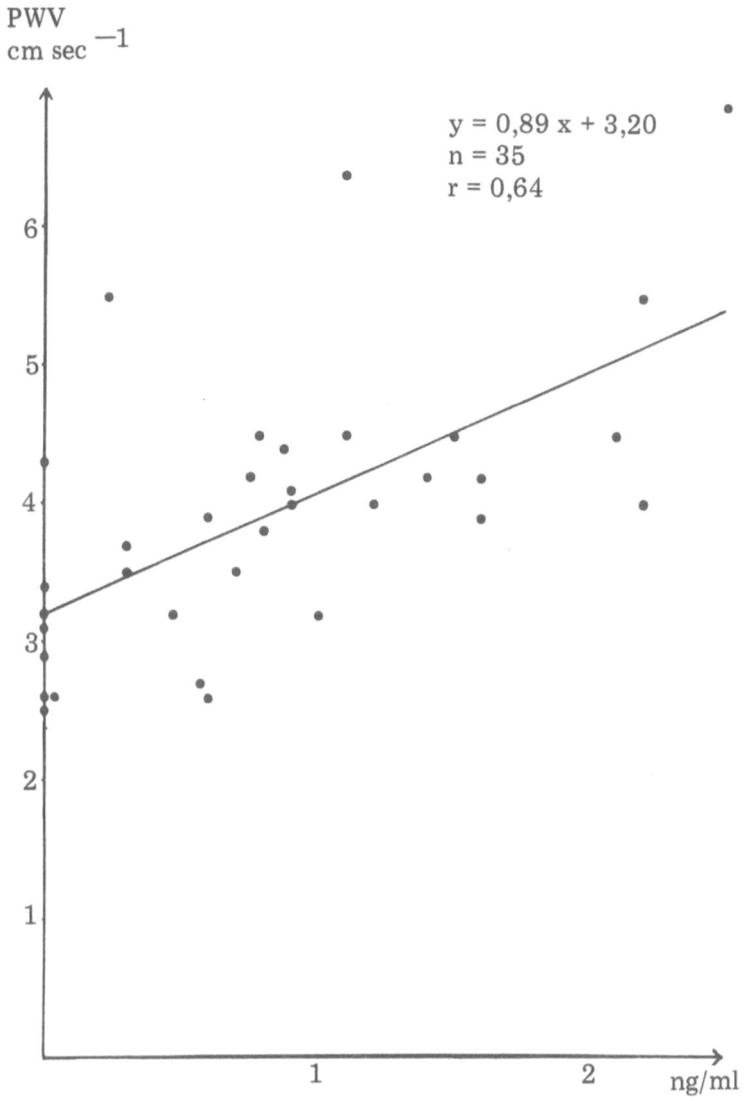

Fig. 18. 4. Velocity of posterior-wall movement (determined by echocardiography) vs. digoxin blood levels (Gilfrich, 1974)

Pharmocokinetic studies with digoxin and other cardiac glycosides have added many numerical data to our knowledge of digoxin disposition and have to a certain extent corrected our clinical dosage schedules, particularly in cases of renal failure. Nevertheless, we admire the correctness of clinical observations in digitalis therapy and of the derivation of numerical data by Augsberger.

221

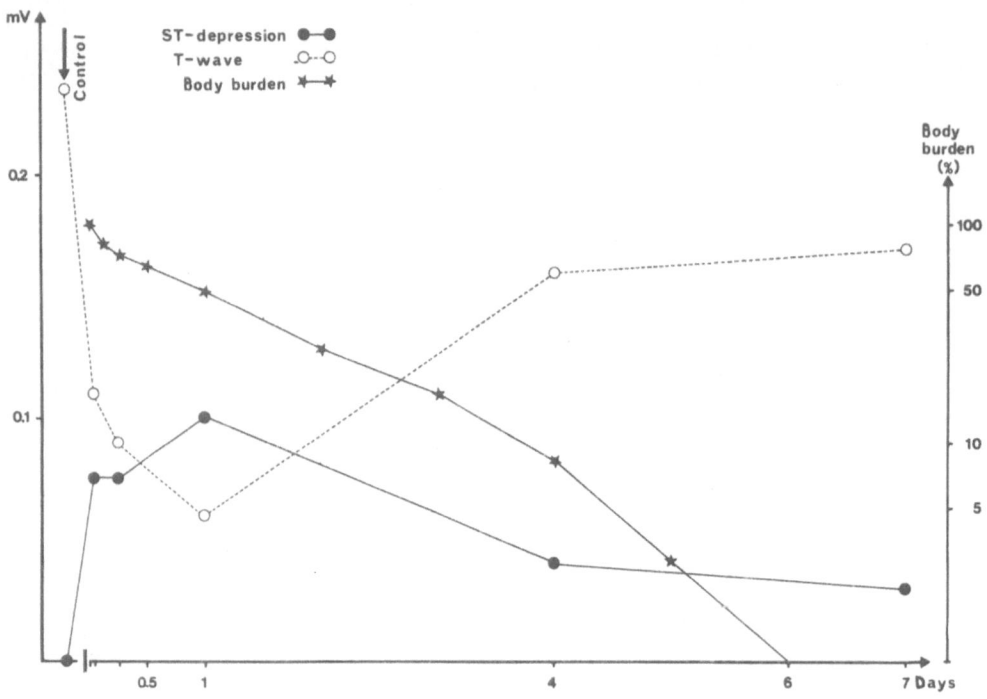

Fig. 18.5. Decay of body burden and changes of electrocardiographic parameters during exercise after a single i.v. dose of 1.5 mg digoxin in nine patients (Otten et al., 1976)

References

Abshagen, U.: Stoffwechsel und Kinetik von Digoxin, α-Acetyldigoxin, β-Acetyl-digoxin and β-Methyldigoxin beim Menschen. Habilitationsschrift. Berlin, 1973

Augsberger, A.: Quantitatives zur Therapie mit Herzglykosiden. I. Mitt.: Die Variabilität von Glykosidbedarf und -toleranz. Med. Welt 20, 1471 (1951)

Augsberger, A.: Quantitatives zur Therapie mit Herzglykosiden. Kumulation und Abklingen der Wirkung. Klin. Wschr. 32, 945 (1954)

Blankart, E., Preisig, R.: Pharmakokinetische Grundlagen der Digitalisdosierung: Eine Studie an Probanden. Schweiz. Med. Wschr. 100, 2163 (1970)

Bodem, G., Gilfrich, H.J., Aulepp, H., Ochs, H.R., Dengler, H.J.: Klinische und pharmakokinetische Untersuchungen zur Digitalisintoxikation. Klin. Wschr. 55, 13 (1977)

Bodem, G. et al.: Unpublished Results

Dengler, H.J., Bodem G., Wirth, K.: Pharmacokinetic and Metabolic Studies with β-Methyldigoxin. Cardiovasc. Res. 4, World Congr. Cardiol. 119 (1970)

Dengler, H.J., Bodem, G., Wirth, K.: Pharmacokinetic and Metabolic Studies with Lanatosid C, α- and β-Acetyldigoxin and Digoxin in Man. Proc. 5th Int. Congr. Pharmacol. 3, 112 (1970)

Dengler, H.J., Bodem, G., Wirth, K.: Pharmakokinetische Untersuchungen mit ^{3}H-Digoxin und ^{3}H-Lanatosid C beim Menschen. Arzneim. Forsch. (Drug Res) 23, 64 (1973)

Doherty, J.E.: The Clinical Pharmacology of Digitalis Glycosides. A Review. Am. J. Med. Sci. 255, 382 (1968)

Gilfrich, H.J.: Untersuchungen zur Pharmakokinetik und Pharmakodynamik von Digoxin während chronischer Anwendung. Habilitationsschrift, 1974

Koup, J.R., Greenblatt, D.J., Jusko, W.J., Smith, Th.W. and Koch-Weser, J. Pharmacokineties of Digoxin in Normal Subjects after Intravenous Bolus and Infusion Doses. J. Pharmacokin. Biopharm. 3, 181 (1975)

Kramer, W.G., Lewis, R.P., Cobb, T.C., Forester, W.F. Jr., Visconti, J.A., Wanke, L.A., Boxenbaum, H.G., Reuning, R.H.: Pharmacokinetics of Digoxin: Comparison of a two- and a three-Compartment Model in Man. J. Pharmacok. Biopharmaceutics 2, 299 (1976)

Lukas, D.S.: Studies of the Metabolism of Digoxin and Digitoxin Using Double Isotope Dilution Derivative Methods. These proceedings

Müller-Schauenburg, W.: A New Method for Multi-compartment Pharmacokinetic Analysis: The Eigenvector Decompostition Principle. Europ. J. Clin. Pharmacol. 6, 203 (1973)

Nüesch, E.: Proof of the General Validity of Dost's Law of Corresponding Areas. Europ. J. Clin. Pharmacol. 6, 33 (1973)

Ohnhaus, E.E., Vozeh, S., Nüesch, E.: Untersuchungen zur Resorption von Digoxin bei Patienten mit dekompensierter Rechtsherzinsuffizienz. Schweiz. Med. Wschr. 105, 1782 (1975)

Otten, H., Ochs, H.R., Konen, W., Bodem, G.: Beziehung zwischen dem Abklingen der Digoxinwirkung im Belastungs-Elektrokardiogramm und pharmakokinetischen Parametern. Verhandlg. Deutsche Gesellsch. f. Innere Med. 82, 1720 (1976)

Rietbrock, N., Kuhlmann, J. Vöhringer, H.F.: Pharmakokinetik von Herzglykosiden und Klinische Konsequenzen. Berliner Seminar 1, Verlag Dr. Straube, Erlangen, 1977

Wagner, J.G.: Linear Pharmacokinetic Models and Vanishing Exponential Terms: Implications in Pharmacokinetics. J. Pharmacok. Biopharmaceutics 4, 395 (1976)

Discussion

Greenblatt: Just to bring up this annoyance about volumes of distribution. I think the term $V_{d(ss)}$ is really a misnomer because with "volume of distribution" we would like it to represent a volume term which relates concentration in the blood to amount of drug in the body. Even during chronic dosage $V_{d(area)}$ is the most universally applicable volume of distribution because after distribution of the most recent dose is complete, then $V_{d(area)}$ is that number. In fact $V_{d(ss)}$ serves as an actual apparent volume of distribution only during continuous intravenous infusion. $V_{d(area)}$ is the most useful volume of distribution even though it's always slightly larger — usually trivially so — than the so-called $V_{d(ss)}$

Dengler: I just wanted to show that the volume of distribution at steady state is not as easy to calculate as many people believe, and the demonstrated equation gives us the opportunity to judge the contribution of different compartments and processes to this factor. For practical purposes, I definitely agree with your statements.

Nyberg: The use of the distribution volume at steady state, $V_{d(ss)}$, is not limited to constant-rate infusions. During maintenance dose treatment, it may be desirable to define an "average plasma concentration," i.e., the plasma concentration during the dosage interval containing both the initial α- and the terminal β-phase. In this situation, $V_{d(ss)}$ is the correct volume parameter.

Greenblatt: After any given dose, whether it is the first dose or at steady state, the volume of distribution changes all the time. The volume of distribution is not the static thing that we would like it to be, it's kinetic and it changes all the time. I think we have to be aware of this limitation in our interpretation of volumes of distribution.

Dengler: I think there is some gap between the theoretic discussion as you already stated and the practical application. I showed the equations on page 219 particularly with respect to considerations about a possible deep compartment. There is no question about the existence of a deep compartment, as Dr. Kuhlmann has shown, but it is so small that it has no discernibel influence on the predominant half-life. In fact I do not believe that any drug is eliminated from the body finally with one slope.

Kuhlmann, Berlin: I agree with your statement that the deep compartment for digoxin is small and influences the elimination rate only in the terminal phase. Fourteen days after cessation of multiple doses, 93%-95% of the total amount of glycoside is excreted.

Dengler: A good example is the retina which stores some psychotropic drugs. The retina of the eye is a deep compartment for these drugs with a long elimination half-life. But does it really make sense to include it in any calculations regarding blood levels?

Grahame-Smith, Oxford: I am very interested in the deep compartment that you speak about because one tends to think of compartment first in mathematic terms, which don't mean anything to me at all, and then in anatomic terms, which may not mean a great deal either. But then one can also think of compartments in biochemical terms when maybe they do mean something. An analysis I saw recently of digoxin pharmacokinetics by Whiting and Sumner from Manchester looked at the third deep compartment and it has quite a high rate constant in and a rather low rate constant out. Is this the same for your compartment, and were you able to analyze that? I'll tell you why I'm interested in that, it signifies to me some kind of binding site with a reasonably high affinity which lets go of the drug rather slowly. This could possibly be the sodium-potassium ATPase and this compartment may, therefore, be of some pharmacologic importance.

Smith: What kind of a dissociation rate constant are you proposing for sodium-potassium ATPase?

Grahame-Smith: No many hours, but certainly half an hour.

Erdmann, München: I would like to comment on this. If you incubate a (Na^+ + K^+)-ATPase preparation with radioactively labeled digoxin and after the binding process has reached equilibrium, you wash off all the nonreceptor-bound digoxin (i.e., you isolate the digoxin-receptor complex), then you add unlabeled digoxin in excess, and you get a rather quick dissociation of the digoxin-receptor complex. The digoxin will dissociate from the membrane preparation with a half-life of some 45 min under those conditions.

Smith: What is the source of your membrane preparation?

Erdmann: I am talking about human cardiac cell membranes. If you do this experiment in a more natural way, which is completely different, that is where you dilute the concentration of the digoxin in the serum continuously. You can do this in an experiment, too, by just diluting the volume, let's say, for instance you dilute it 1:5, 1:10, 1:100, and so on, then in fact you will get different experimental curves. You actually get a curve linear dissociation. I mean, it does not come off in a straight line, if you plot the dissociation in a semilogarithmic way. So, the dissociation of digoxin from the specific binding sites does not follow first-order, but it follows second-order kinetics, and the half-life is somewhere around 14-16 h. It does depend, however, on the dilution. If you dilute the digoxin-receptor complex only 1:2, the half-life is about let's say 30 h or so. If you dilute it 1:10, it is just about 16 h. The so-called deep compartment may, in fact, be the rather slow dissociation of the cardiac glycoside from the receptors. And if there are glycoside binding sites with different affinities for the drug, then there should be several "compartments."

Smith: Could some of this heterogeneity be related to rebinding of material that's dissociated from one receptor and reassociated with another?

Erdmann: We have not looked at this suspected rebinding to the cardiac glycoside receptor yet, but we have done so with the β-receptor and so has Bob Lefkovitz (Lefkovitz, 1975) and he does not think so, either. He has published some experiments showing that there is no rebinding — but this, of course, would take too much time to discuss now.

Reference

Lefkovitz: B.: Biochem. Biophys. Res. Commun. 64, 1160 (1975)

19 Clinical Interpretation of Serum Concentrations of Cardiac Glycosides[1]

T. W. Smith, L. H. Green, and G. D. Curfman

As we enter the third century of the clinical use of digitalis, numerous challenges regarding the optimal use of this class of drugs continue to confront the clinician as well as the research investigator. The narrow margin between therapeutic and toxic doses of digitalis, resulting in a high incidence of digitalis toxicity in clinical practice, has stimulated the development of improved methods for measuring the circulating concentrations of these drugs. To facilitate the interpretation of serum or plasma cardiac glycoside concentrations in the clinical context, we review in the present communication the available data regarding the relationship between serum concentrations of cardiac glycosides and their therapeutic and toxic effects.

Available techniques for measurement of circulating cardiac glycoside concentrations have been reviewed recently (Smith and Curfman, 1977; Smith and Haber, 1973) and will not be dealt with in detail. It should be noted, however, that there are numerous pitfalls associated with each of the assay techniques. With the proliferation of commercial kits for the measurement of cardiac glycoside concentrations, it is particularly important for the clinician and clinical investigator to be certain that the values reported by the laboratory are accurate. Moreover, uncertainty can be introduced if sufficient time has not elapsed since the last previous dose to allow full equilibration of the drug between intravascular and peripheral compartments. In practice, a safe time for sampling of serum or plasma is 6 h or more after the last cardiac glycoside dose.

Rationale for Use of Serum Digitalis Concentration Measurements

Several lines of evidence suggest a potentially useful relationship between serum digitalis concentrations and the pharmacologic effects of these drugs. First, and probably most important, both inotropic and toxic effects of cardiac glycosides are known to be dose-related phenomena. A large number of studies have shown increasing serum digitalis concentrations with increasing dosage (Smith and Haber, 1973) so that at least a statistical correlation should exist between plasma levels and clinical state. Second, at least in the case of digoxin, a number of investigators

1 This work was supported in part by NHLI Award HL-18003, NHLI Program Project Award HL-19259, and NHLI National Research Service Award HL-07049.

have documented a relatively constant ratio of digoxin concentration in serum or plasma to that in the myocardium, both in experimental animal studies and in human subjects (Doherty et al., 1967; Güllner et al., 1974; Härtel et al., 1976; Carroll et al., 1973). The argument can be raised, however, that since total myocardial concentration includes both nonspecifically bound drug and drug specifically bound to myocardial receptors, the total myocardial digitalis content cannot be assumed to bear a direct relationship to effect. Third, evidence continues to accumulate indicating that $(Na^+ + K^+)$-ATPase is involved in at least some of the actions of cardiac glycosides (Schwartz, 1976). This plasma membrane enzyme transport system is influenced by cardiac glycosides only when these agents are present at the outer cell surface (Caldwell and Keynes, 1959; Hoffman, 1966). Thus, at least one putative cardiac glycoside receptor is in close proximity to the extracellular compartment, providing a basis for the translation of plasma concentration to myocardial effect. Finally, experimental studies have documented a highly significant relationship between serum digoxin concentration and electrophysiologic effect on the heart (Barr et al., 1972).

Clinical Studies

The literature continues to expand rapidly with respect to clinical studies of the relationship between serum or plasma digitalis concentrations and clinical effect. Although many techniques have been used to perform the measurements, there is substantial agreement regarding concentrations of digoxin and digitoxin in patients receiving usual maintenance doses of these drugs. Table 19.1 summarizes digoxin concentration data from a number of studies, involving well in excess of 1000 patients. Mean serum or plasma digoxin concentrations in groups of patients without evidence of toxicity average about 1.4 ng/ml. As would be expected, increasing digoxin doses or decreasing renal function are correlated with higher mean serum levels. Table 19.1 also provides data concerning the relationship between serum digoxin concentration and cardiac toxicity. Mean serum digoxin concentrations tend to be two to three times higher in patients with clinical evidence of digoxin toxicity, and the difference in mean levels was statistically significant in the vast majority of studies. It must be emphasized, however, that overlap of levels between groups with and without evidence of toxicity was observed in most series and tends to be more pronounced in prospective, blind studies than in retrospective studies (Beller et al., 1971; Smith et al., 1969; Smith and Haber, 1970)

Analogous data correlating serum digitoxin concentrations with clinical state are summarized in Table 19.2. Although levels average about tenfold higher than those of digoxin because digitoxin is significantly bound to serum proteins, patients with clinical evidence of toxicity again have mean levels about two times higher than those without evidence of toxic response. As in the case of digoxin, substantial overlap occurs in levels among groups of patients with and without evidence of toxicity despite the statistically significant differences in mean serum concentrations. It is thus apparent from our own experience, as well

Table 19.1. Serum or plasma digoxin concentrations: patients with and without toxicity

		Mean concentration		
Source	Method	Patients without toxicity	Patients with toxicity	Statistical significance
Beller et al.	Radioimmunoassay	1.0	2.3	Yes
Bertler and Redfors	[86]Rb uptake	0.9	2.4	Yes
Bertler et al.	[86]Rb uptake	1.4	3.1	Yes
Brooker and Jelliffe	Enzymatic displacement	1.4	3.1	Yes
Burnett and Conklin	ATPase inhibition	1.2	5.7	Yes
Carruthers et al.	Radioimmunoassay	1.21	2.76	
Chamberlain et al.	Radioimmunoassay	1.4	3.1	Yes
Evered and Chapman	Radioimmunoassay	1.38	3.36	Yes
Fogelman et al.	Radioimmunoassay	1.4	1.7	No
Grahame-Smith and Everest	[86]Rb uptake	2.4	5.7	Yes
Hayes et al.[a]	Radioimmunoassay			
Infants		2.8	4.4	Yes
Children		1.3	3.4	Yes
Hoeschen and Proveda	Radioimmunoassay	0.8-1.3	2.8	Yes
Howard et al.	Radioimmunoassay	0.97	0.91	No
Huffman et al.	Radioimmunoassay	1.49	3.32	Yes
Iisalo et al.	Radioimmunoassay	1.2	3.1	Yes
Johnston, et al.	Radioimmunoassay	1.1	2.2	Yes
Krasula et al.[a]	Radioimmunoassay			
Infants		1.7	3.6	Yes
Children		1.1	2.9	Yes
Lader et al.	Radioimmunoassay	1.1	2.2	Yes

	Method			
McCredie et al.[a]	Radioimmunoassay			
Infants		3.45	—	—
Children		1.41	3.81	Yes
Morrison et al.	Radioimmunoassay	0.76	3.35	Not stated
Oliver et al.	Radioimmunoassay	1.6	3.0	Yes
Park et al.	Radioimmunoassay	1.1	3.8	Yes
Ritzmann et al.	^{86}Rb uptake	1.2 (median)	5.5 (median)	Yes
Scherrmann and Bourdon	Radioimmunoassay	1.37	4.58	Yes
Singh et al.	Radioimmunoassay	2.91	4.79	Yes
Smith et al.	Radioimmunoassay	1.3	3.3	Yes
Smith and Haber	Radioimmunoassay	1.4	3.7	Yes
Weissel et al.	Radioimmunoassay	1.38	2.97	Yes
Whiting et al.	Radioimmunoassay	1.4	3.5	Yes
Zeeger et al.	Radioimmunoassay	1.6	4.4	Yes

[a] Pediatric patients.

Table 19.2. Serum or plasma digitoxin concentrations: patients with and without toxicity

Source	Method	Mean concentration		
		Patients without toxicity	Patients with toxicity	Statistical significance
Beller et al.	Radioimmunoassay	25	34	Yes
Bentley et al.	ATPase inhibition	23	39	Yes
Brooker and Jelliffe	Enzymic displacement	31.8	48.8	Not stated
Chiche et al.	Radioimmunoassay	25.4	57	Yes
Dessaint	Radioimmunoassay	26.8	96	Yes
Hillestad et al.	[86]Rb uptake	16.8	28.3	Yes
Lukas and Peterson	Double isotope dilution derivative	20	43-67 (range)	Not stated
Morrison and Killip	Radioimmunoassay	25 (0.1 mg/day) 44 (0.2 mg/day)	53	Yes
Peters et al.	Radioimmunoassay	28.8	56.4	Yes
Rasmussen et al.	[86]Rb uptake	16.6	48.7	Not stated
Ritzmann et al.	[86]Rb uptake	20.5 (median)	37 (median)	Yes
Smith	Radioimmunoassay	17	34	Yes

as that of a number of other investigators, that no serum concentration of digoxin or digitoxin can be selected that cleanly separates toxic and nontoxic states in the usual clinical setting. Judgement of optimal doses and serum concentrations must be based to a large extent on assessment of each individual clinical response.

Factors Influencing Individual Sensitivity to Cardiac Glycosides

Many factors must be taken into account in the clinical evaluation of individual responses to cardiac glycosides. Detailed assessment of the studies referred to in Tables 19.1 and 19.2 clearly indicates that symptoms consistent with digitalis intoxication frequently occur at serum levels below the range usually associated with toxicity, while other patients are without evidence of toxicity at serum levels usually considered to be in the "toxic" range. In some instances, discrepancies between serum concentration and clinical state may be due to analytic problems in the assay procedure, but variation in individual sensitivity to the effects of cardiac glycosides for any given dose has long been appreciated on clinical grounds. Even though serum concentration data take into account variations in absorption and excretion of digitalis glycosides by individual patients, factors including metabolic derangements, interactions with other drugs, severity and type of underlying heart disease, and certain concurrent disease states further modify individual response at any given serum concentration of the drug. These factors are of considerable clinical importance and deserve the attention of the clinician in every instance where the cardiac glycoside dosage regimen is in question.

Before discussing factors that may influence individual sensitivity, it should be noted that assigning a diagnosis of digitalis toxicity is at best a difficult and imprecise undertaking. Digitalis toxicity is usually inferred from the occurrence of certain characteristic disturbances of cardiac impulse formation or conduction that disappear when the drug is withdrawn (Beller et al., 1971). Other systemic symptoms such as nausea, anorexia, and neurologic manifestations further support the diagnosis. Neither these systemic complaints nor the occurrence of rhythm disturbances are specific for digitalis excess, however, and these phenomena commonly occur independently with a variety of disease states including congestive heart failure, myocardial ischemia, respiratory insufficiency, and acid-base or electrolyte imbalance. Discontinuation of cardiac glycosides simultaneous with effective management of such underlying problems may lead to a mistaken diagnosis of digitalis toxicity. With these limitations in mind, factors influencing individual sensitivity to cardiac glycosides will now be considered. These are summarized in Table 19.3.

Electrolyte and Acid-Base Disturbances

Disturbances of potassium homeostasis are well-known to influence the action of cardiac glycosides (Enselbert et al., 1950; Sampson et al., 1963). Cardiac uptake of digoxin is influenced by serum potassium concentrations, tending to increase with decreasing serum potassium. This appears to be related to an allosteric ef-

Table 19.3. Factors influencing individual sensitivity to the
toxic effects of digitalis glycosides

---

1. Type and severity of underlying cardiac disease

2. Serum electrolyte derangements
    a) Hypokalemia or hyperkalemia
    b) hypomagnesemia
    c) hypercalcemia
    d) hyponatremia

3. Acid-base imbalance

4. Concomitant drug administration
    a) Anesthetics
    b) Catecholamines and sympathomimetics
    c) Antiarrhythmic agents

5. Thyroid status

6. Renal function

7. Autonomic nervous system tone

8. Respiratory disease

---

fect on cardiac glycoside binding to $(Na^+ + K^+)$-ATPase (Schwartz et al., 1968). In addition, hypokalemia has a direct arrhythmogenic effect (Fisch, 1973). Atrioventricular conduction disturbances can be caused or exacerbated by markedly elevated serum potassium concentrations (Davidson and Surawicz, 1967). Diuretic therapy, insulin administration or carbohydrate loading, renal disease, and acid-base imbalance are all potential causes of significant alterations in potassium homeostasis and deserve particular attention in patients receiving digitalis.

Disturbances in serum concentrations of other electrolytes may also influence individual sensitivity to digitalis. Administration of magnesium ion is known to suppress digitalis-induced arrhythmias (Ghani and Smith, 1974), and there is evidence that digitalis-induced K^+ efflux from the myocardium is reduced by magnesium ion (Neff et al., 1972). Hypomagnesemia has been reported to predispose to digitalis toxicity (Seller et al., 1970). Although the epidemiologic importance of magnesium depletion as a cause of enhanced digitalis sensitivity remains unresolved, the frequent occurrence of Mg^{2+} depletion with diuretic therapy should keep the clinician alert to the potential interactions of magnesium ion and digitalis.

Hypercalcemia tends to increase ventricular automaticity, and this effect may be additive to or even synergistic with the effect of digitalis (Nalbandian et al., 1957) Conversely, patients with digitalis intoxication have been reported to respond successfully to calciumchelating agents (Surawicz, 1959-60). Although animal experiments have yielded somewhat variable results (Lown et al., 1960; Smith et al., 1939), one should be alert to the possibility of reduced digitalis tolerance when treating patients with elevated serum calcium levels or when administrating calcium intravenously to digitalized patients. Experimental hyponatremia has been shown to reduce myocardial binding of digoxin (Harrison and Wakim, 1969) but the significance of this phenomenon within the range of serum sodium concentrations encountered clinically is uncertain.

There are reports in the literature that acid-base disturbances may cause enhanced digitalis sensitivity. Certainly, alterations in potassium homeostasis that follow shifts in hydrogen ion concentration will affect myocardial binding of digitalis glycosides. Although disturbances of acid-base balance have not been convincingly shown to precipitate digitalis toxicity in clinical studies, the experimental literature suggests caution in the use of digitalis in patients with marked acidosis or alkalosis.

Drug Interactions

Concomitant administration of other drugs can affect the response to digitalis glycosides through several mechanisms. Certain drugs including cholestyramine, neomycin, antacids, and kaolin-pectin can decrease gastrointestinal absorption of digoxin, thereby altering the serum and myocardial levels ultimately achieved (Binnion 1973; Koch-Weser, 1975). Other drugs including phenobarbital, phenytoin, and phenylbutazone have been reported to diminish serum digoxin concentrations in some patients, presumably through induction of hepatic drug-metabolizing enzyme systems (Koch-Weser, 1975). The magnitude of this effect at usual therapeutic doses of these drugs is often insignificant, but in certain sensitive subjects may lead to inadequate levels of digitalization. Diuretic agents potentially enhance the occurrence of digitalis toxicity both through diminution in glomerular filtration rate and through the various electrolyte disturbances that result from their use.

Underlying Heart Disease

Listed first in Table 19.3 because of its overriding importance is the type and severity of underlying heart disease. This is dramatically demonstrated in otherwise healthy subjects who ingest massive doses of cardiac glycosides with suicidal intent (Smith and Willerson, 1971). Toxicity in this clinical setting is usually apparent as disturbances of atrioventricular conduction or sinoatrial exit block, rather than by enhanced automaticity of ectopic pacemakers as commonly seen in patients with underlying heart disease. Common causes of heart disease including ischemia, cardiomyopathy, and valvular lesions may result in an electrophysiologic instability that will decrease tolerance to cardiac glycosides. The more severe and advanced the heart disease, the more likely the appearance of myocardial fibrosis, focal ischemia, and ventricular dilatation with stretching of Purkinje fibers and thus an attendant increase in automaticity.

The issue of altered cardiac glycoside sensitivity in acute myocardial infarction remains controversial. Although animal models of experimental myocardial infarction have shown some reduction in digitalis tolerance, recent clinical studies suggest that the incidence of arrhythmias is not appreciably increased at moderate drug doses (Lown et al., 1972; Rahimtoola and Gunnar, 1975). Nevertheless, there is a consensus that digitalis has no well-defined role in the management of acute myocardial infarction without congestive heart failure (Karliner and Braunwald, 1972) or supraventricular tachyarrhythmias. Additional research is clearly needed to define the subclasses of patients who may be at increased risk, or who stand to gain increased benefit from the judicious use of cardiac glycosides.

Concurrent Disease States

Several concurrent disease states have been reported to be associated with an increased frequency of digitalis toxicity. Some authors have considered advanced age itself as a risk factor, but recent studies suggest that diminished glomerular filtration rate with age is probably responsible for most of the apparent increase in cardiac glycoside sensitivity (Evy et al., 1969). Renal failure, particularly in patients requiring hemodialysis, can also cause considerable difficulties in the clinical use of digitalis, both because of the decreased elimination of digoxin with reduced renal function, and also because of the electrolyte shifts that are prone to occur in this patient group.

Thyroid disease has long been known to exert a substantial effect on cardiac glycoside sensitivity. Hypothyroid patients tend to have a prolongation of serum digoxin half-life while hyperthyroid patients tend to have relatively reduced serum digoxin levels (Doherty and Perkins, 1966). Changes in elimination rates and distribution space may both contribute to these alterations (Croxson and Ibbertson, 1975; Doherty and Perkins, 1966). In addition, there is a strong clinical impression that thyrotoxic patients tend to respond less well to any given serum concentration of digoxin, particularly with regard to the slowing of ventricular response in the presence of supraventricular tachyarrhythmias such as atrial fibrillation or atrial flutter. Conversely, there is an impression that hypothyroid patients have a higher incidence of overt toxicity at cardiac glycoside concentrations that are usually well tolerated.

The autonomic nervous system plays an important part in the mediation of the effects of cardiac glycosides, both through the parasympathetic (Moe and Farah, 1970) and sympathetic arms of the autonomic nervous system. It therefore follows that underlying autonomic tone will have an important influence on the clinical response to digitalis. Recent research suggests a permissive or even triggering role for the nervous system in digitalis-induced arrhythmias characterized by increased automaticity of ectopic pacemakers (Gillis et al., 1972). Thus, drugs or clinical states that influence sympathetic or parasympathetic tone might be expected to cause alterations in apparent digitalis sensitivity.

The relationship of cardiac glycoside sensitivity to pulmonary disease is a particularly complex area. Recent epidemiologic studies (Beller et al., 1971; Chung, 1969; Mason et al., 1971) indicate that the frequency of digitalis toxicity is increased in patients with pulmonary disease. Clinical reports are often difficult to interpret, however, since respiratory failure and hypoxemia frequently provoke arrhythmias indistinguishable from those associated with digitalis toxicity (Hudson et al., 1973). Indeed, it is by no means certain that the association of lung disease with an increased incidence of digitalis toxicity can be attributed to the disturbance in pulmonary function, but rather may result from such associated predisposing factors as excessive cardiac glycoside dosage, hypokalemia, or concomitant renal failure. Although many patients with acute or chronic respiratory disease receive sympathomimetic drugs that might tend to enhance the likelihood of ectopic rhythm disturbances suggestive of digitalis toxicity, there is no direct evidence of such a deleterious effect from these agents. Experimental studies of the influence of arterial oxygen tension suggest that hypoxemia is more likely to predispose to toxicity when present acutely than when it is a chronic condition (Beller and Smith, 1973; Beller et el., 1975). It is apparent that further investigation is needed to define the epidemiology of digitalis intoxication in patients with pulmonary disease, with particular attention to the type of lung disease present, the severity and chronicity of disease, and the influences of factors such as hypoxemia, hypokalemia, and sympathetic tone.

Conclusion

A review of our own clinical experience and of the available literature indicates that knowledge of serum cardiac glycoside concentrations can be quite helpful to the clinician in defining the state of digitalization and in assigning certain broad probabilities to the likelihood of digitalis intoxication. However, the multiplicity of factors that bear on individual response to digitalis require that serum concentration data be interpreted in the overall clinical context and that an isolated serum concentration not be used as a sole arbiter of the presence or absence of toxicity. Finally, much further investigation is needed to define the clinical states likely to result in increased or decreased cardiac glycoside sensitivity. Appropriate identification of such subgroups will greatly facilitate the use of serum digitalis concentration measurements to improve the risk:benefit ratio of this important class of drugs.

References

Barr, I., Smith, T.W., Klein, M.D., Hagemeijer, F., Lown, B.: Correlation of the electrophysiologic action of digoxin with serum digoxin concentration. J. Pharmacol. Exp. Ther. 180, 710 (1972)

Beller, G.A., Smith, T.W.: Digitalis toxicity during acute hypoxia in intact conscious dogs. J. Pharmacol. Exp. Ther. 193, 963 (1973)

Beller, G.A., Smith, T.W., Abelman, W.H., Haber, E., Hood, W.B., Jr.: Digitalis intoxication: a prospective clinical study with serum level correlations. N. Engl. J. Med. 284, 989 (1971)

Beller, G.A., Giambo, S.R., Saltz, S.B., et al.: Cardiac and respiratory effects of digitalis during chronic hypoxia in intact conscious dogs. Am. J. Physiol. 229, 270 (1975)

Binnion, P.F.: Absorption of different commercial preparations of digoxin in the normal human subject, and the influence of antacid, anti-diarrheal, and ion-exchange agents. In: Storstein, O. (ed): Symposium on Digitalis. Oslo: Gyldendal Norsk Forlag 216-224 (1973)

Caldwell, P.C., Keynes, R.D.: The effect of ouabain on the efflux of sodium from a squid giant axon. J. Physiol. (Lond.) 148, 8 P (1959)

Carroll, P.R., Gelbart, A., O'Rourke, M.F., Shortus, J.: Digoxin concentrations in the serum and myocardium of digitalized patients. Aust. N.Z.J. Med. 3, 400 (1973)

Chung, E.K.: Digitalis-induced cardiac arrhythmias: A report of 180 cases. Jap. Heart J. 10, 409 (1969)

Croxson, M.S., Ibbertson, H.K.: Serum digoxin in patients with thyroid disease. Br. Med. J. 1975/III, 566

Davidson, S., Surawicz, B.: Ectopic beats and atrioventricular conduction disturbances. Arch. Intern. Med. 120, 280 (1967)

Doherty, J.E., Perkins, W.H.: Digoxin metabolism in hypo- and hyperthyroidism: studies with tritiated digoxin in thyroid disease. Ann. Intern. Med. 64, 489 (1966)

Doherty, J.E., Perkins, W.H., Flanigan, W.J.: The distribution and concentration of tritiated digoxin in human tissues. Ann. Intern. Med. 66, 116 (1967)

Enselbert, C.D., Simmons, H.C., Mintz, A.A.: The effects of potassium upon the heart, with special reference to the possibility of treatment of toxic arrhythmias due to digitalis. Am. Heart J. 39, 713 (1950)

Ewy, G.A., Kapadia, G.G., Yao, L., et al.: Digoxin metabolism in the elderly. Circulation 39, 449 (1969)

Fisch, C.: Relation of electrolyte disturbances to cardiac arrhythmias. Circulation 47, 408 (1973)

Ghani, M.F., Smith, J.R.: The effectiveness of magnesium chloride in the treatment of ventricular tachyarrhythmias due to digitalis intoxication. Am. Heart J. 88, 621 (1974)

Güllner, H.-G., Stinson, E.B., Harrison, D.C., Kalman, S.M.: Correlation of serum concentrations with heart concentrations of digoxin in human subjects. Circulation 50, 653 (1974)

Gillis, R.A., Raines, A., Sohn, Y.J., et al.: Neuroexcitatory effects of digitalis and their role in the development of cardiac arrhythmias. J. Pharmacol. Exp. Ther. 183, 154 (1972)

Harrison, C.E., Jr., Wakim, K.G.: Inhibition of binding of tritiated digoxin to myocardium by sodium depletion in dogs. Circ. Res. 24, 263 (1969)

Härtel, G., Kyllönen, K., Marikallio, E., Ojala, K., Manninen, V., Reissell, P.:

Human serum and myocardial digoxin. Clin. Pharmacol. Ther. 19, 153 (1976)

Hoffman, J.F.: The red cell membrane and the transport of sodium and potassium. Am. J. Med. 41, 666 (1966)

Hudson, L.D., Kurt, T.L., Petty, T.L., et al.: Arrhythmias associated with acute respiratory failure in patients with chronic airway obstruction. Chest 63, 661 (1973)

Karliner, J.S., Braunwald, E.: Present status of digitalis treatment of acute myocardial infarction. Circulation 45, 891 (1972)

Koch-Weser, J.: Drug interactions in cardiovascular therapy. Am. Heart J. 90, 93 (1975)

Lown, B., Black, H., Moore, F.D.: Digitalis, electrolytes and the surgical patient. Am. J. Cardiol 6, 309 (1960)

Lown, B., Klein, M.D., Barr, I., et al.: Sensitivity to digitalis drugs in acute myocardial infarction. Am. J. Cardiol. 30, 388 (1972)

Mason, D.T., Zelis, R., Lee, G., et al.: Current concepts and therapy of digitalis toxicity. Am. J. Cardiol. 27, 546 (1971)

Moe, G.K., Farah, A.E.: Digitalis and allied cardiac glycosides. In: Goodman, L.S., Gilman, A. (ed.): The Pharmacological Basis of Therapeutics, New York: The MacMillan Company 1970, pp. 677-708

Nalbandian, R.M., Gordon, S., Campbell, R., et al.: A new quantitative digitalis tolerance test based upon the synergism of calcium and digitalis. Am. J. Med. Sci. 233, 503 (1957)

Neff, M.S., Medelssohn, S., Kim, K.E., et al.: Magnesium sulfate in digitalis toxicity. Am J. Cardiol. 29, 377 (1972)

Rahimtoola, S.H., Gunnar, R.M.: Digitalis in acute myocardial infarction: Help or hazard? Ann. Intern. Med. 82, 234 (1975)

Sampson, J.J., Albertson, E.C., Kondo, B.: The effect on man of potassium administration in relation to digitalis glycosides with special reference to blood serum potassium, the electrocardiogram and ectopic beats. Am. Heart J. 26, 692 (1963)

Schwartz, A.: Is the cell membrane NaK-ATPase enzyme system the pharmacologic receptor for digitalis? Circulation Res. 39, 2 (1976)

Schwartz, A., Matsui, H., Laughter, A.H.: Tritiated digoxin binding to $(Na^+ + K^+)$-ATPase: possible allosteric site. Science 160, 323 (1968)

Seller, R.H., Ramirez, O., Brest, A.N.: Digitalis toxicity and hypomagnesemia. Am. Heart J. 79, 57 (1970)

Smith, P.K., Wintler, A.W., Hoff, H.E.: Calcium and digitalis synergism: The toxicity of calcium salts injected intravenously into digitalized animals. Arch. Intern. Med. 64, 322 (1939)

Smith, T.W., Haber, E.: Digoxin intoxication: the relationship of clinical presentation to digoxin concentration. J. Clin. Invest. 49, 2377 (1970)

Smith, T.W., Haber, E.: The current status of cardiac glycoside assay techniques. In: Tai, P.N., Goodwin, J.F. (eds.): Progress in Cardiology. Philadelphia: Lea and Febiger, 1973, Vol. II

Smith, T.W., Curfman, G.D.: Radioimmunoassay of cardiac glycosides. In: Strauss, H.W., Pitt, B. (eds.): Cardiovascular Nuclear Medicine, 2nd ed. St. Louis: Mosby Co. 1977

Smith, T.W., Willerson, J.T.: Suicidal and accidental digoxin ingestion: report of five cases with serum digoxin level correlations. Circulation 44, 29 (1971)

Smith, T.W., Butler, V.P., Jr., Haber, E.: Determination of therapeutic and toxic serum digoxin concentrations by radioimmunoassay. N. Engl. J. Med. 281, 1212 (1969)

Surawicz, B.: Use of the chelating agent, EDTA, in digitalis intoxication and cardiac arrhythmias. Prog. Cardiovasc. Dis. 2, 432 (1959-60)

Discussion

Binnion, Philadelphia: There is one little comment I'd like to make about the second slide. There is some controversy about that "midwife and the witch" business — and some people think that she was in fact a beautiful lady of the aristocracy. I don't know whether this is true or not. I don't know whether Dr. Shaw would like to reply to those comments about digitalization at all.

Shaw: I don't think there is a great deal of disagreement on this point. I was trying to emphasize yesterday that, particularly when beginning digitalization in a new patient, one should work upward, starting off with a dose which is on the safe side and increasing it later if needed. It's obviously true that digitalis has a beneficial effect in cardiac failure and this can be usefully added to that of the diuretics.

Binnion: I think the point of Dr. Shaw is a good point for the younger doctors in hospital - that maybe the use of intravenous digitalis should be forbidden them, just to teach them that you can take it orally and it is absorbed promptly.

v. Bernuth, Ulm: I would like to make a comment. It is certainly well-known to you but has not been mentioned here yet that what one considers to be a therapeutic digoxin level is higher in newborns than in older children and adults. Figure 1 shows the plasma digoxin concentrations in premature and mature newborns, infants, children, and adults. As you can see, the digoxin concentration in premature and mature newborns is higher than in the other age groups. This difference is statistically significant and has been found by other investigators also. In the groups of premature and mature newborns there are several with clinical evidence of digoxin intoxication. The plasma digoxin concentration in these infants was 5 ng/ml or higher. On the other hand, there are some infants with plasma digoxin concentrations between 3 and 5 ng/ml without any evidence of intoxication. It appears that infants may be more tolerant to digitalis than adults, but it is not the place here to speculate why this might be so.

Binnion: I think your nice columns imply of course that you can define digitalis toxicity. That's not a very easy thing to do.

Smith: I agree with Dr. Binnion, and I think that's one of the reasons why there is inevitably overlap. There is no arrhythmia that's unique to digitalis toxicity, and any set of criteria that are set up will be met by many patients who have

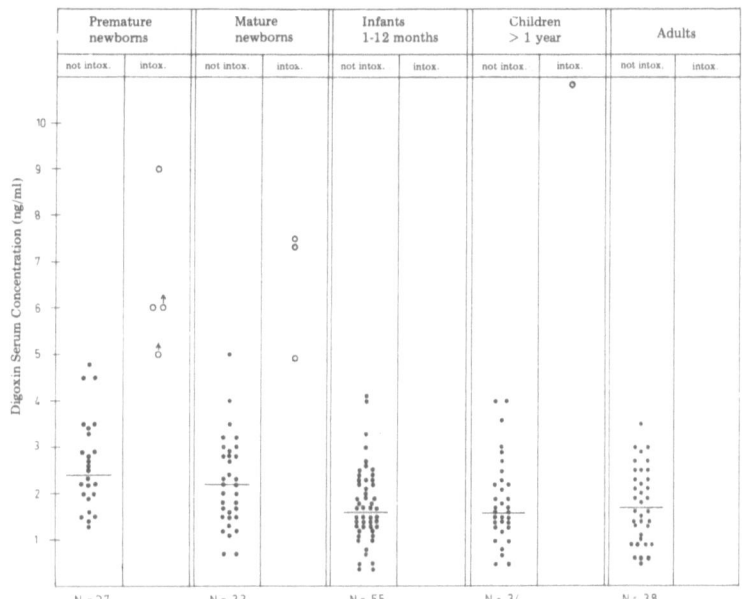

Fig. 1

never received digitalis. The data shown are in keeping with our own experience. Experimental work also bears out the fact that there are differences in volume of distribution and differences in pharmacodynamics as a function of age.

Lukas: It has impressed me that we have really learned how to use digoxin properly only within the past few years. Formerly 1.5 mg of digoxin, even when given intravenously, was considered the dose to initiate therapy. That is now, I think, considered a fairly large dose. What is your notion about the appropriate dosage to achieve a therapeutic body pool and plasma concentration of the drug in a patient, both for the intravenous and the oral route?

Smith: Our own recommendations are below 1.5 mg as an initial loading dose, although many patients will require that ultimately. Much depends on exactly what patients you are talking about. There are certainly patients in whom rapid digitalization is indicated, but with the availability of potent diuretics, in many clinical settings large doses of digitalis given intravenously in a short period of time are not required to effectively manage the immediate crisis. Our own recommendations are to start out with a loading dose more of the order of 0.75 mg, and to proceed with the digitalization in small increments given intravenously as indicated by the clinical response.

Lukas: Would you adjust the oral dose on the basis of our knowledge of bioavailability? If 0.75 mg is given orally as one bolus or in divided doses of 0.5 mg and 0.25 mg given 4-6 h apart, what plasma concentration would you see 24 h later? I am talking about patients now, because your own data show that there is a difference between patients and normal subjects.

Smith: My guess would be that at the end of 24 h you probably would see levels of about 1 ng/ml or so in most of those patients.

Reissell, Helsinki: I think that we are too much emphasizing the value of the serum digoxin determinations. Though they are valuable in many patients, the majority should be treated by monitoring carefully the clinical state of the patient. This is the method which the cardiologists in my clinic are practicing.

Kramer, Göttingen: We are glad to have the routine determination of plasma digoxin and we are convinced that it gives us some information about our digoxin therapy. I noticed that in one of your slides the concentration in the plasma water instead of the total plasma concentration was displayed. The concentration in the plasma water, however, is more likely to correlate with myocardial concentration. My question concerns therapy control using digitoxin, which is highly bound to plasma proteins. The unbound fraction of digitoxin is only about 6%, but by radioimmunoassay we measure the total plasma concentration. Do you think that the measurement of the total plasma concentration is of any help, if there is a high interpatient variation in the unbound fraction as found in uremic patients?

Smith: I think Dr. Lukas can answer that better than anyone else. His equilibrium dialysis studies show that about 3% of the drug is free, 97% is bound, but it takes a large change in the serum albumin concentration to vary that percentage much. There are higher average total digitoxin levels in general in patients who show manifestations of toxicity. The kinds of toxicity we are talking about are dose-related phenomena. If you double a patient's digitoxin dose, other things being equal, you will just about double the serum level. I would, therefore, consider it likely that in a large group of patients there would be some statistical correlation between serum levels and clinical state. I would agree with you if you are saying that you can't simply take a single level in a given patient and say whether that indicates toxicity or the lack of it. I think that you can only interpret that issue in patient groups and assign broad probabilities. A patient with a serum digitoxin level of 75 ng/ml is more likely to be toxic than a patient with a serum level of 25 ng/ml, I think we'd all agree on that. I think we probably also agree that the patient with the level of 75 ng/ml might conceivably have no manifestations of toxicity whereas the patient with the serum level of 25 ng/ml might. There is a lot of overlap in the intermediate range.

Lukas: I think the issue is pretty clear. There is no question that plasma albumin concentration must be considered in interpreting the significance of a plasma concentration of an agent that is heavily bound to plasma albumin. Although even with a decrease of serum albumin concentration to 1 g/100 ml, digitoxin is 92% bound, nevertheless the ratio of bound to free drug is decreased. With 97% binding at a serum albumin level of 4 g/100 ml the ratio is 97:3 or approximately 32:1 for bound to free drug, whereas at 92% binding, the ratio is approximately 11:1. So for the same free concentration of drug, the plasma concentration of digitoxin at the lower albumin concentration will be only one-third of that at the normal plasma albumin content. With digoxin, the effect of albumin concentration on plasma level is less important because digoxin is bound only to the extent of 23%. I believe that Dr. Storstein has some data on protein binding in the serum of digitoxin and some metabolites of digitoxin.

Storstein, Norway: I'll be talking about the protein binding of digitoxin later on. I would just like to say that the protein binding of the digitoxin metabolites are all above 90% and the protein binding of the digoxin metabolites are lower than digoxin.

Belz, Koblenz: Dr. Smith, I was very much impressed by your slide showing the decrease of coronary blood flow after the injection of digoxin and by your interpretation about a possible influence on the coronary arteries mediated by the CNS. I don't know if you are aware of the results of Dr. Fleckenstein in Freiburg. He has shown in experiments with strips of coronary arteries that very low concentrations of cardiac glycosides, equivalent to so-called therapeutic levels in man, increase the tone. Would you like to comment on that?

Smith: The work of Powell and his colleagues at the Massachusetts General Hospital in Boston also indicates that bolus doses of digoxin in an isolated canine gracilis muscle preparation causes increases in vascular resistance. These are rapid, transient increases, whereas more sustained pressor responses seem to have, in that preparation, an important neural component. There is a direct effect on the vascular tone in all probability, but at least some data suggest that this may be a fairly rapid transient and that the more sustained pressor effects may have a CNS component which can be blocked with α-blockers.

20 Assessment of Digoxin Action by a Pharmacodynamic Biochemical Method

D. G. GRAHAME-SMITH and J. K. ARONSON

The sequence of events occurring between the administration of digoxin and its therapeutic effect is very complex. The generalities of this sequence which can be applied to any drug are depicted in Figure 20.1. Ignoring bioavailability and patient compliance, the sequence can be broken down into three phases:

Pharmacokinetic Phase

This phase involves the processes of absorption, distribution, metabolism, and excretion, and it may be described through the measurement of drug and metabolite concentrations in blood and/or urine over periods of time after dosing. By study of the pharmacokinetic phase, interindividual variability and variations in individual status in regard to the factors determining the pharmacokinetic phase can be defined , and there is no doubt about the contribution such studies have made to our understanding of the clinical pharmacology of digoxin. Measurements of plasma (or serum) digoxin concentrations have been widely used as an aid in the diagnosis of digitalis toxicity. Recently, Ingelfinger and Goldman (1976) have critically reviewed these studies, and they concluded that the place of plasma glycoside concentrations in the diagnosis of digitalis toxicity has not yet been properly defined. A major difficulty lies in the considerable overlap between "therapeutic" and "toxic" concentrations, and it is evident that in many studies there is a wide range of concentrations apparently compatible with a "therapeutic" status.

Most workers studying the plasma level of digoxin in relationship to its therapeutic or toxic effects use for this measurement blood taken 6 h or more after the last dose, i.e., during the phase of slow decline of the plasma level. However, no one as far as I know, has satisfactorily explained the pharmacologic or therapeutic significance of the characteristics of the time course of the plasma concentrations after doses of digoxin. Do we know the exact meaning in pharmacodynamic terms of the "6 h plus" plasma level after a dose of digoxin? Is the amount of digoxin bound to tissues more influenced by peak plasma levels? This is important because digoxin is not an "on-off" drug as far as its interaction with receptors is concerned — it is a "hit and stick" drug, i.e., binds to receptors from which is dissociates rather slowly. It was this unease with the pharmacologic

242

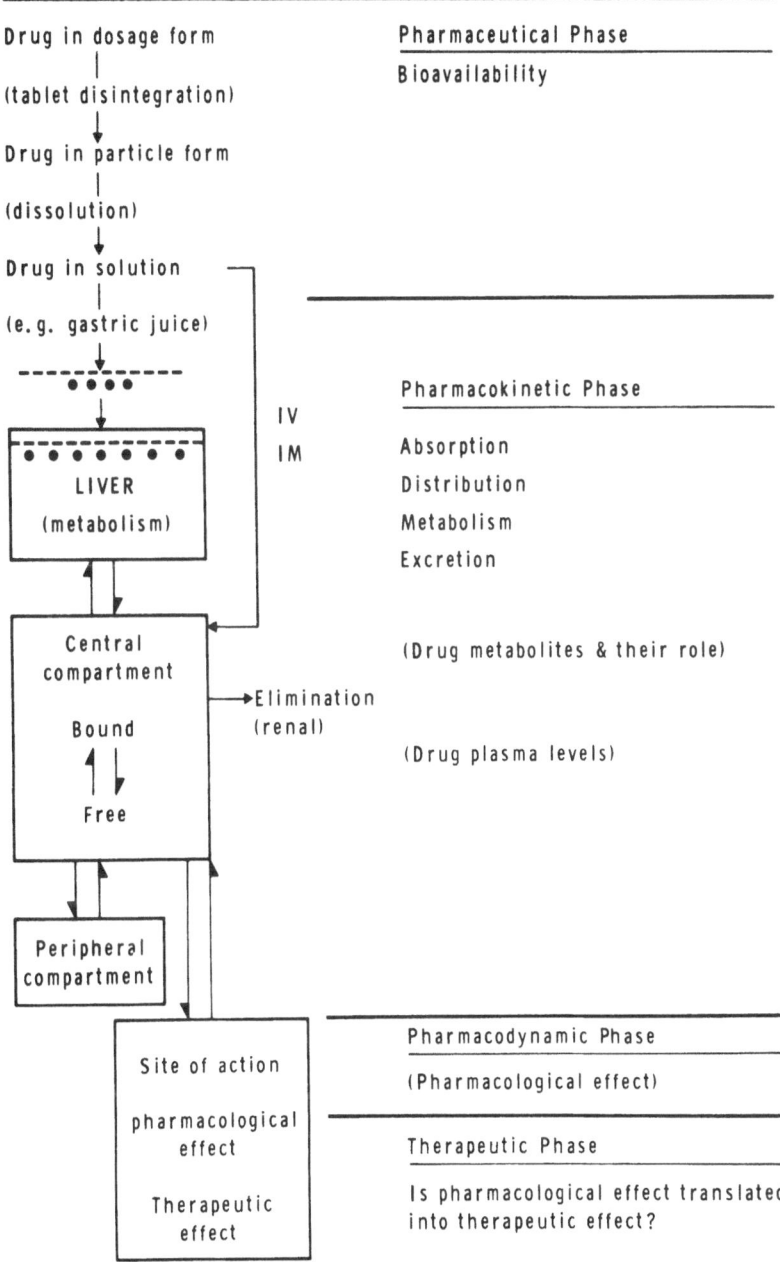

Fig. 20.1. Processes occuring on drug administration

meaning of spot plasma digoxin levels which caused us to initiate studies of a pharmacodynamic nature on digoxin in the clinical situation.

Pharmacodynamic Phase

Theoretically, as one passes from the pharmacokinetic phase into the pharmaco-dynamic phase, the first consideration is the extent of binding of digoxin at specific cardiac sites, of which we have little knowledge in the clinical situation. Nor are we in a position yet to measure in the heart the pharmacologic effect through which the electrophysiologic or positive inotropic effects are mediated, whether these be mediated through inhibition (Schwartz, Lindenmayer and Allen, 1975) or stimulation (Cohen, Dant and Noble, 1975) of the $(Na^+ + K^+)$-ATPase.

We chose, for practical reasons, to explore the effect which cardiac glycosides have to inhibit the ability of red cells to transport potassium inward (Schatzmann, 1953). We have used ^{86}Rubidium (^{86}Rb) to monitor this process as ^{86}Rb has a longer radioactive half-life than ^{42}K (Wang and Willis, 1965) and is handled like ^{42}K by the red cell (Love and Burch, 1953). Inhibition of ^{86}Rb uptake by red cells has previously been used to assay plasma digoxin concentrations (Grahame-Smith and Everest, 1969).

We have, therefore, studied the ability of the individual patients' own red blood cells to accumulate ^{86}Rb both before and during therapy with digoxin and com-pared it with the patients' plasma digoxin concentration and with the clinical response to the drug. This leads to consideration of the therapeutic phase.

Therapeutic Phase

Because of the need for a simple and precise means of monitoring clinical pro-gress in the initial stages of assessing this technique, we have chosen to study the response of the ventricular rate in patients with atrial fibrillation being treated with digoxin, and we have compared this situation with patients being treated with the drug for other supraventricular arrhythmias. These results are presented here. Recently, we have instituted studies on the relationship between plasma digoxin levels, inhibition of ^{86}Rb uptake by the patients' own red cells, and the positive inotropic effect as measured by systolic time intervals, in patients in heart failure in regular rhythm.

Methods

The detailed methodology is described elsewhere (Aronson, Grahame-Smith, Hallis, Hibble and Wigley, 1977). Briefly, before digoxin therapy is begun, blood is taken and plasma separated from red cells which are washed in iso-osmotic sa-line. ^{86}Rb uptake is then measured in these washed cells (washing does not re-move digoxin-H^3 from binding sites on red cell membranes nor does it reverse the effect of digoxin to inhibit ^{86}Rb uptake by the cells once digoxin is bound). Blood samples are taken sequentially during digoxin therapy; plasma digoxin measurements are made in the separated plasma and ^{86}Rb uptake by the red cells estimated. All blood samples during digoxin therapy were taken at least 6 h after doses of digoxin.

Effect of Digoxin on Patients' Red Cell [86]Rb Uptake

In Figure 20.2 are shown the results on a patient with atrial fibrillation and depicted are:
1. Digoxin dosage
2. The time course of the effect of digoxin therapy on red cell ^{86}Rb uptake
3. The time course of the slowing of ventricular rate
4. The plasma digoxin levels

The fall in red cell ^{86}Rb uptake is gradual and usually reaches its nadir within 5 days. Within 3-11 days, however, ^{86}Rb uptake begins to fluctuate. In Figure 20.2 it should be noted that the fall in ventricular rate is accompanied para passu by a fall in red cell ^{86}Rb uptake.

Figure 20.3 shows the case of a patient in whom, during the first 3 days of digoxin therapy, there was no fall in red cell ^{86}Rb uptake and no fall in the ventricular rate (the patient was in atrial fibrillation). By day 4 there was some slowing of the ventricular rate and at this time, for the first time, a clear fall in red cell ^{86}Rb was seen. The dose of digoxin was then increased, the ventricular rate fell further, as did the red cell ^{86}Rb uptake. On day 7, the atrial fibrillation converted to sinus rhythm and on day 10 fluctuations in ^{86}Rb uptake began.

The Relationships Among Plasma Digoxin Concentrations, Red Cell [86]Rb Uptake, and the Therapeutic Response

A total of 15 patients have been studied to date. In 13 of these, there was a definite fall in ^{86}Rb uptake of the patients' own red cells, prior to the onset of fluctuations. In the two patients who had no fall in red cell ^{86}Rb uptake, one had no clinical response, treatment was stopped, and sinus rhythm achieved with DC cardioversion. The other patient responded to therapy without a change in red cell ^{86}Rb uptake.

The patients have been divided into three groups for analysis. Group I consisted of those who remained in atrial fibrillation throughout. Group Ia were those who were initially in atrial fibrillation but who reverted to sinus rhythm during treatment. Group II were those with other supraventricular tachyarrhythmias.

Figure 20.4 shows the relationship between the percentage change in individual values of red cell ^{86}Rb uptake from the pretreatment values and the percentage change in ventricular rates at corresponding times. The values shown are those obtained before the onset of fluctuations in red cell ^{86}Rb uptake and in the case of patients in Group Ia, before reversion to sinus rhythm. Figure 20.5 shows the relationships between plasma digoxin concentrations and the percentage changes in ventricular rates.

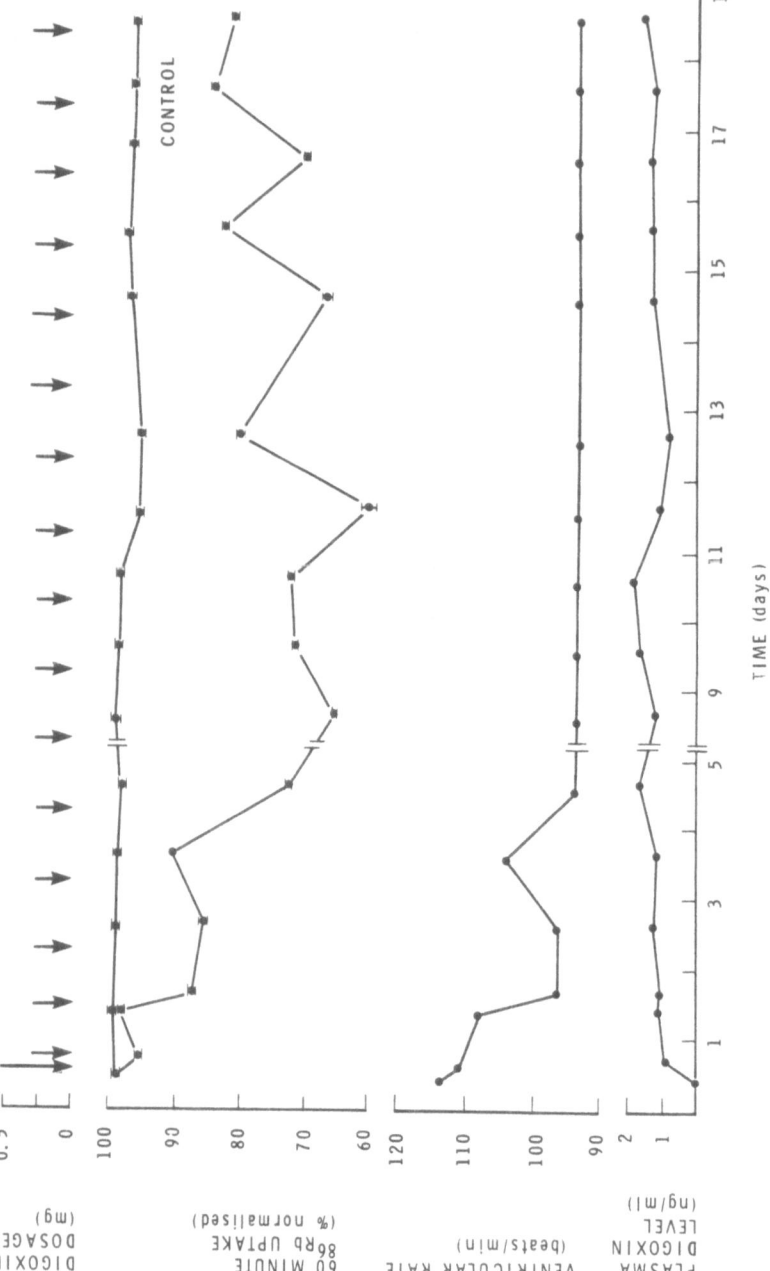

Fig. 20.2. Patient with atrial fibrillation. Response of ventricular rate, change in RBC ^{86}Rb uptake, and plasma digoxin concentrations during digitalization with Digoxin. For description see text

246

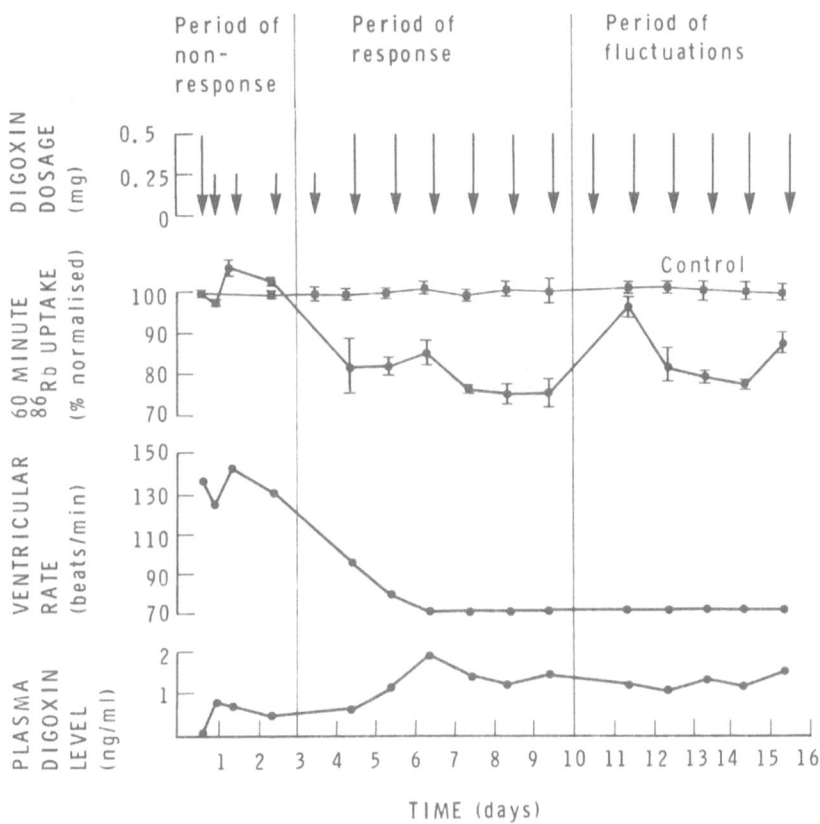

Fig. 20.3. Patient with atrial fibrillation whose ventricular rate did not slow over first 3 days of digoxin therapy but which subsequently responded. Response of ventricular rate, change in RBC ^{86}Rb uptake, and plasma digoxin concentrations. For description see text

Discussion

During the initial stages of digoxin therapy, in all but two of the patients studied, red cell ^{86}Rb uptake fell. We cannot yet say whether this was due to inhibition of red cell $(Na^+ + K^+)$-ATPase or indirectly to changes in intracellular ionic concentrations (Astrup, 1974), though the former is by far and away, the most likely.

Red cell ^{86}Rb uptake values before the onset of fluctuations correlated better with the clinical response in Groups I and Ia than did plasma digoxin concentrations. The regression lines of correlation between changes in ventricular rate and changes in ^{86}Rb uptake illustrated in Figure 20.4 for Groups I and Ia differ significantly from one another in regard to slope ($p < 0.001$) but not with respect to the intercept on the y-axis. This suggests that when reversion to sinus

247

rhythm occurs in patients with atrial fibrillation it does so in association with less inhibition of red cell ^{86}Rb than in patients who do not revert. One wonders whether in patients who revert to sinus rhythm there is increased sensitivity of the $(Na^+ + K^+)$-ATPase to inhibition by digoxin.

The lack of correlation between changes in ventricular rate and red cell ^{86}Rb uptake in Group II (patients with supraventricular tachyarrhythmias other than

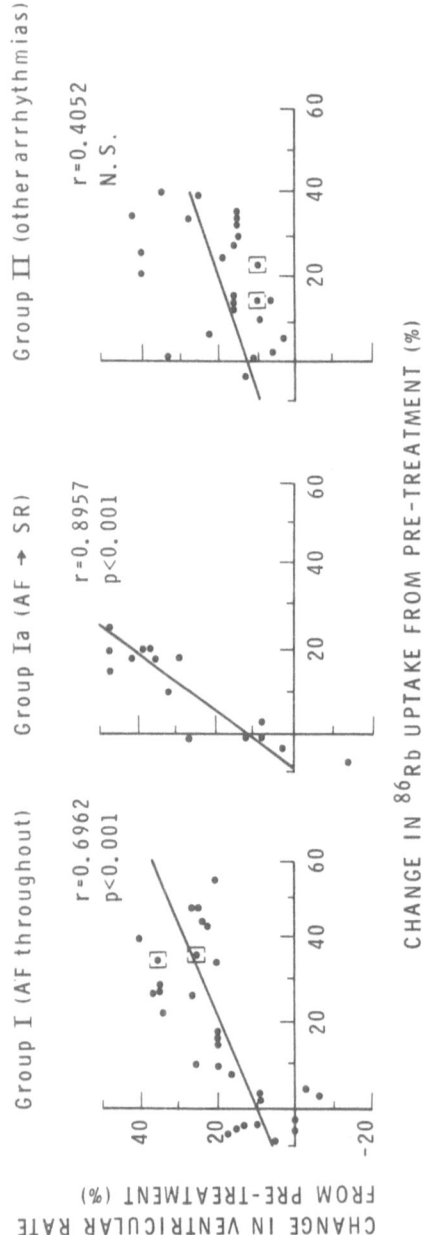

Fig. 20.4. Relationship between change in RBC ^{86}Rb uptake and ventricular rate

248

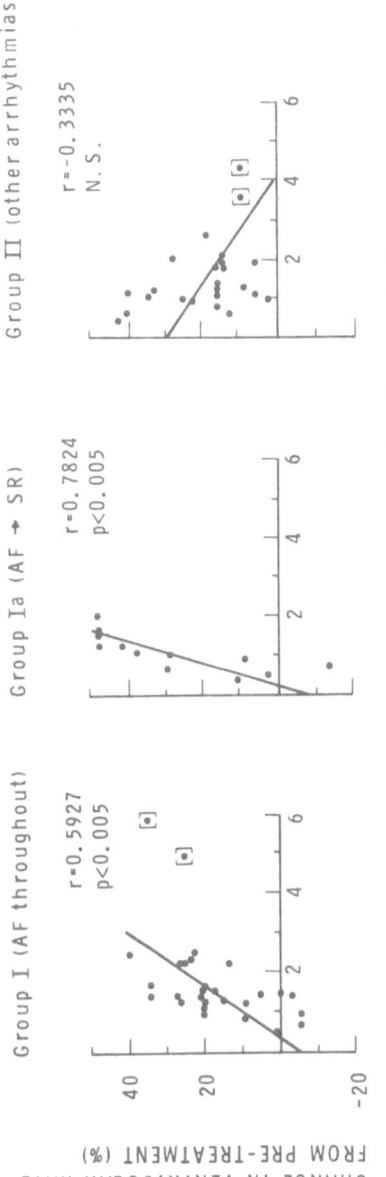

Fig. 20.5. Relationship between plasma digoxin concentration and change in ventricular rate

atrial fibrillation) is not surprising. Cardiac glycosides do not cause appreciable gradual slowing of the ventricular response in such arrhythmias and one would not, therefore, expect a correlation with the gradual fall in ^{86}Rb uptake which occurred in these patients.

In the full paper describing this work, several other points of interest are considered (Aronson, Grahame-Smith, Hallis, Hibble and Wigley, 1977). Multivariate analysis of the values for plasma digoxin, red cell ^{86}Rb uptake, and the response of the ventricular rate in atrial fibrillation shows that combined measurement of plasma digoxin concentrations and red cell ^{86}Rb uptake gives a better index of response than either measurement alone. The correlations between plasma digoxin concentrations and red cell ^{86}Rb uptake (Group I r = 0.516, p < 0.01; Group Ia r = 0.635, p < 0.05; Group II r = 0.282, NS) show that the degree of ^{86}Rb uptake inhibition is related only in small part to plasma digoxin concentrations measured 6 h after the last dose.

The fluctuations in red cell ^{86}Rb uptake seen 3-11 days after starting digoxin therapy are a puzzle. They are of interest in their own right and may reflect changes in intracellular cation concentrations produced in the red cell by the action of digoxin (Astrup, 1974), which themselves may lead to changes in the binding of digoxin to red cell $(Na^+ + K^+)$-ATPase. The phenomenon is being studied further because at present these fluctuations make it difficult to use ^{86}Rb red cell uptake as an index of the pharmacologic action of digoxin in patients chronically on digoxin therapy.

We are hopeful that by understanding the changes in digoxin binding to the red cell, ^{86}Rb uptake, and red cell intracellular $Na^+ + K^+$ concentrations which occur during digoxin therapy, it may be possible to define a peripheral pharmacologic effect of digoxin which will reflect the effect of digoxin on the heart. The effect digoxin has on the red cell does not have to be the effect through which digoxin produces its therapeutic effects on the heart; for monitoring digoxin therapy in the clinical situation it is only necessary that the two go hand in hand.

References

Aronson, J.K., Grahame-Smith, D.G., Hallis, K.F., Hibble, A., Wigley, F.:
    Monitoring digoxin therapy: I. Plasma concentrations and an in vitro assay
    of tissue response. Br. J. Clin. Pharmacol. (in press) (1977)
Astrup, J.: Sodium and potassium in human red cells: Variations among centri-
    fuged cells. Scand. J. Clin. Lab. Invest. 33, 231-237 (1974)
Cohen, I., Dant, J., Noble, D.: The influence of extracellular potassium ions on
    the action of ouabain in membrane currents in sheep Purkinjee fibres. J.
    Physiol. (Lond.) 249, 42-43 (1975)
Grahame-Smith, D.G., Everest, M.S.: Measurement of digoxin in plasma and its
    use in the diagnosis of digoxin intoxication. Br. Med. J. 1969/i, 286

Ingelfinger, J., Goldman, P.: The serum digitalis concentration — does it diagnose digitalis toxicity. N. Engl. J. Med. 294, 867-870 (1976)

Love, W.D., Burch, G.E.: A comparison of [42]potassium, [86]rubidium, and [134]caesium as tracers of potassium in the study of cation metabolism of human erythrocytes in vitro. J. Lab. Clin. Med. 41, 351-362 (1953)

Schatzmann, H.J.: Herzglycoside als Hemmstoffe für aktiven Kalium und Natriumtransport durch die Erythrocytenmembran. Helv. Physiol. Acta 11, 346-354 (1953)

Schwartz, A., Lindenmayer, G.E., Allen, J.C.: The sodium-potassium adenosine triphosphatase: pharmacological, physiological and behavioural aspects. Pharmacol. Rev. 27, 3-134 (1975)

Wang, C.H., Willis, D.L.: In: Radiotracer Methodology in Biological Science. New Jersey: Prentice-Hall 1965, p. 31

Discussion

Belz, Koblenz: We use the ^{86}Rb uptake assay to measure digoxin plasma levels. Have you looked at the reticulocyte content of the blood? I think that may be important and influence your correlations. We have shown in a study, not published, that reticulocytes have much greater pumping function for the rubidium uptake and this may influence your results. For instance, in patients with hemolytic anemias who have reticulocyte percentages of 50% or so, the uptake may be the three- or fourfold of normal people.

Grahame-Smith: That's a very good point which has worried us. Astrup showed that when you subject red cells to differential centrifugation, then you can separate old red cells, not so old red cells, and young red cells, and when you look at the cation concentration within those cells they are different. This is something that we have looked at. We have subjected red cells to the differential centrifugation that he described, and we have looked at the rubidium uptake of the different layers and we didn't find any differences between them. We haven't done a lot of work on it, but at least it didn't stand out as a big error. But it's a very good point because I believe the reticulocyte has more ATPase activity in it than the older red cell.

Marcus, Tucson: I notice that you took each patient's blood prior to the determinations. Was there great variation of rubidium uptake from one patient to another before digitalis was administered? Also, was there any correlation of these data with the rubidium uptake?

Grahame-Smith: There is variation in predigitalization rubidium uptake from patient to patient. Normally, with our method, red cells take up about 35% of rubidium from the medium but it varies between about 40% and 30%. This poses a problem because consequent decreases seen on digitalization are not very great. In real terms, the amount of rubidium taken up in the medium may decrease from 35% to as much as 25% but often only to 30%. This means that in regard to chronic digitalis treatment, ignoring for a moment the fluctuations, unless you know the patient's initial uptake, it is not possible to properly assess the effect of digitalis on that patient's red cell ^{86}Rb uptake. In the slides I showed, initial rubidium uptake is indicated as 100% for each patient in order to equal all the patients up. There does not seem to be any correlation between any particular patient's pretreatment red cell rubidium uptake and his clinical response.

Marcus: In relation to the variation that you see after 5 days, could this be due to any other drugs which were given to the patient? It has been reported that triamterene has an effect on ATPase activity, and I wonder if this type of interaction might have affected your results?

Grahame-Smith: We have looked at that. Many patients had to receive other drugs and we have tried to look at as many drugs as we can. In large concentrations, frusemide can affect ^{86}Rb uptake, but in doses usually given in clinical situations, it does not seem to affect rubidium uptake very greatly. In addition, red cell rubidium uptake is decreased in normal volunteers not on other drugs at all. So, we are confident that the decreased rubidium uptake occurring during the initial phase of digitalis therapy is a digitalis-induced phenomenon in its own right. There is one point I would like to amplify. You will have seen that during the initial phase of therapy there is undoubtedly inhibition of the patient's own red cell rubidium uptake. After a time the fluctuations start to occur. So, superficially this looks as if the red cell is trying to overcome some homeostatic mechanism. Gradually, in spite of the fluctuations, one can see that the rubidium uptake is climbing back up to normal, i.e., the predigitalization level. We have recently been studying the binding of tritiated digoxin to red cell membranes, and in some patients we have seen that tritiated digoxin binding, which indicates the number of receptors available to digoxin on the red cell, fluctuates in time with the ^{86}Rb uptake. In addition, although the number of receptors available for binding digoxin decrease during the initial phase of digoxin therapy, as time goes on, more receptors become available, and this goes hand in hand with the return of rubidium uptake toward normal. It is worthwhile considering that the red cell ATPase is not a stable receptor. To bind digoxin, ATPase has to be in a certain state, and it seems to me not unlikely that when digoxin binds to the cell and sodium concentration within the cell is altered that more ATPase binding sites may be turned on and that this may be responsible for fluctuations in rubidium uptake and digoxin binding. We are investigating more carefully this phenomenon at the moment.

Dengler, Bonn: A question regarding this fluctuation is the possibility of something in the plasma acting either as an inhibitor or activator of ATPase. If, for instance, you incubate normal cells in the serum of a patient showing this fluctuation, what happens?

Grahame-Smith: What we have done is to take the plasmas from patients who are in fluctuation or not in fluctuation. We have incubated them with normal cells and looked to see whether that alters the rubidium uptake in the normal cells and it doesn't. So, we have not been able, so far, to show that the fluctuations are due to a circulating factor of some sort influencing ATPase activity.

252

Jahrmärker, München: Have you excluded the possibility that the fluctuations are the result of repeated bleeding, have you considered replacing the blood you have taken every time?

Grahame-Smith: Yes, we have considered that, but I don't think bleeding is responsible because in normal individuals the same sort of bleeding doesn't produce fluctuations, and repeated bleedings from other patients not taking digitalis doesn't produce fluctuations. I doubt very much whether repeated bleeding is responsible, it is only at the most 10 ml of blood each time, not a large amount.

Erdmann, München: I have a short comment. There is a paper by Chan and Sanslone (Chan and Sanslone, 1969) who have put rats on a potassium-deficient diet. Their $(Na^+ + K^+)$-ATPase content in the erythrocytes went up by some 70%. Last year I had the chance to have seven patients with severe chronic hypokalemia, and they had almost twice as many ouabain binding sites or digoxin binding sites on their erythrocytes. The affinity, however, of the receptors toward the drug had not changed. And there is another paper by Greeff (Greeff, 1976) who has shown that in heart muscle after chronic treatment with digitalis the binding sites and ATPase had increased as well. Apparently, the receptor concentration may be regulated in some states of disease or after chronic administration of drugs.

References

Chan, Sanslone: Arch. Biochem. Biophys. 134, 48 (1969)
Greeff, K.: Eur. J. Pharmacol. 37, 189 (1976)

21 Relationships Between Doses, Plasma Levels and Cardiac Effects Under Digitalis Treatment

G. G. BELZ and R. ERBEL

The aim of the present study was to elucidate two problems concerning digitalis therapy.

1. Generally, dose-effect curves are necessary to characterize pharmacodynamic properties of drugs, especially to compare various drugs (Goth, 1972; Moe and Farah, 1975). Following single injections, in a relative narrow dose range, some attempts have been made to establish dose-effect relationships of cardiac glycosides in man (Apter et al., 1944; Matos et al., 1975; Weissler et al., 1966). However, the dose-response relationship should be based on the effects attained under steady-state conditions (Fingl and Woodbury, 1975).

2. The relations between plasma glycoside concentrations an cardiac effects are not yet well-established in respect to their extent and manner.

Therefore, these two problems should be cleared up using and interindividual controlled randomized double-blind design with different oral maintenance doses of digitoxin (Dt) and β-acetyl-digoxin (D). Plasma levels were measured with a ^{86}Rb erythrocyte assay. Cardiac effects were determined noninvasively with systolic time intervals and ECG.

Methods

The study was carried out in 120 healthy male volunteers. All participants received the drugs daily for 7 days. The applications were performed as an interindividual controlled randomized double-blind study. Each volunteer exclusively took part for a single application period. Groups of 10 volunteers each received the following daily maintenance doses of D: placebo, 0.1, 0.2, 0.3, 0.4, 0.5, or 0.6 mg, whereas the daily Dt doses were: placebo, 0.04, 0.08, 0.12, or 0.16 mg. The following loading scheme was used:

Day	1	2	3	4 7	
D	3	2	1	1	1	-fold of
Dt	6	6	3	1	1	maintenance dose

The last dose on day 7 was given exactly 24 h before the control registrations.

The digoxin preparation used was a β-acetyl derivative (0.1 mg tablets = Nov-odigal mite®). This derivative is completely desacetylated after absorption (Ruiz-Torres and Burmeister, 1972) and shows a high absolute biovailability of ~ 80% compared to an intravenous standard (Flasch, 1975); 0.12 mg (for the loading period) and 0.04 mg Dt tablets were used. The different tablets had identical galenics and showed the same rapid dissolution rate (> 90% solution within 1 min under standardized conditions (Kwee and Ulex, 1974).

Recordings of STI and ECG were done in constant room temperature (24°C) between 6:30 and 8:30 a.m. in the fasting state (= 12 h) after the volunteer had been recumbant for exactly 15 min. According to the original method described by Blumberger (Blumberger, 1942), the following registrations were done simul-taneously using a six-channel jet recorder (Cardirex 6-T, Siemens) at a paper speed of 100 mm/s: ECG in bipolar chest wall lead A (Nehb, 1938), phono-cardiogram in the fourth left intercostal space near sternum, and carotid arte-rial pulse tracing was recorded by means of a pulse receptor (Brecht and Boucke, 1952). Twenty consecutive heart cycles were evaluated each time and their arithmetic mean utilized for the subsequent analysis.

The following variables were measured. QS_2 : the total electromechanical systole. LVET: the left ventricular ejection time. RRI: the RR interval, and QT duration in ECG. The amplitude of the T-waves was measured using five consecutive beats in the leads V2-V6 of the standard ECG and averaged as follows:

$$\overline{T_{V_2-6}} = \sum_{n=5} T_{V_2} + \sum_{n=5} T_{V_3} \ldots + \sum_{n=5} T_{V_6} /25$$

Corrections for influence of heart rate were performed as follows. From QT the QTc was calculated:

$$QTc = \frac{QT}{\sqrt{RRI}} \quad \text{(Bazett 1920)}$$

Corrections of STI were done using the method of Weissler et al. (Weissler et al., 1968): The predicted normal STI for the observed heart rate was calculated from the appropiate regression equation and substracted from the measured interval for this value. This difference was defined as QS_2 c and LVETc. Changes in STI and ECG induced by treatment, were obtained by substracting the values before and after drug application, which resulted in the respective Δ-values (≙ effect).

Immediately following the second registration (a) of STI and ECG, 70 ml of venous blood was drawn from an antecubital vein. Plasma glycoside concentra-tions were measured using a ^{86}Rb erythrocyte assay (Belz et al., 1973; 1974; Lowenstein, 1965).

Calculations and statistics were done using analysis of variance Bartlett test, and Duncan test (multiple t-test) (Weber, 1967).

Results

The original results of the measurements of STI, ECG and plasma glycoside concentrations are documented elsewhere (Belz et al., 1978).

Compared to placebo, both glycosides reduced heart rate. This effect was not clearly dose related and not statistically significant. With the highest D doses, mean heart rate was depressed by 4.6 (SD = ± 6.8) beats/min, the respective value for Dt was 6.9 (SD = ± 6.7).

Both glycosides prolonged the PQ interval dose dependent, but statistically insignificant. The highest doses of D led to a lengthening of 8.1 (SD = ± 6.7) ms, Dt 16.8 (SD = ± 28.5) ms.

Figure 21.1 demonstrates the dose-dependent shortening of QTc. In the semilogarithmic system, a parallel run of the curves for D and Dt is obvious. The highest doses of both glycosides induced a nearly identical shortening of QTc. A plateau of maximum efficacy of the glycosides appeared not to be reached in the curves, as they were still demonstrating an upward slope in the last portion. A shortening of 24 ms (i.e., 50% of maximum effect of D) was attained at 0.3 mg daily for D and at 0.077 mg daily for Dt. From these values, it was calculated that Dt is 3.9 times as potent as D in shortening QTc.

Dt induces a statistically significant dose-related flattening of T (Fig. 21.1). The curve is similar to that of QTc. With the highest dose, the plateau of maximum efficacy was apparently not reached. The curve for D is flatter. The maximum effect with the highest D dose was only 65% of the highest Dt effect. The doses necessary to reach a flattening of the T-wave by 0.17 mV (i.e., 50% of the maximum effect of Dt) was 0.51 mg for D and 0.07 mg daily for Dt. Dt is therefore 7.2 times as potent as D in flattening T at this degree.

Figure 21.2 demonstrates the parallel run of changes of QS_2 c. The highest doses of the glycosides shortened this parameter for an average of ~ 25 ms (Maximum effect: D = 85% of Dt). From the digitoxin curve, one may infer that maximum efficacy is nearly reached. The values for half maximum effect (100% = maximum Dt effect) are: 0.2 mg daily for D and 0.052 mg daily for Dt. Hence, Dt is 3.8 times as potent as D in shortening QS_2 c. Shortening of LVETc revealed a plateau of maximum efficacy (-12.5 ms) for both glycosides. Half maximum effects occur at: 0.22 mg daily for D and 0.06 mg daily for Dt. Thus, Dt is 3.8 times as potent as D in shortening LVETc.

Correlations Between Plasma Glycoside Concentration and Cardiac Effects

Generally, the correlation coefficients for Dt are somewhat higher than those for D. Plasma concentration versus heart rate or PQ show only poor correlations for either glycoside. In Figure 21.3 the interdependence between plasma digitoxin and pharmacodynamic parameters Δ QTc and Δ QS_2 c are shown. Both intervals show the same behavior: significant shortening of the respective parameters with increasing plasma concentration. Similar results were obtained for D (r = 0.7).

256

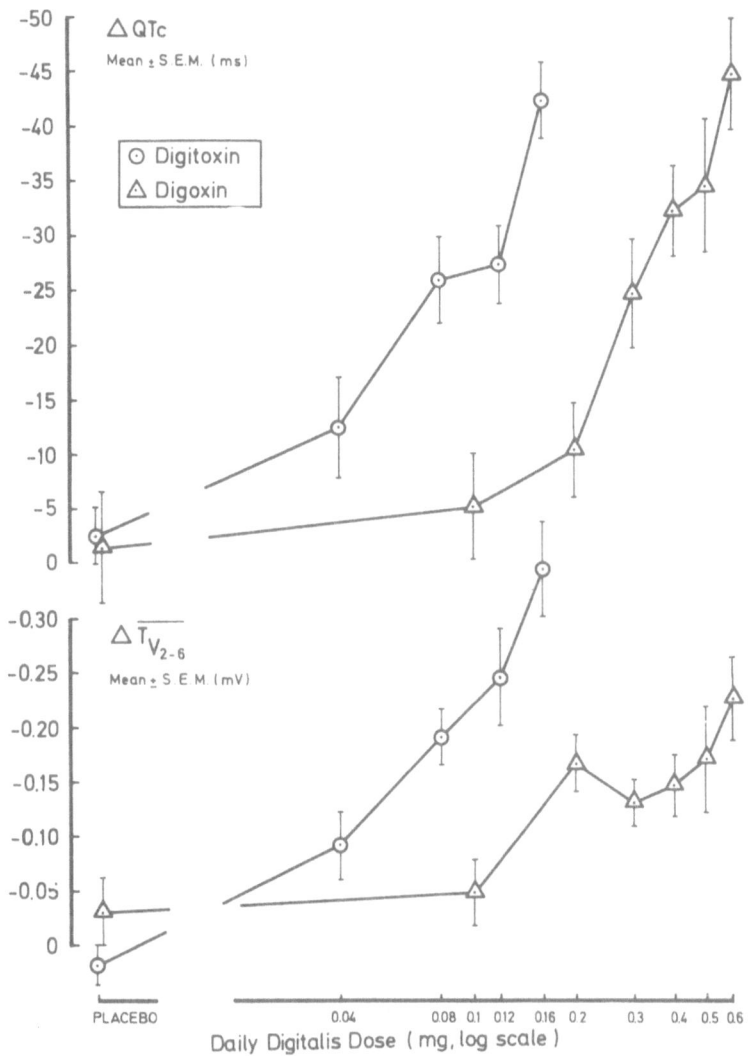

Fig. 21.1. Digitalis versus change of electrocardiographic parameters. Daily oral maintenance doses of the glycosides are given on the abscissa (β-acetyl-digoxin = D; digitoxin = Dt). Each point of the log dose-response curves represents the mean of ten different individuals (total collectives for D: n = 70; for Dt n = 50). The differences (Δ-values) of measurements before and after 7 days of treatment, the latter 24 h after the last dose, are shown. QTc = duration of electric systole corrected for heart rate; $T_{V2\text{-}6}$ = mean amplitude of the T-waves from leads V2-V6. The mean values of the following treatment groups (mg daily mainten-ance doses) differed significantly at a 5% level in analysis of variance and multiple t-test (0 = placebo): Δ QTc - D: 0 vs. 0.2-0.6; 0.1 vs. 0.2-0.6.
  - Dt: 0 vs. 0.04-0.16; 0.04 vs. 0.12-0.16.
  $\Delta \overline{T_{V2\text{-}6}}$ - D: 0 vs. 0.2, 0.4, 0.5, 0.6.
  - Dt: 0 vs. 0.08-0.16; 0.04 vs. 0.12-0.16;
      0.08 vs. 0.12-0.16; 0.12 vs. 0.16

257

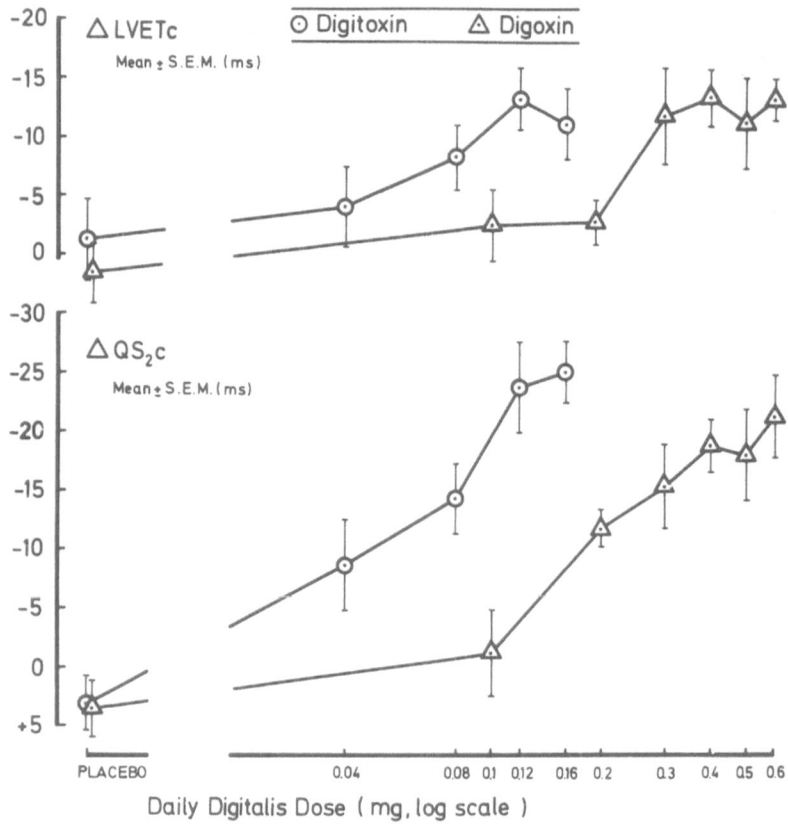

Figure 21.2. Digitalis dose versus change of systolic time intervals. Plot analogus as in Figure 21.1. LVETc = left ventricular ejection time corrected for heart rate QS_2c = total electromechanical systole corrected for heart rate. The following groups differed significantly:

Δ LVETc - D: 0 vs. 0.3-0.6; 0.1 vs. 0.3-0.6.
             - Dt: 0 vs. 0.12-0.16.
Δ QS_2c - D: 0 vs. 0.2-0.6; 0.1 vs. 0.2-0.6.
             - Dt: 0 vs. 0.04-0.16; 0.04 vs. 0.12-0.16; 0.08 vs. 0.16

In Figure 21.4, correlations between plasma levels and Δ T are shown. In principle, there seems to be no difference between the two glycosides: T-flattening with increasing plasma concentration. However, whereas for Dt the degree of correlation is the same as with STI and QTc, the correlation for D is much poorer than those for changes of cardiac performance.

The absolute slope of the correlations of the two glycosides cannot be compared since the plasma concentrations have different ranges. However, a relative comparison is possible. For this purpose Δ QS_2c was assumed to be the most suitable variable representing glycoside effect on cardiac performance. For D and Dt, respectively, the slopes of the correlations between plasma levels and Δ QS_2c were

258

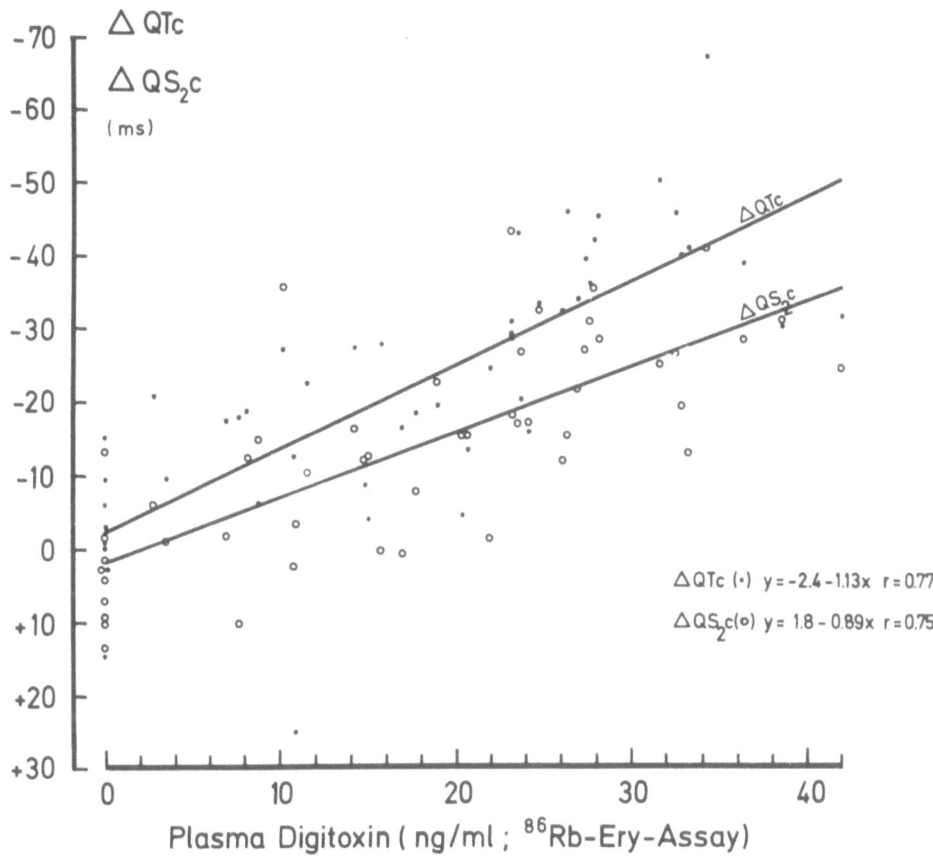

Fig. 21.3. Correlation between individual plasma digitoxin and changes of QTc and QS$_2$c.

Abscissa: plasma glycoside concentration 24 h after the last dose.

Ordinate: differences of the measurements of QTc and QS$_2$c before and after treatment with D (Δ-values).

Analysis revealed the slopes to be significantly (p < 0.001) different from zero

set 1.0 as reference slopes. The relative slopes for the other parameters were calculated dividing their absolute slopes by the absolute slope of Δ QS$_2$c. With D, the following slopes result: Δ LVETc = 0.7, Δ QTc = 1.7, Δ T$_{V2\text{-}6}$ = 6.0 $\times$ 10^{-3}. With Dt, the respective values are: ΔLVETc = 0.6, Δ QTc = 1.3, Δ $\overline{\text{T}_{V2\text{-}6}}$ = 11.3 $\times$ 10^{-3}. The ratio of the relative slopes D/Dt demonstrate now the following values: Δ QS$_2$c = 1.0, Δ LVETc = 1.2, Δ QTc = 1.3, and Δ $\overline{\text{T}_{V2\text{-}6}}$ = 0.5.

Discussion

In this study with D and Dt, sigmoid-shaped log dose-response curves for glyco-side-induced changes of STI and ECG parameters could be demonstrated in man

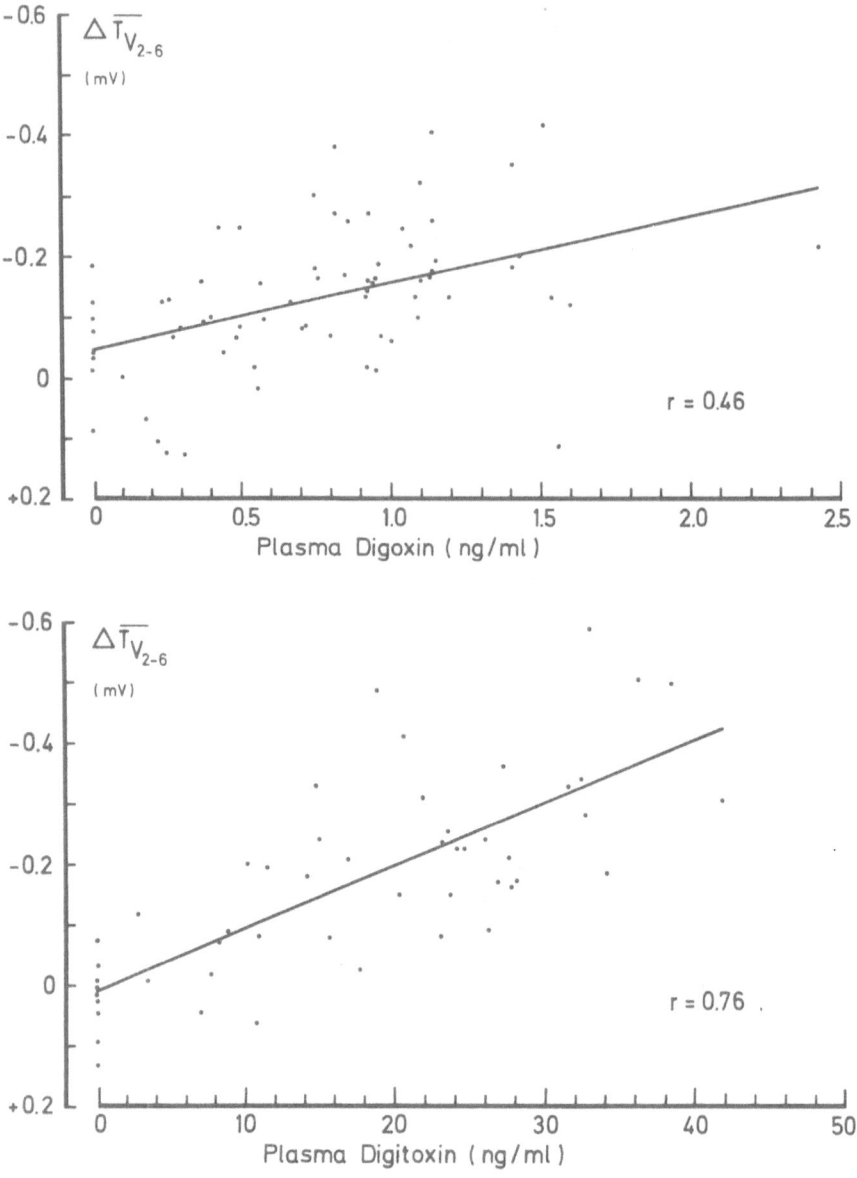

Fig. 21.4. Correlations between individual plasma glycoside and changes of the amplitude of the T-waves for digoxin (upper part) and digitoxin (lower part). Plot analogous as in Figures 21.3. Ordinate: changes of the amplitudes of the T-waves in leads V2-V6 (ΔT_{V2-6}). The slopes of the two regression lines differ significantly from zero ($p < 0.001$)

during maintenance therapy. With the applied doses, a plateau of the effect (maximum efficacy) was observed for Δ LVETc; for Δ QS$_2$c this aim was attained approximately, whereas for the electrocardiographic parameters (Δ QTc, Δ-amplitude of T-waves) the highest doses still appeared too low to induce maximum efficacy. Higher daily maintenance doses (> 0.6 mg of D, > 0.16 mg of Dt), necessary to reach this goal, seem untenable for an experimental procedure in man. A factor 3-6 between the lowest effective and the minimal dose producing maximum efficacy can be estimated for both glycosides from our curves with Δ LVETc and Δ QS$_2$c. This range corresponds well with the results of Greeff and Schlieper (Greeff and Schlieper, 1967) using human atrial strips in vitro.

In the present interindividual study on D and Dt, relatively high correlations were found between plasma glycoside concentrations and Δ QTc and Δ QS$_2$c. For Δ LVETc, Δ HR, and Δ PQ, only lower correlation coefficients were observed. A noteworthy discrepancy is the relatively great difference between the correlation coefficients of D and Dt in respect to the flattening of T. For Dt a distictly higher correlation exists than for D.

We conclude from the results of our correlation analysis that there exists a statistically good relation between plasma glycoside and influence of glycosides on the concentration of the heart. The results support the usefulness of plasma glycoside measurements in digitalis therapy not only for diagnosis of digitalis intoxication. The generally accepted concept states that there are nor pharamacodynamic differences between the various cardiac glycosides, although they differ in respect to their pharmacokinetic properties (Goth, 1972; Moe and Farah, 1975). In the present study, in regard to their influence on the mechanical, electromechanical, and electric phases of ventricular systole, we observed a completely analogous behavior of D and Dt. The only striking difference in respect to their influence on ventricular function is seen in the relative potency of the two glycosides. This is mainly due to pharmacokinetic differences. However, from the dose-effect curves as well as from the degree and the relative slope in plasma level-effect correlations, one observed that Dt induces a more pronounced effect in flattening the T-wave in ECG than does D. This observation confirms older findings of Aravanis and Luisada (Aravanis and Luisada, 1958). These authors observed that the S-T-depression and lowering or inversion of T was much more evident with Dt than with D or other cardiac glycosides. The assumption of a greater relative vagomimetic potency of D compared to Dt could give an explanation of this noteworthy fact which is now evident from two independent studies using quite different techniques. Whether or not the more relevant electrophysiologic properties of varying cardiac glycosides will also show such differences, should be the aim of further research.

Conclusion

Since our studies were done in normal man, a rendering to clinical conditions should be only done with certain reserve. A principally indentical influence of cardiac glycosides on STI in normal subjects and patients suffering from heart failure was, however, shown by Weissler and Schoenfeld (Weissler and Schoenfeld, 1970).

1. Changes in cardiac performance induced by digitalis reach a plateau of maximum effect, where a further increase of dose will not result in a further increase in effect.
2. Plasma glycoside levels within a range of 0-2 ng/ml for D and 0-40 ng/ml for Dt correspond well with the glycoside effects on the heart.
3. At identical level of influence on the cardiac systole with Dt, a more pronounced effect on the T-wave in ECG can be expected than with D. This may indicate that various cardiac glycosides do exert different effects on the electrophysiologic properties of the heart.
4. Dt is about four times as potent as D in influencing cardiac performance, i.e., to induce the same level of inotropic effect with D the four fold maintenance dose is needed.

References

Apter, L., Ashman, R., Hull, E.: A quantitative study of the effects of ouabain upon the electrocardiogram. J. Pharmacol. Exp. Ther. 82, 227-238 (1944)

Aravanis, C., Luisada, A.A.: Clinical comparison of six digitalis preparations by the parenteral route. Am. J. Cardiol. 1, 706-716 (1958)

Bazett, H.C.: An analysis of the time relations of the electrocardiogram. Heart 7, 353-370 (1920)

Belz, G.G., Stauch, M., Belz, G., Kurbjuweit, H.G., Oberdorf, A.: The effect of various cardenolides and bufadienolides with different cardiac activity on the ^{86}Rubidium-uptake of human erythrocytes. Naunyn Schmiedebergs Arch. Pharmakol. 280, 353-362 (1973)

Belz, G.G., Stauch. M., Rudofsky, G.: Plasma levels after a single oral dose of proscillaridin. Eur. J. Clin. Pharmacol. 7, 95-97 (1974)

Belz, G.G., Erbel, R., Schumann, K., Gilfrich, H.J.: Dose — effect — plasma concentration relations of digitalis glycosides in man. Europ. J. Clin. Pharmacol. (in press)

Blumberger, K.J.: Die Untersuchung der Dynamik des Herzens beim Menschen. Ihre Anwendung als Herzleistungsprüfung. Ergeb. Inn. Med. Kinderheilk. 62, 424-531 (1942)

Brecht, K., Boucke, H.: Neues elektrostatisches Tiefton-Mikrophon und seine Anwendung in der Sphygmographie. Pflügers Arch. 256, 43-54 (1952)

Fingl. E., Woodbury, D.M.: General Principles. In: The Pharmacological Basis of Therapeutics, 5th ed. Goodman, L.S., Gilman, A., (eds.) New York: Mac Millan 1975, p. 25

Flasch, H.: Die biologische Verfügbarkeit von β-Acetyldigoxin and Digoxin. Klin. Wochenschr. 53, 873-877 (1975)

Goth, A.: Medical Pharmacology, 6th ed. Saint Louis: C.V. Mosby 1972, p. 8; p. 370

Greeff, K., Schlieper, E.: Artspezifische Wirkungsunterschiede des k-Strophanthins und Prednisolonbisguanylhydrazons: Untersuchungen an isolierten Vorhofpräparaten und Erythrozyten des Menschen, Meerschweinchens und der Ratte. Arch. Int. Pharmacodyn. Ther. 166, 350-361 (1967)

Kwee, H.G., Ulex, G.A.: Die Bestimmung der Auflösungsgeschwindigkeit mit einer neuen Durchflußzelle. Pharm. Ind. 36, 576-582 (1974)

Lowenstein, J.M.: A method for measuring plasma levels of digitalis glycosides. Circulation 31, 228-233 (1965)

Matos, L., Bekés, M., Polák, G., Rausch, J., Török, E.: Comparative study of the cardiac and peripheral vascular effects of strophanthin K and lanatoside C in coronary heart disease. Eur. J. Clin. Pharmacol. 9, 27-37 (1975)

Moe, G.K., Farah, A.E.: Digitalis and allied cardiac glycosides. In: The Pharmacological Basis of Therapeutics, 5th ed. Goodman, L.S., Gilman, A. (eds.) New York: Mac Millan 1975, p. 675

Nehb, W.: Zur Standardisierung der Brustwandableitungen des Elektrokardiogramms. Klin. Wochenschr. 17, 1807-1811 (1938)

Ruiz-Torres, A., Burmeister, H.: Stoffwechsel und Kinetik von β-Acetyldigoxin. Klin. Wochenschr. 50, 191-195 (1972)

Weber, E.: Grundriß der biologischen Statistik, 6th ed. Stuttgart: G. Fischer 1967

Weissler, A.M., Harris, W.S., Schoenfeld, C.D.: Systolic time intervals in heart failure in man. Circulation 37, 149-159 (1968)

Weissler, A.M., Schoenfeld, C.D.: Effect of digitalis on systolic time intervals in heart failure. Am. J. Med. Sci. 259, 4-20 (1970)

Weissler, A.M., Snyder, J.R., Schoenfeld, C.D., Cohen, S.: Assay of digitalis glycosides in man. Am. J. Cardiol. 17, 768-780 (1966)

Discussion

Dengler, Bonn: Dr. Belz, may it be that the better correlation coefficient for digitoxin is due to the fact that the rubidium assay is more suitable for assessing glycoside concentrations after the application of digitoxin than after digoxin? You have a greater amount of metabolites after giving digitoxin which may influence your assay.

Belz: That is one possible explanation. Another explanation could be a lower variance in the plasma levels for digitoxin. In fact, there is not a very great difference between digitoxin and digoxin, the correlation coefficients were 0.77 and 0.7, respectively, as I mentioned. But nevertheless there is some difference.

Scholz, Hannover: There is no evidence at all that different cardiac glycosides have any different effects on action potentials, membrane currents, etc. in electrophysiologic microelectrode studies. Is it possible that the difference in the amplitude of the T-waves merely reflects the fact that the T-wave in the ECG is not a good parameter for changes you can measure with microelectrodes?

Belz: Indeed, that seems to be possible. We know that the amplitude of the T-wave is not only influenced by cardiac glycosides but also by a lot of other factors, as for instance the tone of the sympathetic and parasympathetic nervous system, or by the inotropic state of the heart, etc. You will not measure this kind of influence in experiments on isolated hearts or on muscle fibers. Another question is if in addition to the observed electrophysiologic difference between digoxin and digitoxin there may also be differences in respect to other electrophysiologic properties (e.g., the refractory period of AV-node, etc.).

Marcus: I wondered if you had looked at the correlation between the pre-ejection period (PEP)/left ventricular ejection time (LVET) and some of the other parameters. Weissler found that this ratio was valuable in his studies. Perhaps this ratio may result in a better correlation than was obtained.

Belz: We have done these calculations and did not find better correlations. But there is a difference between the systolic time intervals in healthy volunteers and in patients with cardiac failure. In cardiac failure, the influence of the glycosides on the PEP is greater than in healthy people. We determined PEP and the quotient $\frac{PEP}{LVET}$. But in our experience the QS_2 is the most suitable parameter for an analysis in healthy man. It would be very desirable to achieve dose-effect curves in patients with cardiac failure as we have done in healthy volunteers.

Lukas, New York: Dr. Belz, that is a very fascinating study tome, because I can remember many discussions in our laboratory about whether one could give increasing doses of glycoside and expect an increasing inotropic effect. Of course your subjects were normal persons, but it is interesting that you did reach a maximum effect with what seem to be therapeutic dosages. I'm concerned about your relating dose to effect and your equating the two glycosides by a 1:4 ratio. If you look at the data in another way and examine the relationship of effect to plasma concentration, I thought you were getting a peak somewhere around 1 ng/ml with digoxin and about 20 ng/ml with digitoxin. That is not quite equivalent to a 1:4 ratio.

Belz: Of course I am aware of this fact. I think a main question with the correlations between plasma levels and effects is: why do we not reach a plateau with the plasma concentration versus effect, as we do with the dose versus effect? I have no explanation for this observation, but you have to consider that in the plot effect:plasma concentrations there are two variables and in the other relationship the dependence of certain interindividually constant doses on the effect was correlated.

22.1 Therapeutic Implications of Digoxin Kinetics in Impaired Renal Function[1]

W. J. JUSKO[2]

Although digoxin is largely excreted unchanged by the kidneys, many clinical and pharmacokinetic imperfections exist in calculation of digoxin dosage regimens based on renal function. Some primary concerns regarding digoxin kinetics are its variability in volume of distribution in relation to age and renal function, variability in renal clearance, the role of secondary clearance mechanisms, and the appropriateness of the pharmacokinetic methodology being employed. This report will focus on these concerns as well as the benefits of utilizing "clearance concepts" in characterizing digoxin kinetics in impaired renal function.

Variability in Digoxin Disposition

The apparent or total volume of distribution (V_D) serves as a proportionality constant between serum concentrations of a drug and the amount in the body and provides a means of determining the appropriate loading dose, viz:

$$\text{Loading Dose (mg)} = V_D \times C_p^\circ / F \qquad \qquad \text{(Eq. 1)}$$

where C_p° is the initial desired postdistributive serum concentration and F is bio-availability. With digoxin, the loading dose — if employed — is generally administered in three portions at 6-h intervals because of the relatively slow rate of uptake by tissues and for assessing initial patient tolerance of the drug. We have found V_D values ranging from a mean of 330 liters in patients with severe renal impairment (Koup et al., 1975a) to 590 liters in young healthy adult subjects (Koup et al., 1975b). The data of Ohnhaus et al. (1974) also exhibit the extreme variability in V_D (range 3.0 - 17.1 liters/kg) in patients with various degrees of renal function. This variability may partly be an artifact resulting from the mode of drug administration and the method of calculation of V_D. For example, greater consistency in V_D values is found in cross-over studies when digoxin is given by infusion rather than by intravenous bolus injection (Koup et al., 1975b). However, the change in distribution noted in relation to renal function is also re-

1 Supported in part ·by Grant GM 20852 from the National Institutes of General Medical Sciences, NIH.

2 Unfortunately, Dr. Jusko was not able to present his paper at the symposium.

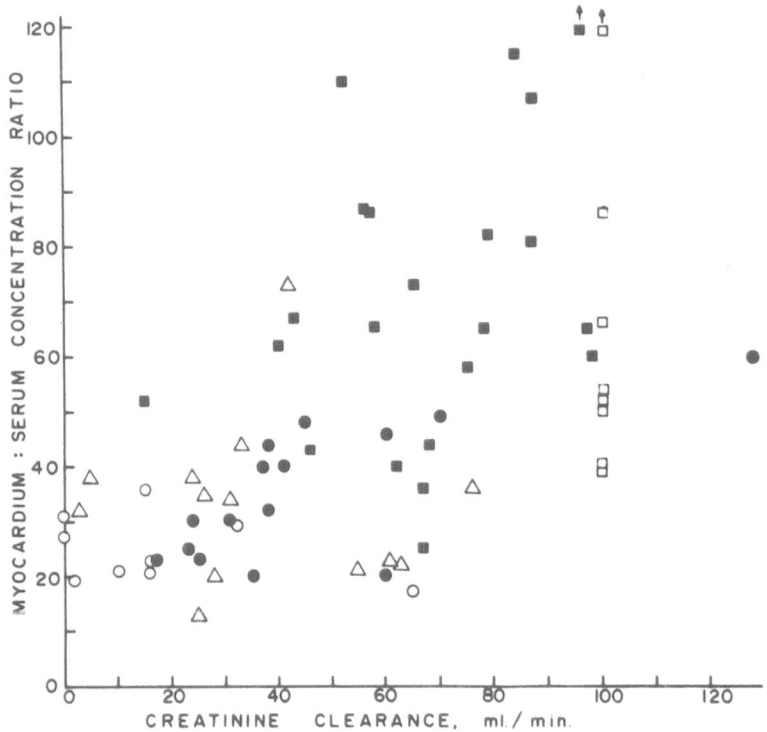

Fig. 22.1. Relationship between myocardium: serum concentration ratio of digoxin and the endogenous creatinine clearance of individual patients. Data are from Jusko and Weintraub (1974)

flected by differences in actual concentrations as a function of age and creatinine clearance (Cl_{CR}). Figure 22.1 shows the myocardium:serum concentration ratio in relation to Cl_{CR} in a large group of patients (Jusko and Weintraub, 1974; Jusko, 1974). Substantiated are both the decreased tissue uptake in patients with poor renal function and the considerable variability in tissue uptake at any degree of renal function. Newborn infants exhibit an even larger V_D than adults, and we have also demonstrated greater uptake of digoxin in myocardial tissue of babies in comparison with adults (Goridischer et al., 1976).

The variability in V_D has led to uncertainties in deciding loading dosages of digoxin in uremic patients. The problem is whether to aim for equal serum levels or equal myocardial levels of the drug. To err on the safe side and to remain consistent with the concept of a "therapeutic serum concentration" range, we usually recommended that similar initial serum concentrations (0.7 - 1.5 ng/ml) be sought in various types of patients. However, the findings of Kramer (this symposium) may clarify the situation in suggesting that uremic patients tolerate higher serum levels of digoxin.

The half-life ($t_{1/2}$) and one-compartment elimination constant (k_{el}) are commonly employed as indices of the rate of elimination of digoxin in patients with various degrees of renal function. This is only approximately correct for a drug such as digoxin which exhibits the characteristics of multiple-compartment distribution. As will be demonstrated, the terminal $t_{1/2}$ for such drugs is a better reflection of the rate of release of drug from tissues than elimination from the body.

We have observed two fundamental difficulties in characterizing the disposition of digoxin. One is the considerable variation in $t_{1/2}$ of digoxin in patients with severe renal impairment. Such patients showed apparent $t_{1/2}$ values ranging from 1.6 - 5.2 h whereas the commonly employed nomograms for dosing digoxin utilize a $t_{1/2}$ of about 4 days in these patients (Koup et al., 1975a). This variation can partly be attributed to altered tissue distribution as can be noted from the relationship:

$$t_{1/2} = \frac{0.693 \cdot V_D}{Cl_B} \qquad \text{(Eq. 2)}$$

where Cl_B is the body clearance. This relationship shows that the $t_{1/2}$ is a function of both distribution and clearance and is subject to the effects of modifications of each basic parameter.

The second problem with many reported $t_{1/2}$ values is the inadequate measurement of β-phase serum concentrations for a period long enough to be certain of the $t_{1/2}$ value. A "rule-of-thumb" is that the β-phase should be followed for a sufficient period of time to allow at least two half-lives to elapse. Alternatively, examination of urinary excretion data allows more precise quantitation of the terminal rate of digoxin elimination (Koup et al., 1975b). The body clearance should serve as the preferred index of digoxin elimination. The area of physiologic pharmacokinetics provides insight into the utility of this parameter.

Physiologic Pharmacokinetics

The utilization of physiologically realistic pharmacokinetic models for drug disposition is based on actual organ volumes and blood perfusion rates of the species examined. These models permit the prediction of drug concentrations in any tissue at any time and allow the effects of various pathophysiologic conditions to be examined including changes in organ blood flow, drug clearance, or binding to tissues.

An extremely important advance in the state-of-the-art of both physiologic pharmacokinetics and digoxin disposition has been the efforts of Harrison and Gibaldi in characterizing digoxin disposition in the rat (Harrison and Gibaldi, 1977) and the dog (Harrison and Gibaldi, 1975) and extension of these efforts to man. These investigators found that tissue binding data from the dog, typical blood flow values for man, average renal, hepatic, and biliary clearance values for man, and the application of a GI secretion and reabsorption process provided predicted plasma concentrations of digoxin which were in excellent agreement with measured values in patients with normal and moderately impaired renal function. However, plasma digoxin concentrations were underestimated in patients with severe renal impairment. The latter finding is consistent with our earlier observation (Fig. 22.1) that such patients have diminished tissue binding of digoxin which elevates serum concentrations of the drug. These efforts in physiologic pharmacokinetics indicate that digoxin kinetics, while exhibiting highly variable disposition in man, is describable by fundamental principles of organ perfusion, clearance, and binding.

The effect of intrinsic physiologic factors on typically measured pharmacokinetic factors such as $t_{1/2}$, V_D, and Cl were examined using a similar physiologic model (Jusko, 1975). For a drug which exhibits multiexponential disposition kinetics, the following observations are important:

1. While the $t_{1/2}$ is only partly affected by alterations in intrinsic hepatic metabolic (or renal) activity, the Cl_B value changes directly in proportion with the activity of the elimination process.
2. The $t_{1/2}$ is only slightly affected by modifications in blood flow to the eliminating organ, but the Cl_B value is more directly altered and serves as a better measure of drug disposition.
3. Tissue binding or partition capability markedly affects both $t_{1/2}$ and V_D but has no affect on Cl_B.

These simulations are relevant to digoxin disposition indicating that the $t_{1/2}$ is a poor index of alterations in drug elimination in comparison with Cl_B and that $t_{1/2}$ may be markedly affected by the distribution characteristics of the patient. On the other hand, the V_D is totally independent of drug elimination and serves as an excellent index of tissue distribution as might be anticipated.

Digoxin Clearance

The foregoing section establishes body clearance (Cl_B) as the optimum measure of drug elimination. The employment of "clearance concepts" in drug disposition is a rapidly enlarging area of pharmacokinetics (Rowland et al., 1973) which deserves further application to digoxin therapy (Koup et al., 1975a; Sumner et al., 1976). The Cl_B parameter should serve as an ideal factor to utilize quantitating digoxin disposition and predicting drug dosage regimens for several additional reasons:

1. It can be generated from experimental serum concentration data without recourse to a pharmacokinetic model because it is simply calculated as:

$$Cl_B = F \cdot \text{dose/area} \qquad \text{(Eq. 3)}$$

where area is the area under the serum concentration versus time curve either over one dosing interval at steady state or from time zero to infinity following a single dose.

2. Its application to devising a dosage regimen allows direct estimation of serum concentrations (C_p^{ss}) and obviates inclusion of the V_D value:

$$\text{dose} / \Upsilon = C_p^{ss} \cdot Cl_B/F \qquad \text{(Eq. 4)}$$

where Υ is the dosing interval. Other techniques which are based on k_{el} values require a more complicated series of computations.

3. The Cl_B is linearly related (slope = b_1) to creatinine clearance (Cl_{CR}), metabolic clearance (Cl_M), and other clearance mechanisms which allows its direct estimation without including body size except in estimating Cl_{CR} from a nomogram:

$$Cl_B = Cl_M + b_1 \cdot Cl_{CR} \qquad \text{(Eq. 5)}$$

For example, the data of Koup et al. (1975a) based on RIA measurements of digoxin yielded the function: $Cl_B = 41 + 1.3\ Cl_{CR}$, while the equation: $Cl_B = 46 + 1.9\ Cl_{CR}$, can be calculated from the data of Ohnhaus et al. (1974) who administered tritiated digoxin to patients with various degrees of renal function.

4. Finally, additional factors which affect digoxin elimination can be incorporated by multiple linear regression analysis, viz:

$$Cl_B = Cl_M + b_1 \cdot Cl_{CR} + b_2 \cdot CHF + \ldots \qquad \text{(Eq. 6)}$$

For example, Koup et al. (1975a) included a reduction in digoxin body clearance in patients with moderate to severe congestive heart failure (CHF) in recognition of the effect of this condition in diminishing hepatic perfusion. This yielded somewhat better agreement between measured and predicted C_p^{ss} values than use of equation 5 or previous techniques (Table 22.1). Optimum prediction of C_p^{ss} values requires use of actual digoxin renal clearances (Cl_{dig}) rather than Cl_{CR}. Many patients exhibit appreciable differences between Cl_{dig} and Cl_{CR} values which limits the accuracy of equations 5 or 6 (Jusko et al., 1974a).

Table 22.1. Performance of predictive techniques for digoxin dosages

Method	Correlation r	In ± 30 % Range[a]
$C_p^{ss} = \dfrac{F \cdot D_0 \cdot t_{1/2}}{V_D \cdot 0.693 \cdot \Upsilon}$	0.79	6/17
$C_p^{ss} = F \cdot D_0/Cl_B \cdot \Upsilon$	0.92	12/17
$Cl_B = 36 + 1.1\ Cl_{dig} - 18$ CHF (0,1)		

[a] Measured versus predicted C_p^{ss} values.
Data are from Koup et al. (1975a).

Body Clearance, ml/min

Normal CVP	Increased CVP		Creatinine Clearance (ml/min)		Weight (kg)		Serum creatinine (mg/100ml)
223	202	- - - - - -	150 / 130				
170	149	- - - - - -	110 / 100		120 / 110 / 100		
145	124	- - - - - -	90 / 80		90 / 80	R	50
119	98	- - - - - -	70 / 60		70 / 60		40
106	85	- - - - - -	50		50	Age (years)	30
92	71	- - - - - -	40		40	♂ | ♀	20 / 17
80	59	- - - - - -	30		30		15 / 13 / 12 / 10 / 09 / 08 / 07 / 06 / 05
66	45	- - - - - -	20				04
53	32	- - - - - -	10				

Nomogram for rapid evaluation of endogenous-creatinine clearance.

With a ruler, join weight to age. Keep ruler at crossing-point of line marked R. Then move the right-hand side of the ruler to the appropriate serum-creatinine value and read the patient's clearance from the left side of the nomogram

40   20 - - - - - anephric patients

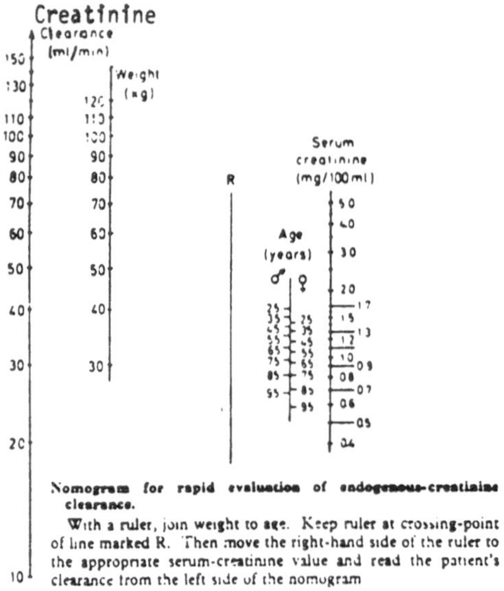

$$\text{Oral Maintenance Dose (mg/day)} = \frac{\text{Serum Conc. (ng/ml)} \times \text{Body Cl (ml/min)}}{417 \text{ (tablet) or } 590 \text{ (elixir)}}$$

Fig. 22.2. Estimation of digoxin body clearance (Cl_B) from creatinine clearance (Cl_{CR}) using the Siersbaek-Nielsen (1971) nomogram and the equation: $Cl_B = 40 + 1.3 \cdot Cl_{CR} - 20 \cdot CHF$ (0,1) where the presence ($CHF = 1$) and absence ($CHF = 0$) moderate to severe CHF is included

The application of these clearance principles to digoxin dosing has been reduced to nomogram format for simplicity of clinical application. The method, shown in Figure 22.2, includes the Siersbaek-Nielsen et al. (1971) nomogram for creatinine clearance from which the Cl_B of digoxin is estimated using equation 6. A correction of Cl_B for the presence of moderate to severe CHF (increased central venous pressure, CVP) or impaired liver function is given. This nomogram works reasonably well for predicting dosages or for checking uncertain measurements of serum digoxin concentrations. Its utility is limited by the facts that Cl_{dig} is somewhat variable and unpredictable (Jusko et al., 1974a), the nomogram estimation of Cl_{CR} is imperfect (Jusko et al., 1974a), secondary factors which affect digoxin Cl_B such as thyroid disease are not included, and mean bioavailability values are included which may not always be appropriate (Jusko et al., 1974b).

Summary

The pharmacokinetics of digoxin in patients with impaired renal function are complicated by the considerable variability in volumes of distribution, half-lives, and clearances of the drug which limits the accuracy of predictive techniques. Part of this difficulty is resolved by recognizing the inherent problems in pharmacokinetic methodology which are partly resolved by utilizing clearance concepts. Because of these uncertainties in digoxin kinetics, the combined use of nomogram predictions with feedback serum concentration measurements are needed to provide optimum therapeutic use of digoxin.

References

Gorodischer, R., Jusko, W. J., Yaffe, S. J.: Tissue and Erythrocyte Distribution of Digoxin in Infants. Clin. Pharmacol. Ther. 19, 256—263 (1976)

Harrison, L. I., Gibaldi, M.: Physiologically-Based Pharmacokinetic Model for Digoxin Disposition in the Dog and its Application to Man. J. Pharm. Sci. (in press) (1975)

Harrison, L. I., Gibaldi, M.: A Physiologically-based Pharmacokinetic Model for Digoxin Distribution and Elimination in the Rat. J. Pharm. Sci. 66, (in press) (1977)

Jusko, W. J.: Clinical Pharmacokinetics of Digoxin. In: Clinical Pharmacokinetiks: A Symposium. Levy, G. (ed.) Washington: Academy of Pharmaceutical Sciences 1974, pp. 31—43

Jusko, W. J.: Factors Affecting the Pharmacokinetics of Some Psychoactive Drugs, In: Clinical Pharmacology of Psychoactive Drugs. Sellers, E. M. (ed.) Toronto: Alcoholism and Drug Addiction Research Foundation 1975, pp. 55—72

Jusko, W. J., Weintraub, M.: Myocardial Distribution of Digoxin and Renal Function. Clin. Pharmacol. Ther. 16, 449—454 (1974)

Jusko, W. J., Szefler, S. J., Goldfarb, A. L.: Pharmacokinetic Design of Digoxin Dosage Regimens in Relation to Renal Function. J. Clin. Pharmacol. 14, 525—535 (1974a)

Jusko, W. J., Conti, D. R., Molson, A., Kuritzky, P., Giller, J., Schultz, R.: Digoxin Absorption from Tablets and Elixir: The Effect of Radiation-Induced Malabsorption. J. A. M. A. 230, 1554—1555 (1974b)

Koup, J. R., Jusko, W. J., Elwood, C. M., Kohli, R. K.: Digoxin Pharmacokinetics: Role of Renal Failure in Dosage Regimen Design. Clin. Pharmacol. Ther. 18, 9—21 (1975a)

Koup, J. R., Greenblatt, D. J., Jusko, W. J., Smith, T. W., Koch-Weser, J.: Pharmacokinetics of Digoxin in Normal Subjects After Intravenous Bolus and Infusion Doses. J. Pharmacokin. Biopharm. 3, 181—192 (1975b)

Ohnhaus, E. E., Spring, P., Dettli, L.: Eliminationskinetik und Dosierung von Digoxin bei Patienten mit Niereninsuffizienz. Dtsch. Med. Wochenschr. 99, 1797—1803 (1974)

Rowland, M., Benet, L. Z., Graham, G. G.: Clearance Concepts in Pharmaco-kinetics. J. Pharmacokin. Biopharm. $\underline{1}$, 123–136 (1973)

Siersbaek-Nielsen, K., Molholm Hansen, J., Kampman, J., Kristensen, M.: Rapid Evaluation of Creatinine Clearance, Lancet 1971/I, 1133

Sumner, D. J., Russell, A.J., Whiting, B.: Digoxin Pharmacokinetics: Multicom-partment Analysis and its Clinical Implications. Br. J. Clin. Pharmacol. $\underline{3}$, 221–229 (1976)

As Dr. Jusko was not able to deliver his paper personally, Dr. Johnson and Dr. Klotz presented data on cardiac toxicity in relation to digoxin plasma levels and the biliary excretion of β-acetyl-digoxin.

22.2 Peak Plasma Digoxin Concentration and Cardiotoxicity

B. F. JOHNSON, D. J. CHAPPLE, R. HUGHES, J. LABROOY, and I. SMITH

Cardiotoxicity remains a significant problem limiting the clinical usefulness of the cardiac glycosides. Many recent studies have demonstrated that patients showing clear evidence of digitalis toxicity have significantly higher plasma digoxin levels than patients without such signs. Although two studies (Fogelman et al., 1971, Howard et al., 1973) failed to demonstrate any relation between the incidence of cardiotoxicity and level of plasma digoxin, the vast majority of such studies have shown some degree of overlap but significant differentiation between toxic and nontoxic patients (Smith and Haber, 1973). It is important to stress that in all these studies, plasma digoxin concentration was determined during continued administration of digoxin, with the blood sample being obtained a minimum of 6 h after the last dose. It is widely accepted that such determination, usually termed the steady-state plasma concentration, are reasonably well correlated with the risk of developing cardiotoxic phenomena.

However, the plasma concentration of digoxin shows quite marked diurnal fluctuations with customary regimes of continued treatment. The variation is particularly marked when oral preparations of high bioavailability are used. Figure 22.3 illustrates a typical plasma concentration profile seen in a subject with normal renal function taking 0.25 mg digoxin every 12 h. With tablets of high dissolu-

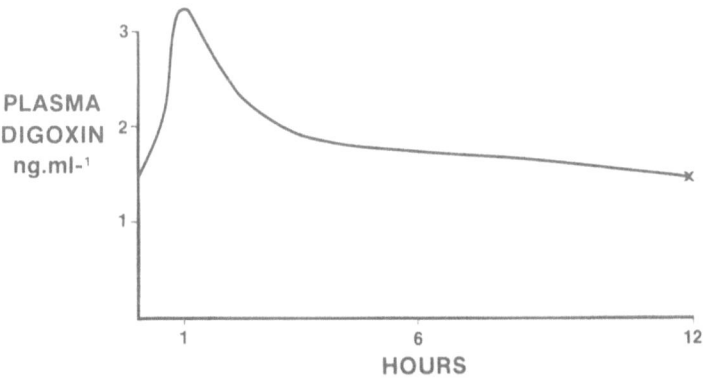

Fig. 22.3. Typical profile of variation in plasma concentration during one dosage interval in a patient taking 0.25 mg digoxin twice daily

tion rates, digoxin elixir, or soft gelatin capsules containing digoxin in solution, marked peak concentrations are apparent about 1 h after ingestion of each dose. In the example illustrated in Figure 22.3., the fluctuations in plasma concentrations are repeated every 12 h. Concern has been expressed (Harter, Skelly and Steers 1974, Reissell et al., 1974) that the pharmacodynamic effects of digoxin might parallel the changes in plasma concentrations and that there might be an increased incidence of transient toxicity associated with the high peak concentrations.

It appears well-established that clinically desirable cardiac effects do not show wide fluctuations in association with transient changes in plasma concentration (Chamberlain, 1974). After either oral or intravenous administration of digoxin in man, there is a considerable time delay before the development of maximum positive inotropic or chronotropic effects (Ganz et al., 1957, Shapiro et al., 1970). In the above studies, the time of maximal effect ranged from 4—12 h after digoxin administration, whereas peak concentrations would have been anticipated within 90 min of administration.

The most obvious explanation for the lack of correlation between cardiac effects and transient changes in plasma concentration is that digoxin concentration at the cardiac receptor differs from that in plasma. The characteristics of the curve

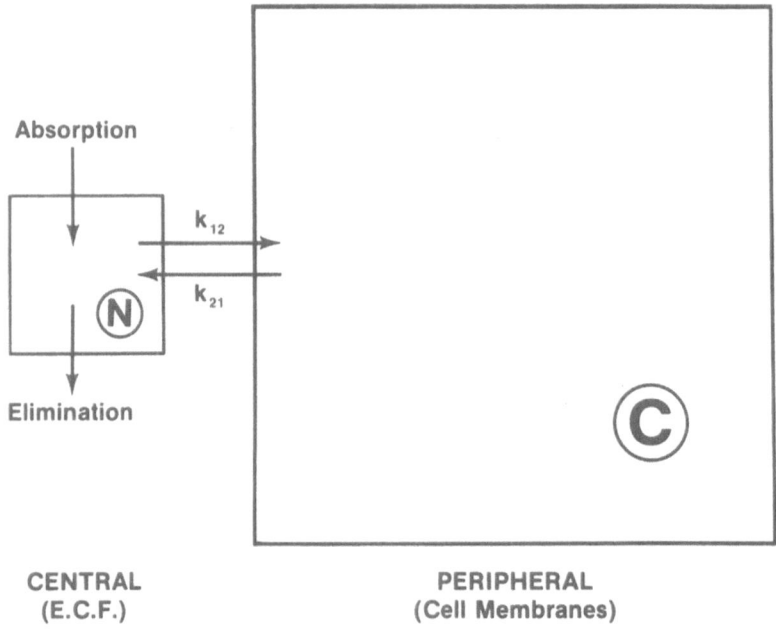

Fig. 22.4. Two-compartment open model of digoxin pharmacokinetics. Digoxin is absorbed into and eliminated from the small central compartment. The speed of transport into and back from the larger peripheral compartment is associated with respective rate constants k_{12} and k_{21}. N and C represent postulated receptor sites mediating the nausea-producing and cardiac effects

of decline of plasma digoxin concentration cannot be adequately explained mathematically unless at least two body compartments are postulated. In the simplest possible model, illustrated in Figure 22.4. the small central compartment into which digoxin is either injected or absorbed might be considered to be extracellular fluid. The much larger peripheral compartment in this two-compartment open model might then represent digoxin bound to cell membranes in various tissues. Transfer of digoxin between these two compartments is controlled by processes with can be considered to have rate constants k_{12} and k_{21} as illustrated. After digoxin enters the central compartment, there will be delay in attainment of peak concentration in the peripheral compartment. Several hours are required for the ratio of digoxin concentrations in the two compartments to reach equilibrium. It is important to note that equilibrium must be established before plasma concentratheidin has any value as an indirect measure of the concentration in the peripheral compartment. By postulating that the receptor for desired clinical effects is within this peripheral compartment, the delayed development of maximal effect and the correlation of steady-state plasma concentration with cardiac effect can be explained.

It would be expected that cardiotoxic manifestations of digoxin would show a similar lack of relation to transient changes in plasma concentration, if the same cardiac receptor controlled both wanted and unwanted effects. However, recent studies (Levitt et al., 1976) have provided evidence that digoxin-induced dysrhythmias may be partially mediated by a central mechanism of action, as they are associated with increased sympathetic discharge from the CNS. It is known that digoxin penetrates into the CNS, and that this is the predominant factor in the causation of nausea and vomiting. In our own experience, nausea and vomiting have always occurred between 45 and 90 min after an oral dose of digoxin, when plasma concentrations were at their highest. Therefore, we consider it highly likely that the receptor initiating the nausea and vomiting response is situated within the central compartment and that the extent of its stimulation closely follows the changes in plasma concentration. If one receptor system within the CNS is rapidly responsive to transient increases in plasma concentrations, it is justified to suspect that a possible central receptor controlling cardiotoxicity might behave in the same manner.

The experiments to be described were designed to answer two questions. First, is there any direct temporal relation of digoxin cardiotoxicity to transient changes in plasma concentrations, and secondly, is there any indirect relationship, namely an influence of high peak concentrations upon the maximal degree of delayed cardiotoxicity.

Experiment 1

Methods

Studies were performed on eight unanesthetized mongrel dogs, in whom the cardiac tolerance to acetylstrophanthidin was determined by the intravenous infusion of a 100 μg/ml solution in 0.9% saline. The rate of infusion was maintained at 95 μg/min. The ECG (lead II) was monitored continuously and the amount of acetylstrophanthidin required to induce cardiotoxicity determined.

It was accepted that cardiotoxicity had developed when one or more of these ECG changes occurred: 1) multifocal ectopics, 2) ventricular ectopic beats occurring with an equal or greater frequency than normal complexes, 3) supraventricular or ventricular tachycardia, or 4) complete heart block. Tolerance to acetylstrophanthidin was determined on three occasions in each study, namely at 45 (ASI), 180 (ASII), and 360 min (ASIII) after either the beginning of a control experiment or the administration of digoxin. Hartmann's solution (Ringer lactate) was infused to replace fluid losses from vomiting.

Each dog underwent four studies with oral doses of 0.05, 0.1, 0.2, and 0.4 mg/kg digoxin using a randomized sequence of administration; at least 10 days were allowed between each experiment. The digoxin was administered in solution to each dog by an esophageal catheter. At least two control experiments with acetylstrophanthidin alone were carried out, including one at the beginning of the study, and one before the third or fourth dose of digoxin. Venous blood was obtained 0, 15, 30, 45, 60, 90, 120, and 360 min after the administration of digoxin. The plasma levels of digoxin were measured by a radioimmunoassay technique using the Lanoxitest-γ kit (Wellcome Reagents Ltd) with an iodinated tyrosine derivative of digoxin as the tracer, but with the modification that standards were prepared with pooled dog serum.

Results

Treatment with digoxin reduced the amount of acetylstrophantidin required to cause cardiotoxicity, and this increased susceptibility to toxicity was dose dependent. At the lower dose levels of 0.05 and 0.1 mg/kg digoxin, increased susceptibility was apparent at ASII, though not significant. At the two higher dose levels of 0.2 and 0.4 mg/kg of digoxin, reduced acetylstrophanthidin tolerance was maximal at ASII, persisted to ASIII, and differed significantly from the control experiments.

The peak plasma concentration of digoxin was reached at about 60 min after each dose and then declined steadily. In these dogs, vomiting did not occur until the first infusion of acetylstrophanthidin which was started 45 min after administration of digoxin.

Acetylstrophanthidin sensitivity was calculated as the difference between the amounts of acetylstrophanthidin required to induce cardiotoxicity in the digoxin and the control studies. The calculations were carried out from the results for comparable acetylstrophanthidin infusions (ASI, II, or III) for individual dogs. Comparison of the plasma levels of digoxin and acetylstrophanthidin sensitivity showed that there was no correlation between these two variables (Figure 22.5.). This was most evident after the 0.2 and 0.4 mg/kg doses of digoxin.

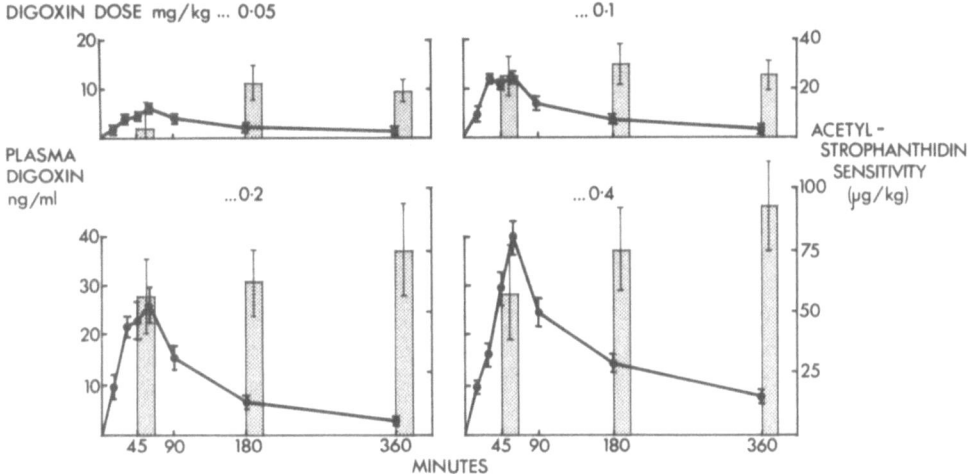

Fig. 22.5. Comparisons of mean plasma digoxin concentration (curves) and mean acetylstrophanthidin sensitivity (columns) for four oral doses of digoxin given to conscious dogs. Bars represent SEM

Experiment 2

Evidence of cardiotoxicity is provided only by assessment of frequency of disturbances in cardiac conduction and rhythm. None of these disturbances is specific, and the most common disturbance is ventricular ectopic beats which are merely seen more frequently during digoxin overdosage. It has been established (Lown and Levine, 1961) that a safe clinical method of uncovering the earliest signs of toxicity is to apply unilateral carotid sinus pressure. This maneuver increases the frequency of rhythm disturbances as the earliest evidence of digoxin cardiotoxicity.

Methods

During a period of 3 months, all patients admitted to six medical wards at Kings College Hospital, London, and who were taking maintenance digoxin treatment were studied. Patients were excluded if they had taken digoxin for less than 4 weeks before admission to hospital, if cardiac, respiratory, or renal function was obviously unstable, or if the patient was over 75 years old. After the patient had been in hospital for at least 4 days, the total daily dosage of digoxin was administered at 9 a.m. on the study day. Electrocardiographic tracings [lead II] were obtained for periods of 3 min immediately before the dose of digoxin was given, and at 1, 4, 8, and 24 h later. During the time that ECG tracings were recorded, carotid sinus massage was performed for 5 s on the left and 5 s on the right side

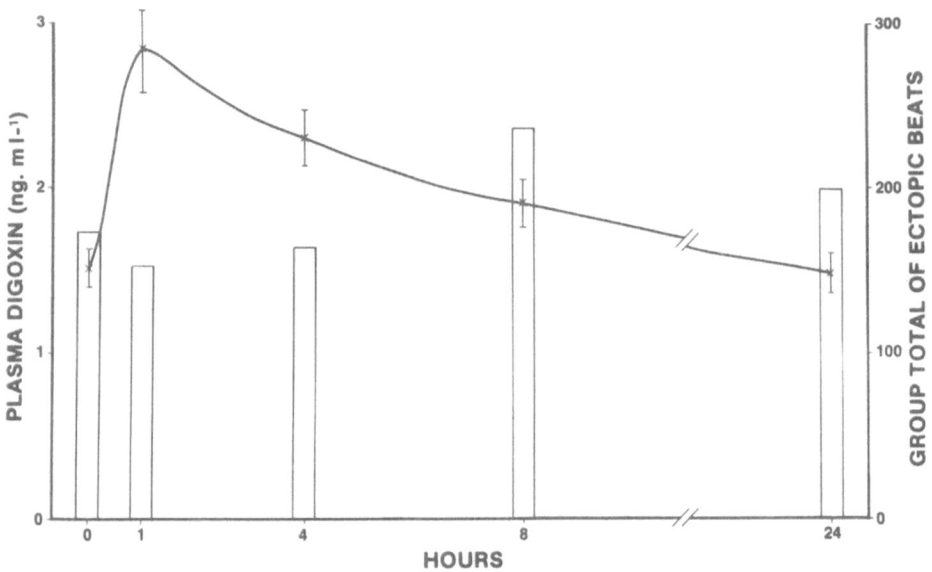

Fig. 22.6. Comparison of mean (± SEM) plasma digoxin concentration (curve) and total number of ectopic ECG complexes (columns) counted in 3-min periods during 1 day in a group of 34 patients

at 1 and 2 min, respectively. Blood samples were collected for determination of plasma digoxin concentration immediately after each ECG tracing had been obtained.

Results

Figure 22.6. illustrates the results obtained in 34 patients. In this group of patients, steady-state plasma concentrations taken immediately before ingestion of digoxin ranged from 0.8 — 3.3 ng/ml. Eight of the subjects had values greater than 2 ng/ml. As shown in Figure 22.6., mean plasma concentration rose to reach its highest level 1 h after digoxin was administered and then fell progressively over the next 24 h. The total number of supraventricular and ventricular ectopic complex occurring during each 3-min ECG tracing were calculated in random sequence by a physician who was blind in relation to the name of the patient or the timing of the tracing. Figure 22.6. illustrates the total number of ectopic complexes seen in the ECG tracings of the total group of 34 patients at each time of determination. By Freedman's nonparametric method of analysis of variance, significant differences were observed between times of determination only for total (i.e., supraventricular plus ventricular) ectopic complexes. The Wilcoxon signed rank sum test confirmed that more ectopic beats were recorded at 8 h than immediately before or 1 h after digoxin had been administered. There was no trend for a greater frequency of either supraventricular or

278

ventricular ectopic beats or of heart block induced by carotid sinus massage during the time when plasma concentrations were at their highest.

Experiment 3

Methods

Further studies were performed on eight unanesthetized mongrel dogs, in whom cardiac tolerance to acetylstrophanthidin was assessed at 150 and 360 min after beginning infusion of 0.1 mg/kg digoxin. In each dog, studies were performed after an infusion of either digoxin over 9 or 90 min, or after infusion of control saline over the same period, with the sequence of administration being randomized. Pertinent samples were collected for determination of plasma digoxin concentration before and 5, 10, 15, 20, 30, 60, 90, 120, 150, and 360 min after beginning the infusion of digoxin. The techniques of assessing acetylstrophanthidin sensitivity and plasma levels of digoxin were as described in experiment 1.

Results

As shown in Figure 22.7., very different profiles of plasma digoxin concentration were obtained over the first 2 h by the different rates of infusion. Acetylstrophanthidin sensitivity tended to be somewhat lower at 360 than at 150 min after beginning the infusion of digoxin. However, at both times, acetylstrophanthidin sensitivity was clearly independent of the rate at which plasma digoxin had been administered, and therefore of the peak plasma concentrations attained.

Conclusions

The results of the first two experiments provide evidence against the concept that transient elevations in plasma digoxin concentration are temporally associated with risk of cardiotoxicity. These conclusions are supported by Larese and Mirkin (1974) who found no relationship between transient elevation in serum digoxin level and either the onset or persistence of cardiac arrhythmias in a group of 15 children with congenital cardiac defects. This appeared true whether the digoxin was administered orally, or by intramuscular or intravenous injection. These results suggest that the risk of cardiotoxicity develops in conjunction with desirable cardiac effects. In man, the greatest risk of cardiotoxicity probably occurs during the period 4—8 h after the last dose administered.

The results of experiment 3 suggest that the tendency to cardiotoxicity is determined solely by the quantity of digoxin entering into the circulation and is unrelated to rate of entry. By inference, neither the speed of intravenous injection nor the rate of intestinal absorption affect the risk of the common types of car-

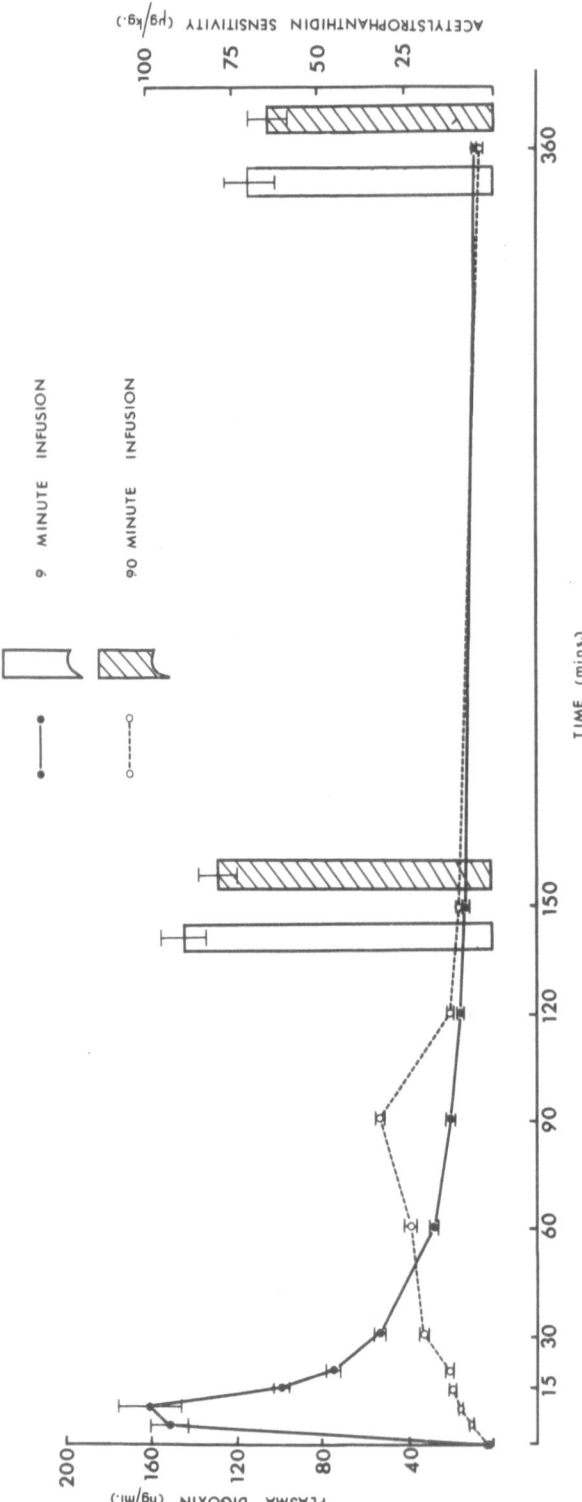

Fig. 22.7. Comparison of mean plasma digoxin concentration (curves) and mean acetylstrophanthidin sensitivity (columns) for two infusion rates of digoxin administrated to conscious dogs. Bars represent SEM

diotoxity. It seems unlikely that oral digoxin preparations of high bioavailability produce any variation in cardiac response due to a qualitative difference in the plasma concentration profile produced. Such products are more efficacious entirely due to increased extent of absorption. These findings are all compatible with the hypothesis that receptors governing both desirable and undesirable cardiac effects all form part of a compartment which is separate from extracellular fluid.

References

Chamberlain, D. A.: The relation of clinical effect to plasma digoxin concentration. Postgrad. Med. J. 50 (Suppl. 6), 29—35 (1974)

Fogelman, A. M., La Mont, J. T., Finkelstein, S., Rado, E., Pearce, M. L.: Fallibility of plasma-digoxin in differentiating toxic from non-toxic patients. Lancet 1971/II, 727

Ganz, A., Fujimori, H., Penna, M., Greiner, T., Gold, H.: Intramuscular administration of digoxin in propylene glycol. Proc. Soc. Exp. Biol. Med. 95, 349—353 (1957)

Harter, J. G., Skelly, J. P., Steers, A. W.: Digoxin — the regulatory viewpoint. Circulation 49, 395—398 (1974)

Howard, D., Smith, C. I., Stewart, G., Vedas, M., Tiller, D. J., Hensley, W. J., Richards, J. G.: A prospective survey of the incidence of cardiac intoxication with digitalis in patients being admitted to hospital and correlation with serum digoxin levels. Aust. N. Z. J. Med. 3, 279 (1973)

Larese, R. J., Mirkin, B. L.: Kinetics of digoxin absorption and relation of serum levels to cardiac arrhythmias in children. Clin. Pharmacol. Ther. 15/4, 387—396 (1974)

Levitt, B., Cagin, N., Somberg, J., Kleid, J.: Neural basis for the genesis and control of digitalis arrhythmias. Cardiology 61, 50—60 (1976)

Lown, B., Levine, S. A.: The carotid sinus: Clinical value of its stimulation. Circulation 23, 766—789 (1961)

Reissell, P., Manninen, V., Ojala, K., Karjalainen, J.: Non-equivalence of digoxin tablets. Ann. Clin. Res. 6, 4—8 (1974)

Shapiro, W., Narahara, K., Taubert, K.: Relationship of plasma digitoxin and digoxin to cardiac response following intravenous digitalization in man. Circulation 42, 1065—1072 (1970)

Smith, T. W., Haber, E.: Digitalis. New Engl. J. Med. 289, 1063 (1973)

Discussion

Butler, New York: Dr. Johnson, why is it that in people on chronic maintenance digoxin we don't often encounter this nausea? Is this just an initial phenomenon in people in single-dose studies, or is it more common than we realize in patients who are on maintenance digoxin?

Johnson: It is difficult to say very much about nausea because it is so idiosyncratic. Most volunteers don't turn a hair when given large single doses, but in occasional experiments almost everybody seems to be vomiting 1 h after digoxin. In the chronic state also, the most common time of nausea is 1 h after the tablet has been given. So I think that there is probably some relation with plasma concentration.

Reissell, Helsinki: I would like to state our opinion later when our paper is presented. As shown in the earlier discussion, the penetration of digoxin in the cerebrospinal fluid is very minimal and I doubt that the amount of digoxin in the cerebrospinal fluid in the early postadministrative phase can cause nausea.

Greenblatt, Boston: We studied steady-state levels of digoxin in plasma and CSF. Even at steady state, the spinal fluid to plasma ratio was about 14 %. So entry into the spinal fluid can't be determined by passive diffusion alone. I should say, Dr. Johnson, that when we studied rapidly dissolving digoxin tablets a few years ago, we found that they tended to cause nausea within 5—10 min after drug administration. We thought that this was at least in part a local phenomenon due . to rapid release and high local concentrations. It considerably preceded the peak plasma concentration, and we didn't see it with the elixir which produced a similar or higher peak.

Johnson: I'm surprised at that rapidity of appearance of nausea. It has been invariable in my experience that nausea never developed before 45 min after oral preparations had been given. Between 45—90 min after ingestion is the time when volunteers may start looking green. It usually lasts for 15—30 min. It hasn't been a problem, fortunately, in bioavailability studies, as where subjects actually have vomited and we've collected the fluid, there's been almost no digoxin in it.

Greenblatt: We observed no instances of vomiting.

Johnson: The cause of the nausea is controversial. Animal pharmacologic evidence suggests that an intact CNS is essential. But I would agree that one sees nausea so much more with oral preparations than after intravenous administration. There must also be some gastrointestinal element in it.

Kramer, Göttingen: Dr. Greenblatt, you have used the term "steady-state plasma concentration" of digoxin. Would you kindly specify this term, because this may be 4 h, 12 h, or 24 h after administration, and one would expect a remarkable change in plasma concentration during this time.

Greenblatt: In general, I mean at least 4 h after the dose. We know that distribution is largely complete within 4 h, and there is not much change in the concentration over the day between say 4—6 and 24 h after the dose.

Kramer: Well, but from 4—24 h I am sure that there is a considerable change of the plasma concentration in patients with normal renal function.

Greenblatt: I was referring to the patients in the CSF study. They were at least 4 h after the last dose, and most of them were 24 h after the last dose, so we felt that they were in steady state. And even so we found a very small CSF to plasma ratio.

Follath, Basel: I should like to make a short comment in support of Dr. Johnson's findings: we have studied 25 patients with acute myocardial infarction at a coronary care unit. They received 0.25—0.75 mg i.v. doses of digoxin; none of them showed acute arrhythmias during a 2-h continuous monitoring.

Schaumann, Mannheim: In a yet unpublished study, Somogyi and co-workers found 18% of the serum concentration in the cerebrospinal fluid both for β-methyl digoxin and for digoxin. That was 24 h after the last dose. And what you said about vomiting after intravenous or oral dosage — well, that's certainly not true for animals. In animals, you always get vomiting with lower intravenous doses than on oral administration, the ratio depending on absorption. I think there is no doubt that vomiting is essentially a central effect.

Johnson: I accept that the animal pharmacologic evidence points that way. But man may be somewhat different. Most clinicians believe that vomiting is rare with intravenously administered digoxin.

Marcus: I wanted to make sure that your remarks regarding very rapid intravenous injection and slow infusion may not be misinterpreted to mean that they are equally safe. Some years ago, when we were doing experiments on the effect of hypokalemia on digoxin toxicity in dogs, we showed that we could give a dose of digoxin over 10—15 min that would not induce ventricular tachycardia, but this same dose would cause a toxic arrhythmia when given over 1 min. I am not sure that these experiments are necessarily clinically relevant, since the dose given was large, but I think that in some patients who are sensitive to digitalis, a rapid bolus injection may not be quite as safe as a slower infusion of the same dose of digoxin.

Johnson: I agree absolutely. I was careful to say that the usual types of cardiac toxicity were uninfluenced by rate of administration. I think that digoxin should never be administered rapidly intravenously, as occasional patients may develop cardiac arrest under these circumstances, possibly via reflex vagal stimulation.

22.3 Biliary Excretion of β-Acetyl-Digoxin in Man

U. KLOTZ

Summary

Biliary excretion of digoxin was measured in one patient after a single i.v. dose of 0.6 mg and in three patients on maintenance therapy with 0.4 mg β-acetyl-dig-oxin/die. From a single dose, 8.8% and 9.2% were recovered in the bile collected via a T-tube within 24 and 36 h, respectively. During steady state, the daily amount excreted with the bile varied between 2% and 10%. In two healthy volunteers, the effect of the intraluminal binding agent cholestyramine on the disposition of digoxin was investigated. The cross-over experiment did not exhibit any difference in the plasma level/time profiles after a single intravenous dose. These results indicate only a minor biliary excretion of digoxin which could contribute only to an insignificant enterohepatic recycling.

Introduction

The polarity of a cardiac glycoside seems to be an important factor for its excretion and its enterohepatic cycling. While the nonpolar digitoxin is significantly recycled with the bile during its metabolism in the liver (Okita, 1967) the biliary excretion of digoxin is considered as insignificant in man (Doherty et al., 1970; Klotz and Antonin, 1977). Doherty and collaborators found that only 4.3%–12.7% of a single dose are excreted into the bile within a collection period of 7 days. In some contrast is the recently published study of Caldwell and Cline (Caldwell and Cline, 1976). These authors found in five subjects an averaged total 24-h recovery in the bile of 30.6%± 6.1% of the administered dose. However, in this study the radioactive digoxin was not measured directly in the bile, but in an intestinal aspirate.

To contribute to this obscure situation, we investigated the biliary excretion of digoxin in four patients with normal kidney and liver function who received a T-tube postoperatively. In addition, the effect of the drug-absorbing agent cholestyramine on the disposition of digoxin was studied in two healthy volunteers. Bile was collected in 4-h intervals during the first 12 h and thereafter in 12-h intervals up to 48 h. Digoxin concentrations in plasma and bile were measured by a specific radioimmunoassay (Klotz et al., 1976). (We thank Dr. Bodem (Bonn) for providing us with antibody).

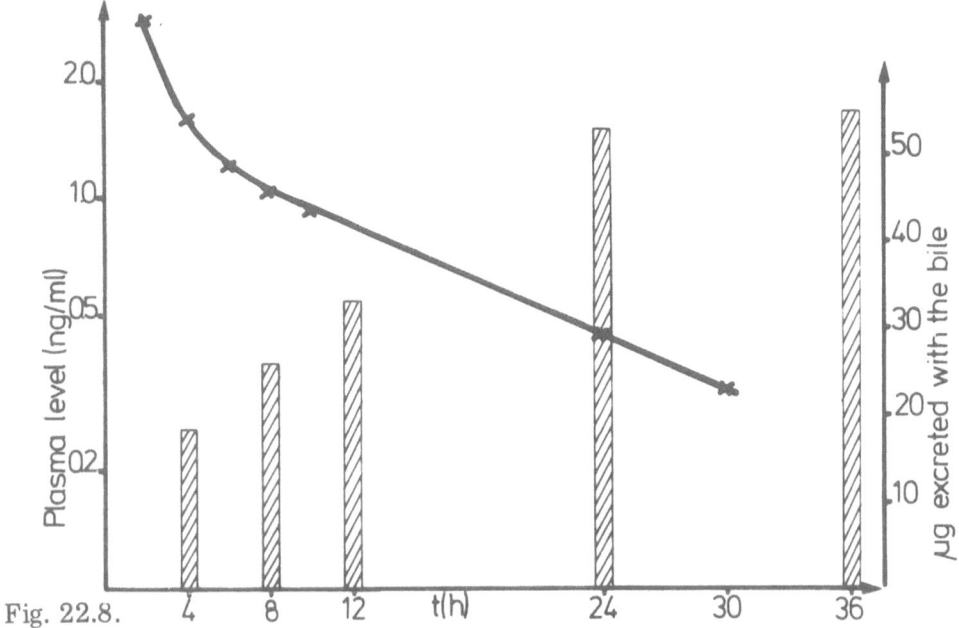

Fig. 22.8.

Results

The results of the one patient who received the single intravenous bolus of 0.6 mg digoxin can be seen in Figure 22.8. Plasma levels ranged within 36 h between 3 and 0.3 ng/ml and the decline was biexponential. The cumulative amount of the digoxin excreted with the bile was 8.8% after 24 h and 9.2% within 36 h. Thereafter, the biliary excretion was insignificant. These numbers confirm the work of Doherty et al. (Doherty et al., 1970).

The results of the three patients on maintenance therapy with 0.4 mg β-acetyl-digoxin administered once daily are summarized in Figure 22.9. Since these patients were on the same digoxin dose for longer than 2 weeks, it can be stated that they were studied under steady-state conditions. This could also be proven by routine plasma level monitoring. The daily loss of digoxin via their biliary T-tube ranged from 2%—10%, if one assumes a bioavailability of 70% of the tablets used. The daily excretion of 2%—10% digoxin of a maintenance dose might be an underestimation, since the total bile fluid cannot be measured by the T-tube technique. But from the bile volume collected, one can calculate the minimal bile flow. This value varied between about 330 and 530 ml per day and is not too much different from a normal daily bile flow of about 600 ml. Also under steady-state conditions, there seems to be ca. 10% biliary excretion of digoxin daily.

The influence of cholestyramine, an effective intraluminal binding agent for various drugs, on the disposition of digoxin was investigated in two healthy subjects. In Figure 22.10. the results in one individual can be seen.

Patient		a.w.	e.f.	e.h.
Excreted amount (μg)	0—24 h	18.1	5.2	24.2
	24—48 h	28.2	6.3	28.5
% of dose excreted	0—24 h	6.4	1.9	8.6
(70% bioavailability	24—48 h	10.1	2.3	10.2
assumed)				
Minimal bile flow		10	19	15
(ml/h)		14	22	16

Fig. 22.9. Biliary excretion of digoxin in man under steady state conditions

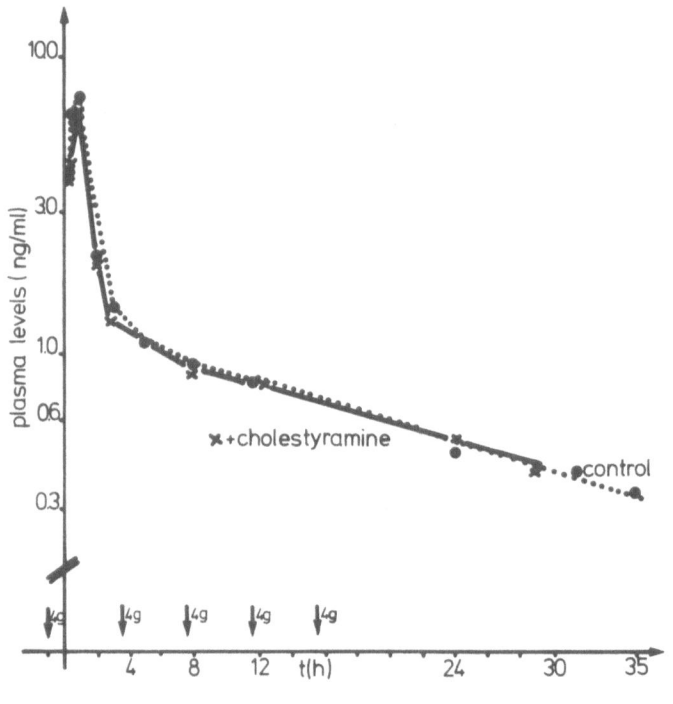

Fig. 22.10

In a cross-over experiment, 0.6 mg digoxin were given by a 1 h infusion, and the digoxin plasma levels were monitored for 30 or 35 h. In one part of the experiment (solid line), 4 g cholestyramine were given five times every 4 h. The oral administration of this agent did not have any effect on the plasma level/time profile of digoxin. Also, in the second individual, both curves were almost identical. In vitro experiments proved a significant binding of digoxin to cholestyramine. These results with cholestyramine support our data about the minor biliary excretion.

From the available data, it can be concluded that for digoxin, biliary excretion and enterohepatic cycling do not play an important role. For this reason, cholestyramine will not be as effective in treating digoxin intoxications as in the comparable case of digitoxin (Caldwell and Greenberger, 1971).

References

Caldwell, J. H., Cline, C. T.: Biliary excretion of digoxin in man. Clin. Pharmacol. Ther. 19, 410–415 (1976)

Caldwell, J. H., Greenberger, N. J.: Interruption of the enterohepatic circulation of digitoxin by cholestyramine. I. Protection against lethal digitoxin intoxication. J. Clin. Invest. 50, 2626–2637 (1971)

Doherty, J. E., Flanigan, W. J., Murphy, M. L., Bulloch, R. T., Dalrumple, G. L., Beard, O. W., Perkins, W. H.: Tritiated digoxin. XIV. Enterohepatic circulation, absorption, and excretion studies in human volunteers. Circulation 42, 867–873 (1970)

Klotz, U., Antonin, K. H.: Biliary excretion studies in man. Intern. J. Clin. Pharmacol. Biopharm. 15, 332-334 (1977)

Klotz, U., Antonin, K. H., Bieck, P. R.: Bioavailability of β-acetyldigoxin tablets and solution after single and repeated administration. Eur. J. Clin. Pharmacol. 10, 417–424 (1976)

Okita, G. T.: Species difference in duration of action of cardiac glucosides. Fed. Proc. 26, 1125–1130 (1967)

Discussion

Scholz, Hannover: Dr. Schaumann, is there a risk of cumulation in *chronic* liver disease with respect to the Lanitop brand?'

Schaumann: There is study in patients with liver cirrhosis. No intrapatient comparison could be made in that case, but there was no difference between the serum concentrations in those patients and in other patients without liver cirrhosis studied by the same investigators and in the same laboratory.

Hahn, Ludwigshafen: I just want to contribute to the question of the effect of cholestyramine on the absorption of β-methyl-digoxin. Several years back, I studied this possible interaction in six volunteers in a controlled single-blind study using a randomized cross-over repetition design. Blood levels of the tritium-labeled compound following the sole or combined intake with cholestyramine were determined in intervals for 48 h. There were no significant differences in the course of the blood levels. A comparison of the areas under the curves yields a 5.8% reduction of drug absorption by the resin, which is not statistically sig-

nificant (Hahn and Reindell, 1974). Accordingly, a therapeutic effect of cholestyramine on the intoxication with methyl-digoxin is not to be expected.

Klotz: We gave the digoxin by intravenous infusion and didn't see any effect,
so we cancelled out an absorption process. But it seems that absorption, too, is
not influenced by cholestyramine.

Ohnhaus, Bern: I would like to make a general comment on studying drugs in
liver disease, because we do not usually have any parameter to measure the extent of liver disease and the transaminases are not a help for us. What we have
tried is to use antipyrine as a substance for measuring the extent of liver damage
in respect to drug metabolism, and we studied this in connection with the β-block-
ing agent pindolol. We found a very good correlation in patients with liver cirrhosis, but in other liver diseases there are other problems as well, and I think we
must be aware if we study drugs and their metabolism that we must have exact
knowledge of the liver function.

Klotz: May I add something, because I have been working in the liver disease
field, too. For instance, most studies with liver disease report half-lives, but half-
life is not a good parameter to characterize the drug-metabolizing enzymes. A
much better expression is clearance, but even clearance is not the key to it, because clearance is dependent on liver blood flow and the extraction ratio. Only
the extraction ratio is the parameter which characterizes your enzymatic activity:

$Cl = Q \cdot E$ (= bloodflow extraction · ratio)
(Clearance)

As the group of Preisig has shown, liver disease can influence liver blood flow so
it's hard to make a prediction if a certain degree of liver disease will influence
the elimination of a drug. Another problem occurs with drugs which are highly
bound to protein, e.g., phenytoin, because you can see two effects in liver disease: one is that by the liver disease the drug-metabolizing enzymes go down,
the other side is that protein binding is decreased and you have much more free
drug available for clearance. The protein binding effect can cancel out the enzymatic effect or can even override it. There is a nice study by Blaschke from San
Francisco showing that in hepatitis phenytoin is eliminated even slightly faster,
and another study by Held and co-workers with an oral antidiabeticum shows
that in some cases the drugs are eliminated even faster. Another example we saw
yesterday is digitoxin — maybe Dr. Storstein will refer to it. Probably the fact
that digitoxin is eliminated faster in liver disease is caused by the decreased protein binding.

Gilfrich, Mainz: A question to Dr. Klotz: did you collect urine in your patients
on and without cholestyramine? It might be easier to realize any difference under both circumstances.

Klotz: We have collected the urine, but so far we didn't analyze it.

Storstein: I would like to comment on the enhanced serum elimination found in patients with chronic active hepatitis. This is probably not due to the small observed decrease in serum protein binding because then one should expect an increase in renal excretion due to an increased free fraction of the drug, this is not the case. The reduction in serum $T_{1/2}$ may rather be due to alternative metabolism in other tissues or an increase in hepatic metabolism.

Kramer, Göttingen: Don't you think that the very low renal clearance of digitoxin is not only a result of high plasma protein binding but also a result of a high tubular reabsorption of the cardiac glycoside?

Storstein: I agree to that.

Lukas: We're back to this issue of how much true glycoside — unaltered glycoside — is excreted in the bile. Your data are quantitatively very similar to those of Doherty and co-workers, but they showed that approximately 50% of the compounds emerging in the bile after a dose of tritiated digoxin were not digoxin itself. Did you distinguish between metabolites and the original compound? You made some implication about the efficacy of cholestyramine in treating digitoxin intoxication. Again, we have to refer to some of the estimates that are available on the amount of digitoxin that undergoes enterohepatic recirculation. The data of Beermann and Rosén indicate that the amount is really quite small. Their similar studies of digoxin show an enterohepatic recirculation of *that* drug that is quantitatively very similar to that of digitoxin. So I'm not clear how cholestyramine is not going to affect either the clearance of digoxin or methyldigoxin and yet is going to affect the clearance of digitoxin from the body.

Klotz: To your first question: we measured the digoxin with the radioimmunoassay and I may give the question to Dr. Bodem. He has given us a specific antibody for digoxin. From our data of other studies, I think that mainly digoxin is recognized from the antibody because we measured the urinary excretion of a single dose with this antibody. Under steady-state conditions, we recovered only about 40%—50% of a dose, which is the amount of unchanged digoxin you expect in urine. But maybe Dr. Bodem can say a little bit more about the specificity of his antibody.

Bodem, Bonn: The antibody detects digoxin and all compounds containing digoxigenin. We determined also the association constants for dihydrodigoxin and digitoxigenin. They were much lower than for the digoxigenin compounds.

Klotz: If the antibody measures digoxin and some of its metabolites, the amount or the numbers which we calculated were even too high, but this may be cancelled out by incomplete collection of the bile by the T-tube techniques. Since in both individuals the curves with and without cholestyramine were superimposable, I think there is not a significant effect, and if there is only a small recirculation with the bile, you can expect that you will not see a significant effect.

Kuhlmann, Berlin: In patients with acute hepatitis, Zilly et al. (1975) found a lower demethylation of methyl-digoxin to digoxin and a rapid increase of the plasma level with toxic side-effects. Therefore, you must reduce the maintenance dose of β-methyl-digoxin in patients with acute hepatitis because of the longer half-life of methyl-digoxin (Rietbrock et al., 1975).

Schaumann: According to the evidence available to me, there is no consistent difference in the half-lives of β-methyl-digoxin and digoxin, and the total body clearance is only 15% higher for digoxin. A decrease in the demethylation can, therefore, have no influence on the total clearance which is the essential factor determining steady-state serum concentrations during intravenous administration. In Zilly's study with β-methyl-digoxin, the renal glycoside clearance was lower in the patients with acute hepatitis than in his controls. To my mind, this cannot be explained by differences in demethylation. In addition to that, Somogyi et al. found identical serum concentrations of digoxin and β-methyl-digoxin in patients during and after acute hepatitis.

Abshagen, Berlin: I will give an indirect answer to Dr. Lukas' question. We have studied the biliary excretion of β-methyl-digoxin in biliary fistula in patients with T-tube drainage, and we found within 48 h about 10% of the given radioactivity in bile. The metabolic excretion patterns in bile showed in addition to the demethylation product digoxin between 20% and 45% water-soluble metabolites, and since after demethylation the metabolism is quite the same as when digoxin is given, this would in part answer your question that about 20%— 45% water-soluble metabolites and very small amounts of mono- and bisdigitoxoside appear in bile.

Marcus, Tucson: Just a few words about cholestyramine in the treatment of digitoxin intoxication. We had the occasion to study one patient who had digitoxin intoxication with levels starting at 65—70 ng/ml. Since the patient had complete heart block, but her hemodynamic state was stable, we obtained daily blood samples for analysis of digitoxin and determined a half-life curve over 3—4 days. We then gave cholestyramine, 16 g a day, and found that the half-life continued unchanged. We discontinued the cholestyramine and administered charcoal without altering the half-life of digitoxin. In this patient, cholestyramine or charcoal did not alter the half-life of digitoxin. This suggests that the enterohepatic circulation of digitoxin was not a major factor in determining the half-life of digitoxin or that these agents were not effective in preventing the reabsorption of digitoxin and its active metabolites.

References

Hahn, K. J., Reindell, K.: No influence of cholestyramine on the absorption of β-methyldigoxin in man. In: Atherosclerosis III, Proceedings of the 3rd. Internat. Symp. Schettler, G., Weizel, A. (eds.), Springer-Verlag, Berlin-Heidelberg-New York: (1974), p. 908

Zilly, W., Richter, E., Rietbrock, N.: Pharmacokinetics and metabolism of digoxin-
and β-methyl-digoxin-12 α-^{3}H in patients with acute hepatitis. Clin. Pharmacol.
Ther. 17, 302-309 (1975)

Rietbrock, N., Abshagen, U., v. Bergmann, K., Rennekamp, H.: Disposition of
β-methyldigoxin in man. Eur. J. Clin. Pharmacol. 9, 105-114 (1975)

23 Digitoxin Pharmacokinetics in Patients With Renal Disease[1]

L. STORSTEIN

William Withering's "An Account of the Foxglove" was translated into German 9 months after its publication by a medical doctor in Leipzig, Christian Friedrich Michaelis (Withering, 1786). This indicates an early German awareness of Withering's important clinical investigations which started in 1775. I find it highly appropriate that's a "Symposium on Cardiac Glycosides" is being held in Bonn some 200 years later to discuss recent advances in our knowledge of the cardiac glycosides.

Digitoxin is the main cardioactive substance in the digitalis purpurea or foxglove. It was the first glycoside to be purified by Claude-Adolphe Nativelle who called it "digitaline cristalisé". The name digitoxin was given it by Schmiedeberg. Digitoxin is thus the oldest glycoside in clinical use although it has been surpassed by digoxin in the last decades in most areas of the western world.

In recent years, attention has been drawn to the influence of renal function on the pharmacokinetics of cardiac glycosides. A reduction of digitalis dosage in patients with renal disease has been strongly recommended. The measurement of serum glycoside levels has confirmed the soundness of this attitude in regard to digoxin (Doherty et al., 1964), acetyl-digoxin (Brass and Philipps, 1970), methyl-digoxin (Kramer et al., 1970), and strophantin (Brass and Philipps 1970; Kramer et al., 1970). The serum half-time ($T_{1/2}$) of digitoxin, however, was not increased in patients with renal disease (Kramer et al., 1970; Rasmussen et al., 1972). Serum levels in uremic patients on maintenance dosage were lower than the corresponding levels in control patients on the same dosage (Rasmussen et al., 1972) as seen in table 23.1. This study initiated further research in patients with uremia, on treatment with hemodialysis, and with nephrotic syndrome. The main findings from these investigations will be summarized in the present review.

1 This work was supported by grants from "The Norwegian Council on Cardiovascular Diseases", The University of Oslo, and "The Norwegian Research Council for Science and the Humanities".

292

Table 23.1. Serum digitoxin levels in patients with impaired and normal renal function on comparable doses

| Dose (mg/day) | Impaired renal function | | | Normal renal function | | | |
	No.	Mean (SE) (ng/ml)	Range	No	Mean (SE)	Range	p
0.05	15	8.5 (0.9)	0 – 12.5	17	12.0 (1.3)	4.0 – 20.5	< 0.05
0.07	12	9.6 (1.5)	0.5 – 16	17	16.7 (1.8)	6.0 – 30.5	< 0.01
0.10	24	16.1 (1.6)	1.0 – 27	32	18.2 (1.1)	10.5 – 40	NS

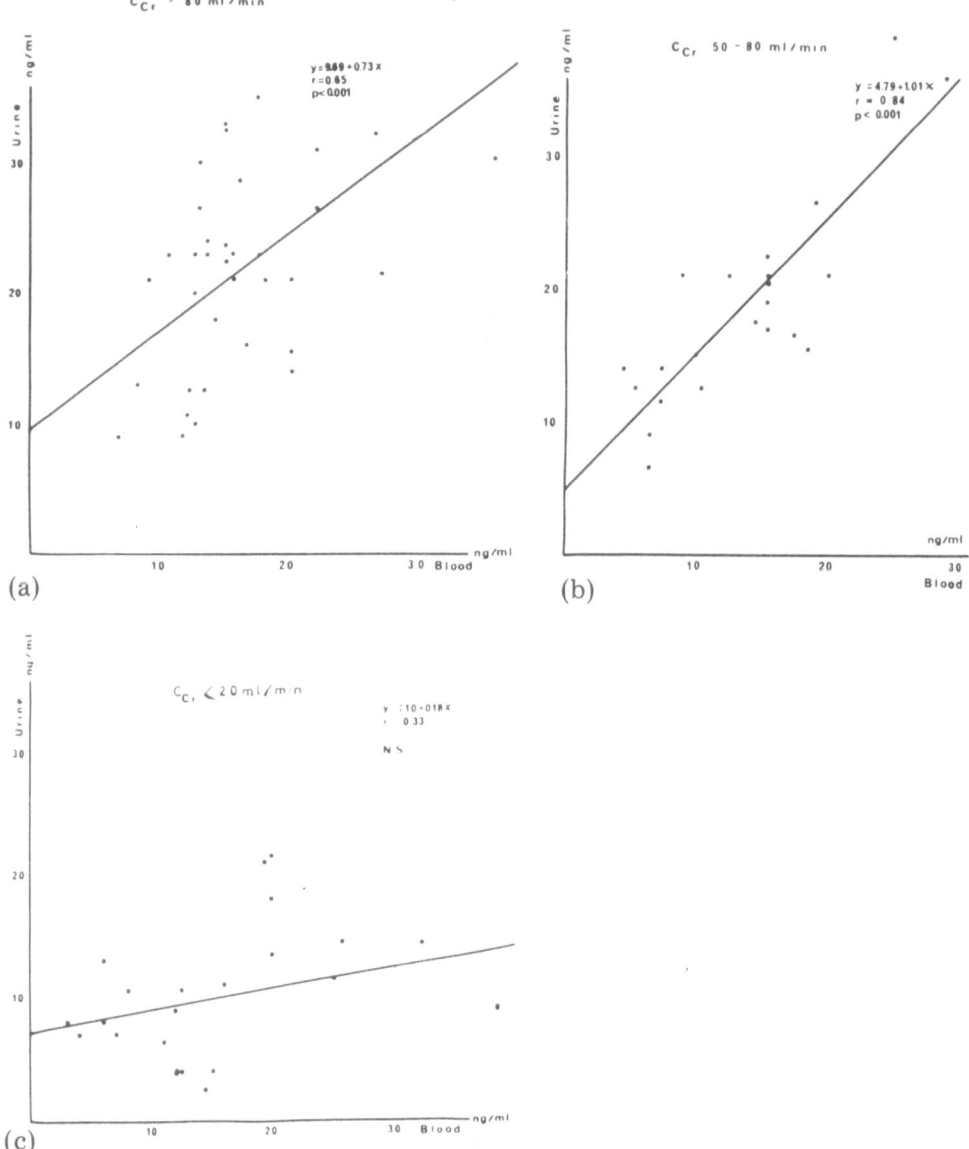

Fig. 23.1. (a) Correlation between serum and urine concentrations of digitoxin and cardioactive metabolites in patients with normal renal function (creatinine clearance > 80 ml/min, (b) a group with slightly impaired renal function (creatinine clearance 50—80 ml/min, (c) a group with severely impaired renal function (creatinine clearance < 20 ml/min. Reproduced with permission from Storstein, L., Clin. Pharm. Ther. 16; 14—24, 1974 and Storstein, L., Clin. Pharm. Ther. 16 : 25—34, 1974

294

Uremia

The serum protein binding of digitoxin was unchanged (97.3%, SD 0.5) in 15 patients with severely impaired renal function (mean serum creatinine 6.7 mg/dl) and serum albumin levels within the normal range (Storstein, 1976a). In the control group, a serum digitoxin protein binding of 97.3% (SD 0.5) was found with equilibrium dialysis. Serum elimination of digitoxin and cardioactive metabolites (measured with a modified ^{86}Rb method) was more rapid in a group of uremic patients (mean serum creatinine 12.3 mg/dl) who had a serum $T_{1/2}$ of 3.9 as compared to 8.1 days in a control group ($p < 0.01$) (Storstein, 1974b). The renal excretion of digitoxin and cardioactive metabolites was lower in uremics than in the control group. Alternative metabolic pathways or excretion routes must thus be operative in uremia.

Digitoxin is a drug with zero-order absorption and first-order elimination kinetics. As can be expected, a significant correlation exists between serum and urine levels in patients with normal renal function defined as a creatinine clearance above 80 ml/min (Fig. 23.1, left panel) (Storstein, 1974a). Such a correlation also exists in a group of patients with slightly impaired renal function defined as a creatinine clearance between 50 and 80 ml/min (Fig. 23.1, middle panel) (Storstein 1974b). In patients with severely impaired renal function and a creatinine clearance below 20 ml/min, however, there is no correlation between serum and urine levels (Fig. 23.1, right panel) (Storstein, 1974b). Table 23.2 shows data from the three patient groups mentioned above who were on main-

Table 23.2. Data from patients with normal renal function (left), slightly impaired renal function (middle), and severely impaired renal function (right) on maintenance treatment with digitoxin

	Se-Cr clearance		
	> 80 ml/min	50—80 ml/min	< 20 ml/min
No	22	11	12
Digitoxin dose (mg/day)	0.08	0.07	0.07
Serum concentration (ng/ml)	20.6	14.2	16.7
Urine concentration (mg/ml)	24.9	17.4	10.3
DT clearance (ml/min)	0.98	1.25	0.58
per cent excreted of dose	32.9	37.9	13.6

tenance treatment with digitoxin. In patients with normal renal function, the uringe levels of digitoxin and cardioactive metabolites are higher than serum levels in patients with slightly impaired renal function. In the uremic group, however, urine levels are lower than those in serum. The percentage of the daily dose excreted in urine as digitoxin and cardioactive metabolites is 14% in uremic patients compared to 33% in patients with normal renal function and 37% in patients with slight impairment of renal function. It is thus apparent that the compensatory mechanisms in digitoxin pharmacokinetics first occur when renal function is severely deranged. Slight impairment of renal function as seen in old age or congestive heart failure can be handled by excreting the same percentage of daily digitoxin dose through the kidneys as when renal function is normal.

Possible explanations for the changed digitoxin pharmacokinetics found in uremia can be:
1. Increased excretion through other pathways.
2. Changes in digitoxin metabolism.

Data on the fecal excretion of digitoxin in patients with renal disease are scarce (Lahrtz et al., 1969) and not conclusive. I have studied the metabolic pattern of cardioactive and inactive, conjugated metabolites (Storstein, in press) in uremic patients on maintenance treatment with digitoxin. The pattern of known inactive metabolites like epi-, keto- and dihydroderivatives has not been investigated nor have I searched for still unknown inactive metabolites. The main findings are the following:

1. Unchanged digitoxin is the main cardioactive substance present in serum and urine of uremic patients.
2. Uremic patients have significantly less unchanged digitoxin than the control group.
3. Uremic patients have significantly more hydroxylated (DG−3: digoxin) and hydroxylated and hydrolyzed (DG−2: digoxigenin-bisdigitoxoside, DG−1: digoxigenin-monodigitoxoside, and DG−0: digoxigenin) metabolites than the control group.
4. The extent of conjugation to glucuronic and sulfuric acid is the same in the two groups.

In conclusion, digitoxin elimination, renal excretion, and metabolism are changed in patients with severely impaired renal function. Serum elimination is enhanced and serum levels on maintenance treatment are reduced in comparison with patients with normal or slightly impaired renal function. Impairment of renal function is no precipitating factor for digitoxin intoxication. In a prospective study on digitoxin intoxication including 650 patients (Storstein et al., in press), toxic patients had a slightly lower mean serum creatinine value than nontoxic.

Hemodialysis

Serum protein binding of digitoxin was significantly reduced in a group of uremic patients on treatment with hemodialysis (92.0%, SD 4.5) (Storstein, 1976a). The blood samples were drawn in the middle of the dialyzing period. Blood samples were then obtained before start and at the end of an 8-h dialyzing period (Fig. 23.2.). Before start of hemodialysis, the serum protein binding was normal, but the free fraction rose significantly toward the end of the dialyzing period. Digoxin protein binding changed in the same manner. This finding was not consistent with uremia-induced changes in protein binding nor were the normal values found before start of hemodialysis. Kinetic studies (Storstein and Janssen, 1976) showed that the change in protein binding had an early maximum after 5—15 min. Patients on hemodialysis get a bolus dose of 5000 IU heparin at start and 1000 IU every hour thereafter. Heparin in vitro did not influence the protein binding of digitoxin. When giving control patients a bolus dose of 5000 IU heparin, the same changes in protein binding occurred as in the patients on hemodialysis. We propose that these changes are caused by an heparin-induced release of free fatty acids which leads to a displacement of digitoxin and digoxin from their binding sites on the albumin molecules. Serum elimination of digitoxin and cardioactive metabolites has not been measured with the [86] Rb method. No change in serum elimination was found after a single dose of radioactive digitoxin to a group of anephric subjects (Kramer et al., 1970). The renal excretion of digitoxin and cardioactive metabolites in hemodialysis patients on

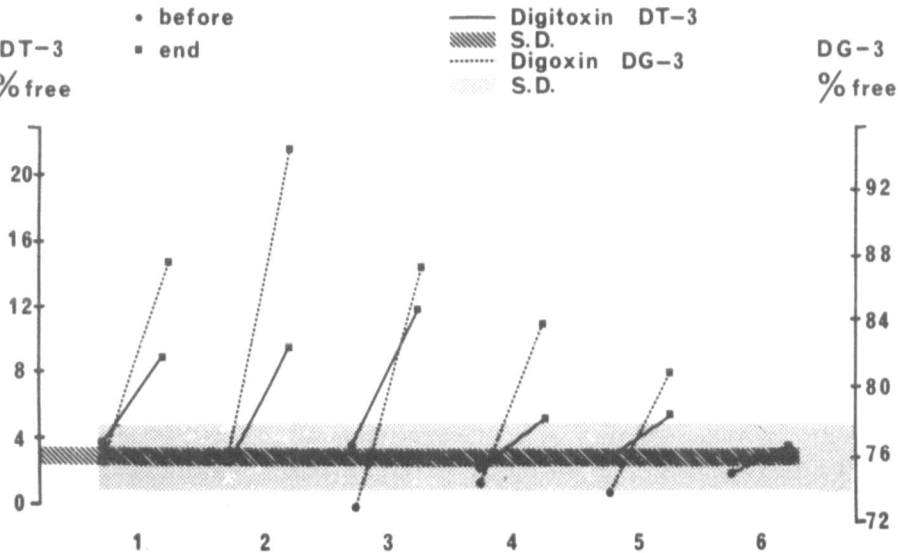

Fig. 23.2. Protein binding of digitoxin and digoxin before start and at the end of an 8-h hemodialysis. The free fraction of both drugs rose significantly toward the end of hemodialysis. Reproduced with permission from Storstein, L., Clin. Pharm. Ther. 20:6—14, 1976

maintenance therapy is only 2% (Storstein, in press) as compared to 33% in the control group and 14% in uremic patients. Serum levels on maintenance therapy are significantly lower in hemodialysis patients than in control patients on comparable doses (8.5 vs. 16.7 ng/ml). The pattern of cardioactive digitoxin metabolites was similar to that found in the control group and differed significantly from the pattern found in uremic patients not on treatment with hemodialysis (Storstein, in press). The extent of conjugation was the same as in the control group.

Treatment with hemodialysis thus normalizes the uremia-induced changes in digitoxin metabolites. It is, therefore, important to distinguish between uremic patients with and without treatment with hemodialysis when discussing digitoxin pharmacokinetics. They differ both in regard to serum protein binding and digitoxin metabolism.

Nephrotic Syndrome

The nephrotic syndrome is characterized by hypoalbuminemia and a high renal protein loss. As could be expected, digitoxin protein binding is slightly decreased (96.2%, SD 1.4) in a group of patients with nephrotic syndrome (Storstein, 1976b). Serum elimination is enhanced with a $T_{1/2}$ of 4.8 days compared to 8.1 days in the control group (p < 0.05). The renal excretion of digitoxin and cardioactive metabolites is increased compared with the control group (138.9 μg during 8 days vs. 94.9 μg during 8 days). It is interesting to note that the renal excretion during one serum half-time is the same for the two groups. The increase in renal excretion can thus explain the fall in serum half-time. The greater part of digitoxin in urine was bound to protein (60.1%, SD 30.6). Preliminary data on digitoxin metabolism in patients with nephrotic syndrome indicate that these patients may have less digitoxin metabolites than control patients 24 h after a single dose of digitoxin. Patients with nephrotic syndrome have lower serum levels of digitoxin than control patients (Peters et al., 1974), the main reason probably being the increased loss of protein-bound drug rather than the minor changes in serum protein binding of digitoxin.

Conclusion

Digitoxin pharmacokinetics is significantly changed in patients with various types of renal disease like uremia with and without treatment with hemodialysis and nephrotic syndrome. Changes occur in digitoxin protein binding, serum elimination, renal excretion, and metabolism. The resultant effect is an enhanced or unchanged elimination rate and lower serum levels on comparable digitoxin dosages. Renal disease is no precipitating factor for digitoxin intoxication. Digitoxin can thus be used safely in patients with renal disease and we recommend the same doses as in patients with normal renal function (mean loading dose 1.0 mg, mean maintenance dose 0.1 mg 6 days a week).

References

Brass, H., Philipps, H.: Die Elimination von a-Acetyldigoxin und k-Strophanthin bei Niereninsuffizienz. Klin. Wochenschr. 16, 972—978 (1970)

Doherty, J. E., Perkins, W. H., Wilson, M. C.: Studies with tritiated digoxin in renal failure. Am. J. Med. 37, 536 — 544 (1964)

Kramer, P., Horenkamp, J., Wilms, B., Scheler, F.: Das Kumulationsverhalten verschiedener Herzglykoside bei Anurie. Dtsch. Med. J. 95, 444 — 454 (1970)

Lahrtz, Hg., Reinhold, H. M., van Zwieten, P. A.: Serumkonzentration und Ausscheidung von ³H-Digitoxin beim Menschen unter normalen und pathologischen Bedingungen. Klin. Wochenschr. 47, 695 — 700 (1969)

Peters, U., Hausamen, T.-U., Grosse-Brockhoff, F.: Therapie mit Digitoxin unter Kontrolle des Serum-Digitoxinspiegels. Dtsch. Med. Wochenschr. 99, 1701 — 1701 (1974)

Rasmussen, K., Jervell, J., Storstein, L.: Digitoxin kinetics in patients with impaired renal function. Clin. Pharmacol. Ther. 13, 6 — 14 (1972)

Storstein, L.: Studies on digitalis. I. Renal excretion of digitoxin and its cardioactive metabolites. Clin. Pharmacol. Ther. 16, 14 — 24 (1974a)

Storstein, L.: Studies on digitalis. II. The influence of impaired renal function on the renal excretion of digitoxin and its cardioactive metabolites. Clin. Pharmacol. Ther. 16, 25 — 34 (1974b)

Storstein, L.: Studies on digitalis. V. The influence of impaired renal function, hemodialysis and drug interaction on serum protein binding of digitoxin and digoxin. Clin. Pharmacol. Ther. 20, 6 — 14 (1976a)

Storstein, L.: Studies on digitalis. VII. The influence of nephrotic syndrome on protein binding, pharmacokinetics, and renal excretion of digitoxin and cardioactive metabolites. Clin. Pharmacol. Ther. 20, 158-166 (1976b)

Storstein, L.: Studies on digitalis. XI. Digitoxin metabilism in patients with impaired renal function. (In press)

Storstein, L., Janssen, H.: Studies on digitalis. VI. The effect of heparin on serum protein binding of digitoxin and digoxin. Clin. Pharmacol. Ther. 20, 15 — 23 (1976)

Storstein, O., Hansteen, V., Hatle, L., Hillestad, L., Storstein, L.: Studies on digitalis. XIII. A prospective study of 649 patients on maintenance treatment with digitoxin. (In press)

Withering, D. W.: Abhandlung vom rothen Fingerhut und dessen Anwendung in der praktischen Heilkunde vorzuglich der Wassersucht Leipzig. In der Johann Gottfried Müllerschen Buchhandlung, 1786

Discussion

Kramer, Göttingen: Concerning the plasma protein binding of digitoxin in patients on intermittent hemodialysis, we have obtained results which differ considerably from your data.

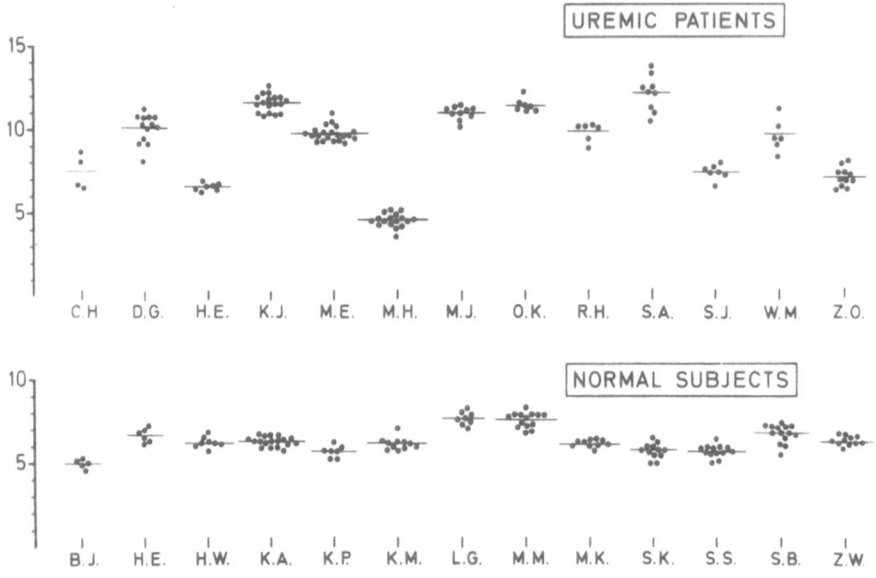

Fig. 1. Unbound plasma digitoxin (% of total concentration)

The unbound fraction of plasma digitoxin was determined repeatedly by means of the unerobic ultrafiltration chamber of Paschen in 13 hemodialysis patients and 13 normal subjects of comparable age, body weight, and sex (Fig. 1). The unbound fraction of digitoxin on an average was twice as high in the uremic patients than in the normal subjects. In addition, there was a considerable inter-patient variation of the unbound fraction in uremia ranging from 5%−13%. The blood samples were taken after the longest dialysis-free interval before onset of hemodialysis.

Storstein: In our study, there was a reduction in plasma protein binding during hemodialysis, but we didn't find any reduction when we took the samples just before start. We had a mean protein binding in hemodialysis patients of 97.4% in one group of 11 patients and 97.1% in another group of 14 patients when the samples were taken before start of an 8-h hemodialysis. The mean value in 51 control patients was 97.3%.

Vöhringer: According to your data, the digitoxin metabolism is significantly changed in uremia toward less unchanged digitoxin and more hydroxylated products. But if you calculate an increase of hydroxylated products from 10% to 20% in renal failure, the patients with a plasma digitoxin level of 10 ng/ml will have a digoxin level of 2 ng/ml, at a digitoxin concentration of 20 ng/ml a digoxin level of 4 ng/ml. This is — according to Dr. Smith — a toxic digoxin concentration. Have you seen any toxic symptoms in your patients?

Storstein: I think that's a very fair and interesting question. I cannot explain the lower serum levels or the enhanced elimination found in uremics by a change in cardioactive metabolites. I think there must either be an increased conversion to cardioinactive metabolites or an increased fecal excretion. The last point has been poorly investigated. We never see levels of 60 ng/ml but we give the therapeutic range to 15—25 ng/ml. If you have a steady-state level of 20 ng/ml, then the mean digoxin level should theoretically be 2.0 ng/ml. I can just say that 51 uremics which we followed very closely (Rasmussen et al., 1972) and in the study on digitoxin intoxication where we studied 650 patients on maintenance treatment with digitoxin, uremia was no predisposing factor for digitoxin intoxication. It is possible that when you have many cardioactive metabolites present in serum, their affinity to tissue will not be the same as when you have one glycoside present. This could be one possible explanation.

Vöhringer: We have measured the "steady-state" plasma concentrations of digitoxin (^{125} J-RIA digitoxin, clinical assays) and of digoxin (^{125} J-RIA digoxin, NEN) in normal patients and in patients with impaired renal function (Fig. 2). As can be seen from the Figure, the differences of the plasma digitoxin as well as of digoxin concentrations, respectively, are not statistically significant between the two groups. The percentage of hydroxylated products amounts to 2% in normal and in uremic patients.

	Control	Renal failure
digitoxin	26.1 ± 3.3	22.4 ± 2.3
digoxin	0.49 ± 0.03	0.49 ± 0.04
% hydroxylation	1.9	2.2

Fig. 2. "Steady state"-plasma concentration of digitoxin (ng/ml) and digoxin in 6 control patients and 11 patients with impaired renal function (creatinine i.S. 1.6—17.0 mg%)

On the other hand, we have studied the relationship between the concentrations of "total" digitoxin in plasma and of the extracted digitoxin after thin layer chromatography in normal patients and in patients with impaired renal function (creatinine i.s. 1.5—12 mg %). The recovery for this procedure accounted for 80%. However, the formation of metabolic products of digitoxin is not altered in patients with renal failure compared to (Vöhringer et al., 1976).

Have you calculated in your study the distribution volume of digitoxin and is it also possible to explain the lower steady-state level of digitoxin in uremic patients by a different volume of distribution?

Storstein: I cannot tell, because I found no significant change in the volume of distribution of digitoxin. When you measured digitoxin and digoxin, did you take the whole serum sample and assay it with the two different antibodies?

Vöhringer: Yes, I did. The cross-reactivity was 0.44%.

Pippig, Gütersloh: May I ask a question relevant to clinical practice? Do you think some patients with marked renal impairment need a higher dosage of digitoxin? Could you relate the clinical effects to the serum levels?

Storstein: I think one can use serum levels in uremic patients in the same way as controls. As the question about the effect of the increased hydroxylation products is not completely solved, I would not want to press them. We use the same therapeutic range for the uremics as for controls and without any special problems.

Klotz: I just want to ask if you see such a dramatic effect in the decrease of protein binding after 5—10 min. What do you think is the reason? Are there interfering lipids or fatty acid? And did you do in vitro experiments to see a displacement of the digitoxin binding by fatty acids or things like that?

Storstein: We think the change in protein binding is probably caused by heparin-induced release of free fatty acids. I have not added free fatty acids in vitro. It has been done for a number of other drugs, for example clofibrate, where a change in protein binding occurred when free fatty acids were added.

Shaw: Sometimes in individual patients, renal function can change very quickly, and over matter of a week or so they can go from near normal renal function to very severe impairment. Do you know if these changes in the handling of digitoxin which you described in people with chronic uremia can appear quickly?

Storstein: No, I do not know. If it is due to an enzyme induction then it usually takes time, but I don't have any data on this.

Lukas: I think the issue of protein binding in uremia is really a very open one. There are several factors to be considered. The concentration of albumin alone is important since a reduced albumin concentration will decrease total digitoxin concentration in the plasma by lowering the bound to free ratio of the drug. Next, there is the question of whether there are substances in the plasma of uremic patients which compete for digitoxin binding sites. I don't believe that that's been solved at all. The affinity of digitoxin for albumin is so very high so these substances would have to possess an enormously great affinity for albumin or exist in high concentrations to affect plasma binding of digitoxin to an appreciable degree. Then there is the issue of whether a conformational alteration in albumin is present that might affect the binding site for digitoxin. I am concerned about the scatter of some of the values that have been reported for binding of digitoxin by plasma albumin. Repeated studies by dialysis in our laboratory revealed that 97% of the drug is normally bound. Dr. Storstein gets a very similar Figure. If one uses tritiated digitoxin as the tracer for binding, it is absolutely essential that the radiolabeled compound be immaculately pure because a small quantity of radioactive impurity that has little affinity for albumin will falsely raise the free concentration very significantly. This may have been a problem with some of the values that have been reported. With regard to displacement of digitoxin from its binding site on albumin by free fatty acid, when we first studied binding of digitoxin to albumin, we had two basic preparations of serum albumin. One had its full complement of free fatty acid, and we reported an association constant at 37°C for it and digitoxin of $9.6 \cdot 10^4$ liter/mol. Another preparation had only about 0.3 mol of free fatty acid bound to the albumin, and its association constant with digitoxin was indeed increased to $11.4 \cdot 10^4$ liter/mol. So there is a very definite effect of free fatty acid, which has an enormous affinity for albumin, on the binding of digitoxin. There is one point that struck me about your half-life data, Dr. Storstein, and that is you're measuring more with the rubidium assay in plasma than digitoxin alone, aren't you? We've not done very many studies of digitoxin half-life in renal disease with the double isotope dilution derivative assay, but in two patients we noted a normal half-life using that specific assay for the compound.

Storstein: I appreciate very much the comment you made on hypoalbuminemia because every time there is a lowering of albumin values, you will get a change in protein binding regardless of what has caused this hypoalbuminemia. You are right when you think that with the rubidium method we measure digitoxin and cardioactive metabolites. And as we have shown in a study, (Storstein and Amlie, 1977) there is a very great change in the metabolic pattern with the time. We have only studied that in urine because we need a large amount of urine for the analysis and we can't take serum that often. But during an 8-day period, there is a change from mostly digitoxin to mostly metabolites so that we will — when we use the rubidium method — also incorporate metabolites. I think it is feasible that the half-time of unchanged digitoxin may be unchanged in the uremic patients but because they have more metabolites, the overall effect on the rubidium method makes the half-time shorter.

References

Rasmussen, K., Jervell, J., Storstein, L.: Clin. Pharmacol. Ther. 21, 255 (1977)
Storstein, L., Amlie, J.: Naunyn-Schmiedeberg's Arch. Pharmacol. Suppl. 294, R 9 (1976)
Vöhringer et al.: Clin. Pharmacol. Ther. 13, 6-14 (1972)

24 Increased Digitalis Tolerance in Uremic Patients[1]

P. KRAMER, E. STROH, D. MATTHEI, F. TEIWES, and F. SCHELER

Introduction

Only a few years ago, the clinicians were still impressed by a decrease of digitalis tolerance in uremic patients with respect to the daily dose required for induction of over dosage symptoms (Jelliffe 1967, 1968; Christiansen et al., 1973; Jelliffe and Brooker, 1974; Dettli, 1971; Ohnhaus et al., 1974; Kramer, 1974). By the introduction of serial radioimmunologic determinations of the plasma digoxin, we have learned to look at digitalis tolerance from a different aspect, which nowadays may be related to the plasma concentration. During the last years, we had accumulated some evidence (Buckesfeld and Bolte 1974; Kramer, 1977) that digitalis tolerance is in fact increased in uremic patients in relation to the plasma concentration. In order to substantiate these preliminary observations, a prospective study was undertaken to determine the incidence of digitalis toxicity in patients with an elevated plasma digoxin in relation to the plasma creatinine.

Materials and Methods

During 1976, we had to determine a total of 4500 plasma digoxin levels in our laboratory by means of commercial radioimmunoassay 125-J kits as supplied from Clinical Assay Inc., Cambridge, Mass. Before the determination of the values, we tried to get information about the creatinine and electrolyte concentration in the plasma, the ECG, and possible cerebral signs of digitalis toxicity by means of questionnaires and direct inquiry. All plasma digoxin values higher than 2.0 ng/ml regardless of signs of digitalis toxicity and all lower values from patients with definite signs of toxicity were analyzed in relation to the plasma creatinine level. In order to avoid misinterpretation and to get a uniform patient material, the plasma digoxin values were not included in the study if the question – aires were not completely filled out, if the patients had a pacemaker or suffered from an irreversible atrial fibrillation (e.g., mitral disease), if the age was less than 20 or more than 70 years, if the plasma potassium was less than 3.6 or higher

---

1 Supported by the Deutsche Forschungsgemeinschaft im Rahmen des SFB 89, Kardiologie, Göttingen.

than 5.4mEq/liter, and if the time interval between the last digoxin administration and the blood withdrawal had been less than 10 or more than 24 h. Finally, there were left 184 elevated values which fulfilled the criteria for entering the analysis. The following criteria were considered to be signs of digitalis impregnation: bradycardia with occasional av-junctional escape beats, first degree av-block, and ST- T-wave depressions, if not combined with signs of digitalis toxicity. The criteria for digitalis-induced toxicity were: bigeminal rhythm, premature ventricular beats (multifocal), av-junctional tachycardia, paroxysmal atrial tachycardia with block, second and third degree av-block, atrial fibrillation, and also nausea, vomiting, blurred or colored vision, if combined with ECG changes, provided that all these signs were reversible after reduction or discontinuation of digoxin administration. The effect of digitalis on the myocardial contraction force was estimated by means of the systolic time intervals as measured from a simultaneous recording of the electrocardiogram, the phonogram, and the indirect carotid artery or direct femoral artery pulse tracing. The durations of the systolic time intervals were determined as follows.

The total electromechanical systole (QS_2) was measured from the initial QRS deflection of the ECG to the initial high frequency vibration of the aortic component of the second heart sound on the PCG; the left ventricular ejection time (LVET) was measured on the pulse tracing from the point of onset of rapid upstroke to the "through" of the incisura; the preejection phase (PEP) was indirectly obtained by substracting the LVET from the QS_2. The time intervals were expressed in per cent of the R-R duration. Each of these intervals was measured in at least five randomly selected cardiac cycles and the mean of each interval was taken as the representative length. The volume of the heart was estimated planimetrically from the cardiac silhouette of x-ray pictures taken in two plains from a distance of 2 m.

Results and Discussion

From 4500 determinations of plasma digoxin, 184 elevated values (> 2 ng/ml) fulfilled the criteria for entering the analysis as shown in Figure 24.1. Another 16 values were selected although the plasma level was lower than 2 ng/ml because these patients had presented clear signs of digitalis-induced toxicity. Without statistical analysis, it is evident from Figure 24.1 that the incidence of digitalis toxicity for high plasma digoxin values was markedly reduced in patients with elevated plasma creatinine. Among those patients with a plasma creatinine of more than 3 mg%, only 5 out of 55 patients manifested signs of digitalis-induced toxicity. On the other hand, among those patients with a plasma creatinine below 1.5 mg%, 50 out of 83 patients with an elevated plasma digoxin had signs of digitalis toxicity or digitalis impregnation. In addition to these findings, the incidence of digitalis-induced toxicity in patients with normal plasma digoxin values was also increased in patients with normal renal function.

From these results, one may conclude that in fact digitalis tolerance is increased with respect to the plasma concentration required for induction of overdosage symptoms. This, however, does not necessarily apply to the maintenance of

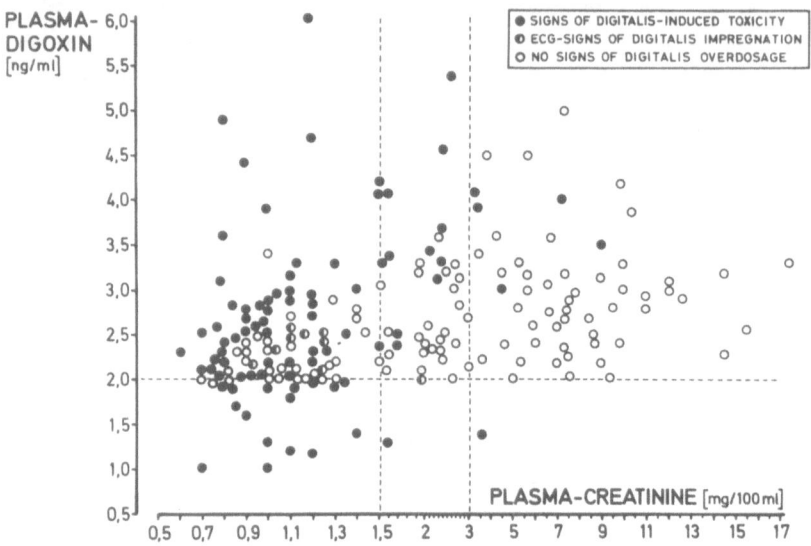

Fig. 24.1. Incidence of digitalis-induced toxicity in relation to the plasma creatinine

a positive inotropic effect. Therefore, during the last months, we have studied
the positive inotropic effect of cardiac glycosides in uremic patients on cardiac
function in relation to the plasma concentration. Thereby, however, we were
confronted with a number of problems:

1. We were not allowed for ethical reasons to study cardiac function by invasive
   methods such as cardiac catheterization.
2. There are only a few patients who manifest uremia and cardiac insufficieny
   without having been treated with cardiac glycosides.
3. The commonly used signs of effective digitalis treatment in patients with
   normal renal function as a decrease of edema are not available in patients
   without urine output. Thus we had to try to estimate the improvement of
   cardiac function by indirect methods.

In Figure 24.2. the effect of plasma digoxin elevation on the PR time in the
ECG, the systolic time intervals, and the estimated cardiac volume is demonstrated for six uremic patients, who exhibited severe cardiac failure intractable
by fluid withdrawal through hemodialysis. As the plasma digoxin level rose from
0.9 to 2.9 ng/ml, the PR interval was prolonged, the PEP was significantly shortened, and there was a slight shortening of the mechanical systole (QS_2). The
estimated cardiac volume decreased from 910 to 790 cm^3, and all these patients
showed a significant improvement of their physical ability.

Figure 24.3. shows the representative clinical course of a 43-year-old patient
with severe cardiac failure who was treated with methyl-digoxin. When the plasma
digoxin rose up to 3.3 ng/ml, the patient developed nausea, vomiting, and intermittent av-block. These signs disappeared after the plasma concentration had

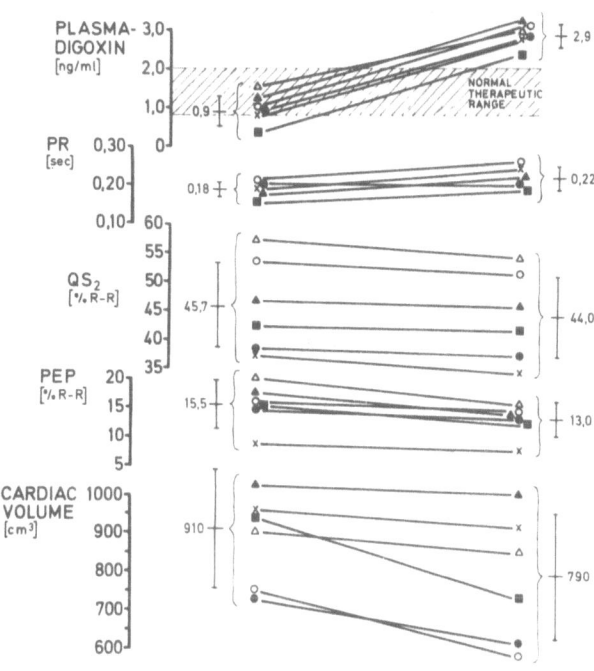

Fig. 24.2. Effect of plasma digoxin elevation on PR time, systolic times intervals, and cardiac volumes in six uremic patients

returned to 2.9 ng/ml. The mechanical systole and the PEP were markedly shortened by digitalization, and this corresponded well with an improvement of the patient's physical ability. In Figure 24.4 the clinical course of a 54-year-old patient who had been on 0.1 mg digitoxin for a long time is demonstrated. The cardiac failure of this patient was so severe that he was almost unable to dress himself without dyspnea. After increasing the daily dose to 0.2 mg/day, the plasma concentration of digitoxin rose from 15 to 30 ng/ml. Thereby, the patient's physical bility improved considerably. Thus, he was able to walk up hill for half an hour without resting. The effect of digitalis on the cardiac contraction force is demonstrated by the shortening of the mechanical systole from 58% to 53% and of the PEP from 21% to 15%. Since in patients with clinical conspicuous congestive heart failure, an abreviation in systolic intervals particularly of the PEP (Büyüközfürk et al., 1971; Weissler et al., 1964; Weissler and Schoenfeld, 1970) proved to be a consistent finding, our results also indicate that high plasma levels may be necessary to obtain an optimal positive inotropic effect, although we have to admit that the number of patients investigated so far is rather small and has to be extended certainly to another 50 patients in the coming years for a final conclusion. Nevertheless, one may conclude that with respect to the plasma concentration, the margin of therapeutic safety is higher in uremic patients than in patients with normal renal function. This finding may be explained at least in part by a combination of hyperkalemia, hypermagnesemia, hypocalcemia,

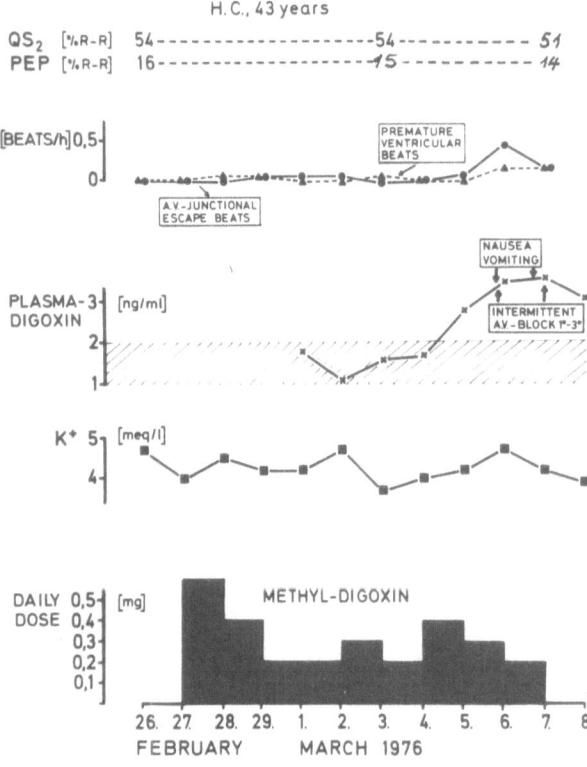

H.C., 43 years

Fig. 24.3. A typical clinical course of an hemodialysis patient with severe cardiac failure who was treated successfully with methyl-digoxin. Signs of digitalis toxicity were observed as the plasma digoxin level rose to 3.3 ng/ml

and acidosis which is found almost exclusively in conjunction with advanced renal insufficiency. All these changes in electrolyte metabolism are known to decrease the sensitivity of the myocardium to digitalis drugs. Prindle et al. (1971) and Goldman et al. (1973) have clearly demonstrated that both the toxic and the contractile actions of digitalis are reduced when the glycoside is administered during hyperkalemia. Whereas hyperkalemia in chronic renal failure sometimes is prevented by a high tubular secretion, so that the clearance of potassium exceeds that of creatinine (Platt, 1952), distinct hypermagnesemia is common in patients with a glomerular filtration rate below 20 ml/min. The antiarrhythmic properties of high extracellular magnesium concentration in digitalis-induced arrhythmias were first recognized by Szekely and Wynne in 1951. According to studies of Neff et al. (1972), there is evidence that extracellular magnesium concentrations may overcome the digitalis-induced inhibition of the sodium-potassium-dependent transport ATPase. Whereas membrane fluxes of sodium and potassium underlie the electric properties of the cardiac glycoside, the fundamentally positive inotropic effect of digitalis apparently rests on an increase of free intracellular calcium (Klaus and Lee, 1969), which again depends on the

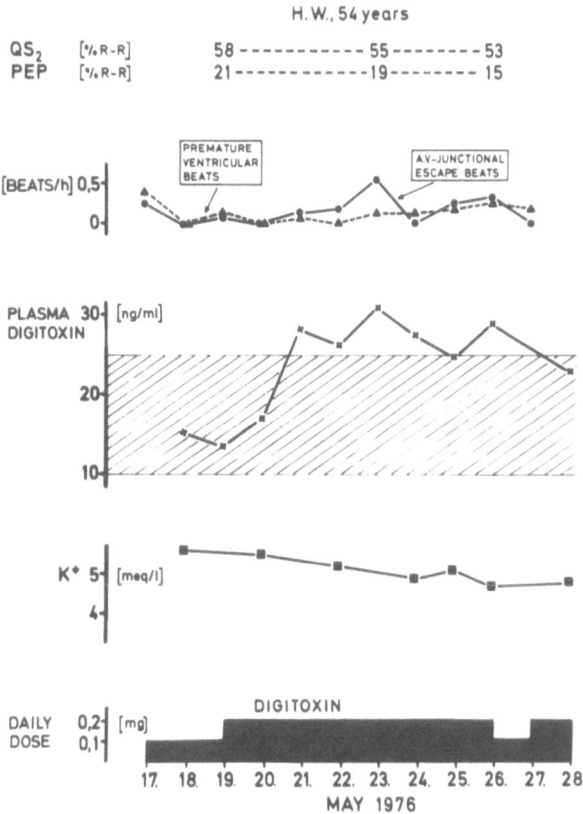

Fig. 24.4. A typical clinical course of an uremic patient with cardiac failure intractable by fluid withdrawal through hemodialysis who had been treated with 0.1 mg digitoxin. Doubling of the daily dose improved his physical ability remarkably

extracellular concentration of this cation. The synergistic relationship between plasma calcium and digitalis was soon generally accepted through painful clinical experience in patients with hypercalcemia (Bower and Mengle, 1936; Gold and Edwards, 1927). In patients with chronic renal failure, hypocalcemia is common due to reduced intestinal aborption (Hesch et al., 1972; Hosking and Chamberlain, 1973; Koppel et al., 1969). According to studies of Coburn (Coburn et al., 1969) not only total plasma calcium but also ionized calcium is diminished in advanced renal failure. Metabolic acidosis adds another explanation for reduced myocardial sensitivity to digitalis in patients with disturbed renal function. According to studies by Bliss et al. (1963) and Schafer et al. (1960), acidosis counteracts the toxic effect of digitalis as a result of cellular potassium efflux. In the presence of metabolic acidosis, there is a shift of hydrogen and sodium from the extracellular fluid to the cell and a concomitant movement of potassium out of the cell. The pH per se apparently has no special effect on digitalis toxicity.

309

Besides all speculations on the cause of increased digitalis tolerance in uremic patients in our opinion, conclusions may be drawn for clinical practice. As a kind of working hypothesis we have suggested a higher therapeutic range for patients with renal insufficiency than for patients with normal renal function. We would think that in patients with normal renal function the therapeutic range is somewhere between 1.0 and 2.0 ng/ml, whereas in patients with severely impaired renal function the therapeutic range is increased to somewhere between 1.6 and 2.8 ng/ml.

If one, however, accepts that in patients with renal failure the plasma concentrations have to be higher in order to obtain the same positive inotropic effect as in patients with normal renal function. Dosage regimens (Fig. 24.5) as proposed by most authors such as Jelliffe and Brooker (1974), Dettli et al. (1971), Ohnhaus et al. (1974), and recently by Gault and co-workers (1976) are no longer useful since these dosage regimens have been derived from the decrease of the creatinine clearance without considering a change in digitalis tolerance. Meanwhile, evidence has accumulated that in clinical practive, dosage regimens for digoxin based on the creatinine clearance are of little help because the body-distribution volume of cardiac glycosides, both interpatient and intrapatient, and the myocardial sensitivity are reduced to a highly varying degree. In addition, there may be interpatient variation in the fraction of digoxin that is absorbed. Peck et al. (1973) reported a randomized prospective clinical trial comparing performance of physicians in their use of digoxin with and without computer assistance. Their results indicated that only 17.6% of the variance of measured

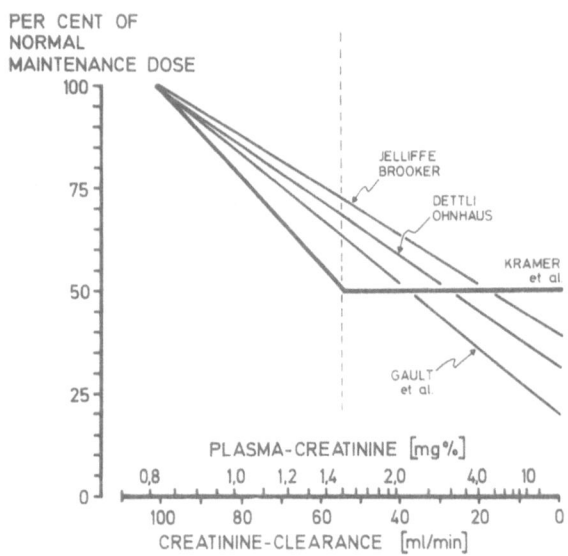

Fig. 24.5. Dosage regimens for digoxin in patients with renal insufficiency. Plasma creatinine calculated for an age of 40 years according to Jelliffe and Brooker. (Ohnhaus, Spring and Dettli 1974; Gault et al. 1976; Jelliffe and Brooker, 1974; Kramer, 1977)

plasma digoxin concentrations could be accounted to computer prediction and 2% by physician prediction. In a similar study, Wagner et al. (1974) have shown that the computer predictability of plasma digoxin in an individual patient from dose of digoxin, sex, body weight, height, age, and creatinine clearance is extremely low. Therefore, we would like to suggest a very simple rule of thumb for dosage regimens in patients with renal failure: *If the plasma creatinine is 1.5 mg% or higher, the daily dose should be reduced to 50% of the normal maintenance dose.* (In a 40-year-old patient, one would give 0.25 mg Lanicor instead of 0.5 mg. As the renal function deteriorates, a further decrease of the maintenance dose is not necessary since the reduction of renal digoxin excretion is compensated by an increase of digitalis tolerance. Thus, as shown in Figure 24.5, even in anuric patients, the daily dose has only to be reduced to 50% of the normal maintenance dose in contrary to the dosage regimens proposed by the other authors. The maintenance dose suggested in mild renal failure is lower than that of the other authors. According to our experience in these particular patients, there is a great interpatient and intrapatient variation of digitalis tolerance due to electrolyte disturbances (treatment with diuretics); thus, it is more safe to start in these patients with a lower maintenance dose and to increase the dose according to the therapeutic effect and ECG signs. Nowadays, with the help of serial measurements of plasma concentration, it may not be necessary to produce evidence of toxicity. The clinician may adjust the maintenance dose to the 12-h steady-state concentration of the plasma digoxin trying to reach the upper level of the therapeutic range which, according to our preliminary experience, is elevated in patients with advanced renal insufficiency from 1.2-2.0 (normal range) to 1.5-2.8 ng/ml.

References

Bliss, H.A., Fishman, W.E., Smith, P.M.: Effect of alterations of blood pH on digitalis toxicity. J. Lab. Clin. Med. 62, 53-58 (1963)

Bower, J.O., Mengle, H.A.K.: The additive effect of calcium and digitalis: A warning with a report of two deaths. J.A.M.A. 106, 1151 (1936)

Buckesfeld, R.P., Bolte, H.D.: Glykosidtoleranz und Glykosidkonzentration im Serum. Klinische Untersuchungen bei herzkranken Patienten unter Digoxintherapie. Verh. Dtsch. Ges. Kreislaufforsch. 40, 315-320 (1974)

Büyüköztürk, K., Kimbiris, D., Segal, B.L.: Systolic time intervals. Relation to severity of coronary artery disease intercoronary collateralization and left ventricular dyskinesia. Am. J. Cardiol. 28, 183-190 (1971)

Christiansen, N.J.B., Kølendorf, K., Siersbaek-Nielsen, K., Mølholm Hansen, J.: Serum digoxin values following a dosage regimen based on body weight, sex, age and renal function. Acta Med. Scand. 194, 257-259 (1973)

Coburn, J.W., Massry, S.G., Popovtzer, M.M., Kleeman, C.R.: The physicochemical state and renal handling of divalent ions in chronic renal failure. Arch. Intern. Med. 124, 302 (1969)

Dettli, L.R., Spring, P., Ryter, S.: Mutiple dose kinetics and drug dosage in patients with kidney disease. Acta Pharmacol. Toxied. (Kbh.) 29, Suppl 3, 211 (1971)

Gault, M.H., Jeffrey, J.R., Chirito, E., Ward, L.L.: Studies of digoxin dosage, kinetics and serum concentrations in renal failure and review of the literature. Nephron 17, 161-187 (1976)

Gold, H., Edwards, D.J.: The effects of ouabain on the heart in the presence of hypercalcemia. Am. Heart J. 3, 45 (1927)

Goldman, R.H., Coltart, D.J., Friedman, J.P.: The inotropic effects of digitalis on hyperkalemia. Circulation 48, 830-938 (1973)

Hesch, R.D., Gerlach, W., Henning, H.V., Emrich, D., Scheler, F., Kattermann, R.: Untersuchungen zur intestinalen ^{47}Ca-Absorption bei Gesunden und Patienten mit chronischer Niereninsuffizienz. Dtsch. Med. Wochenschr. 97, 1735-1742 (1972)

Hosking, D.J., Chamberlain, M.J.: Calcium balance in chronic renal failure. Q. J. Med. N.S. XLII, 167, 467 (1973)

Jelliffe, R.W.: A mathematical analysis of digitalis kinetics in patients with normal and reduced renal function. Math. Bioscience 1, 305 (1967)

Jelliffe, R.W.: An improved method of digixin therapy. Ann. Intern. Med. 69, 703-717 (1968)

Jelliffe, R.W., Brooker, G.: A nomogram for digoxin therapy. Am. J. Med. 57, 63-68 (1974)

Klaus, W., Lee, K.S.: Influence of cardiac glycosides on calcium binding in muscle subcellular somponents. J. Pharmacol. Exp. Ther. 160, 68-76 (1969)

Koppel, M.H., Coburn, J.W., Massry, S.G.: Intestinal calcium absorption in renal failure: effects of dietary calcium, vitamin D, hemodialysis and transplantation. Abstracts Am. Soc. Nephr. 3, 36 (1969)

Kramer, P.: Digitalis pharmakokinetics and therapy with respect to impaired renal function. Klin. Wochenschr. 55, 1-11 (1977)

Kramer, P., Saul, J., Köthe, E., Scheler, F.: Vereinfachte Schnellbestimmung von Plasma-Digoxin. Methodik und klinische Erfahrungen. Klin. Wochenschr. 53, 215-219 (1975)

Neff, M.S., Mendelssohn, S., Kim, K.E., Banach, S., Swartz, C., Seller, R.H.: Magnesium sulfate in digitalis toxicity. Am. J. Cardiol. 29, 377-382 (1972)

Ohnhaus, E.E., Spring, P., Dettli, L.: Eliminationskinetik und Dosierung von Digoxin bei Patienten mit Niereninsuffizienz. Dtsch. Med. Wochenschr. 99, 1797-1803 (1974)

Peck, C., Sheiner, L., Martin, M., Combs, T., Melmon, K.L.: Computer-assisted digoxin therapy. N. Engl. J. Med. 289, 441-446 (1973)

Platt, R.: Structural and functional adaptation in renal failure. Br. Med. J. 1952/I, 1313

Prindle, K.H., Skelton, C.L., Epstein, S.E., Marcus, F.I.: Influence of extracellular potassium concentration on myocardial uptake and inotropic effect of tritiated digoxin. Circ. Res. 28, 337-345 (1971)

Schafer, H.H., Witham, A.C., Burns, J.H.: Digitalis tolerance and effect of acetylstrophanthidin upon serum potassium of dogs with acidosis and uremia. Am Heart J. 60, 388 (1960)

Szekely, P., Wynne, N.A.: The effects of magnesium on cardiac arrhythmias caused by digitalis. Clin. Sci. 10, 241-253 (1951)

Wagner, J.D., Yates, J.D., Willis, P.W., Sakmar, E., Stoll, R.G.: Correlation of plasma levels of digoxin in cardiac patients with dose and measures of renal function. Clin. Pharmacol. Ther. <u>14</u>, 329-338 (1974)

Weissler, A.M., Gamel, W.G., Grode, H.E., et al.: The effect of digitalis on ventricular ejection in normal human subjects. Circulation <u>29</u>, 721-729 (1964)

Weissler, A.M., Schoenfeld, C.D.: effect of digitalis on systolic time intervals in heart failure. Am. J. Med. Sci. <u>259</u>, 4-20 (1970)

Discussion

Dengler, Bonn: Dr. Kramer, I am a little bit concerned about your final recommendation because your regimen might be good if you like to answer the question of the digitalis tolerance in uremia per se. But you don't take into account that these patients often have electrolyte disturbances and quite a number of complications which in practice are very frequently combined with renal insufficiency. If somebody takes your recommendation verbatim — may it not be dangerous to give this advice?

Kramer: I would think that our dosage regimen accounts for this danger. In patients with mild renal insufficiency, the maintenance dose recommended by our dosage regimen is lower than that proposed by all other authors. Great and acute changes in electrolyte metabolism can be elicited by diuretics, particularly in patients with mild renal insufficiency, whereas this is not possible in patients with advanced renal failure. Thus, I would think — if at all — one is more safe with our dosage regimen than with others.

Ohnhaus, Bern: I would like to ask you, Dr. Kramer, how do you explain the study published 1972 in the New Engl. Journal of Medicine about digitalis intoxication where it was found that the main cause of digitalis intoxication was renal function? The second point I would like to make relates to clinical practice. Since we used the dose regimen published by us and other authors, we have reduced digitalis intoxication in our hospital in patients with low kidney function.

Kramer: There is no question that digitalis tolerance is decreased in renal failure with respect to the daily dose required for induction of overdosage symptoms. Thus, you are perfectly right. One has to reduce the daily dose of digoxin in patients with renal failure. It is just a matter of whether the daily dose has to be reduced according to the creatinine clearance — which I think is more or less a pseudoaccuracy — and whether it has to be reduced to 30% in patients with end-stage renal failure. According to our experience, a reduction of the daily dose by 50% and a consecutive adjustment of the maintenance dose with respect to the therapeutic effect and to the ECG signs in all patients with renal failure is a more simple and practical approach. Thus, I don't think that there is great discrepancy between our findings and those of other authors.

Doering, München: Do you know how many of your patients were in advanced chronic renal failure? Because we see digoxin intoxication quite often in patients with mild renal insufficiency when their renal function deteriorates over a short period of time. Then the digoxin concentration rises and these patients do not show a great digitalis tolerance. Perhaps there is a difference when you have patients in advanced chronic renal failure who may show tolerance to high digoxin concentrations or when you have patients with a deterioration of a mild renal insufficiency.

Kramer: I think you are perfectly right. One has to be very careful when using digitalis in acute renal failure or in patients with any other acute changes in the electrolyte metabolism. This may also hold true for changes during hemodialysis. A decrease in digitalis tolerance during hemodialysis may be the result of a change of a high plasma potassium concentration to normal values.

Bodem, Bonn: Dr. Kramer, don't you think your results are influenced by patient selection? It was not a prospective study and as I know our colleagues in the clinic, they are much more ready to take digoxin levels in patients with known renal impairment. So it might have been that the routine demand for digoxin determination was done in more patients not showing any clinical signs of digoxin intoxication, whereas in the other group serum digoxin levels were only demanded if there was a clinical suspicion.

A second question I would like to ask: what were the serum potassium levels of the two patient groups? Finally, I think that serum creatinine alone is a bad criterion for judging renal function.

Kramer: I don't think we used any unnecessary criteria for selection of patients with signs of toxicity. We did exclude those patients who — as I said — had severe electrolyte disorders, who had a pacemaker or irreversible atrial fibrillation, as well as very young and very old patients, because in these patients digitalis tolerance in relation to plasma creatinine is difficult to evaluate. Concerning the plasma potassium, I want to stress again that we excluded all patients with very low or high plasma potassium (3.6 and 5.4 mEq/liter) and there was no significant difference in potassium levels of patients with normal renal function and those with impaired renal function.

Baligadoo, Paris: I am not convinced of the recommendation by Dr. Kramer that the serum glycoside concentrations in patients with renal failure be increased to obtain a therapeutic effect. We have studied in Paris 147 patients (Chiche et al., 1976) on digitoxin — I think the conclusions would be the same as for digoxin — and we have found cases of toxicity in both patient groups in renal failure and in patients with normal renal function. When toxicity develops in patients with renal failure, the serum concentration is in the same range of values as those found in cases of toxicity in patients without renal failure. In another study (as yet unpublished) on 3000 out patients, including patients in renal failure, all of whom are on digitoxin maintenance therapy, we did not find patients with renal failure manifesting toxicity at serum concentrations higher than those found in cases of toxicity in patients without renal failure. These two studies indicate that patients in renal failure are not more resistant than patients without renal failure to the toxic effects of digitoxin and probably of other cardiac glycosides. In my opinion, this should preclude the use in patients with renal

314

failure of serum concentrations higher than those used in patients without renal failure.

I do not know why your results seem to be different. I am asking myself whether the signs that you have used for the diagnosis of toxicity may not be partially responsible. You have noted first-degree av-block as a sign of impregnation and not as a sign of toxicity. In our opinion, first-degree av-block related to maintenance therapy with digitoxin is a sign of toxicity even if that toxicity is mild. First-degree av-block when related to the administration of digitoxin is often associated with ventricular premature beats on the same ECG or in an ECG done on the same day. Both of these signs, associated or not, occur at a serum concentration (32.1 ng/ml) statistically higher than that found in patients with normal renal function (25.4 ng/ml) on digitoxin maintenance therapy. I wonder if your decision not to consider first-degree av-block as a sign of toxicity may not partially explain your results.

I would like to ask you a second question. You state that the inotropic effect of digoxin is manifest in patients with renal failure at higher serum concentrations than in patients with normal renal function, and you use systolic time intervals to prove that point. I think that systolic time intervals are difficult to interpret. We have done a study in 26 patients in heart failure similar to that which was reported this morning by Dr. Belz in normal patients. We could find correlations — increase in "inotropic effect" versus serum concentrations — only in a few patients, mainly with cardiomyopathy. Our studies in patients with valvular heart disease failed to show significant modifications in systolic time intervals with significant increases in digitoxin doses and serum concentrations during maintenance therapy. We feel that Weissler's results concerning the acute ingestion of a fairly large single dose of a cardiac glycoside are highly reproducible. However, under maintenance therapy, the increase in inotropic effect is likely to manifest itself slowly and progressively. Therefore, systolic time intervals should be interpreted with caution, because the increase in ventricular performance which is assessed by systolic time intervals depends not only on contractility but also on other factors. Systolic time intervals may fail to detect a significant inotropic effect especially in certain types of heart disease. Could you please tell us what were the clinical diagnoses in your patients?

Kramer: Concerning your first comment: I have presented results on digoxin and not on digitoxin. I do not know whether the therapeutic range also for digitoxin is elevated in uremic patients. Concerning your second comment. I think you are right that in some cases there might have been signs of toxicity in addition to first-degree av-block, but — as I said — if these patients also exhibited some other signs, they were considered to have digitalis-induced toxicity. Only those patients who had just a first-degree av-block were considered to show digitalis impregnation. Concerning your third comment: we are aware of the fact that it is rather difficult to study the effect of digitalis on cardiac function. Actually there are no noninvasive parameters for repeated studies in these patients except for systolic time intervals. Weissler et al. (1979) found that the most significant change induced by digitalis is shortening of the preejection phase. These authors observed in some cases a prolongation of the left ventricular ejection phase after digitalization, but the preejection phase was frequently shortened in patients who manifested severe cardiac failure. All our patients suffered from severe cardiac failure and had an enlarged cardiac volume.

Grahame-Smith, Oxford: There are two important points that I would like to know about. You say you excluded patients with potassium below 3.6 and above 5.4. But even that range can be significant in terms of binding of digitalis to receptor sites, and I just wonder whether in fact you have looked within that range to see whether there is any correlation with your so-called tolerance.

Kramer: The mean plasma potassium was 0.8 mEq/liter higher in the patient group with a plasma creatinine greater than 3.0 mg% as compared to the patients with normal plasma creatinine, but I don't think this is the explanation for the difference in digitalis tolerance.

Grahame-Smith: There is just one other point and that is that Welt and co-workers showed some time ago that in the red cell the sodium-potassium ATPase activity may be stimulated in renal failure, and in fact you may need higher levels to produce an effect. So that's another possibility.

Larbig, Tübingen: I would like to support Dr. Baligadoo in his observation on the significance of first-degree av-block. We also have seen a good number of patients who developed first-degree av-block being intoxicated by other clinical criteria, e.g., extracardiac symptoms — vomiting, nausea, disturbance of vision, etc. So, we definitely think these patients are intoxicated, and I would not classify them as "impregnated."

We have also measured serum concentrations in patients on digoxin and digoxin derivatives and obtained the same results as Dr. Baligadoo, that in patients with first-degree av-block, steady-state serum concentrations were significantly higher than in those intoxicated patients with frequent ventricular premature beats. So, according to our results, first-degree av-block is a sign of intoxication.

Kramer: In order to avoid any misunderstanding, I think I have to stress again the point that we considered a patient intoxicated when he exhibited other signs of toxicity besides the prolongation of the PR interval.

References

Chiche, P., Baligadoo, S., Laruelle, P., Borgard, J.P.: "Intoxications digitaliques et déviations de l'activité thérapeutique de la digitaline." Coeur Med. Interne 15, 2, 249 (1976)

Weissler, A.M., et al.: Am J. Med. Sci., 259, 4 (1979)

25 Digitoxin and Digoxin in Patients With Chronic Renal Failure and on Hemodialysis

B. GRABENSEE, U. PETERS, T. RISLER, and F. GROSSE-BROCKHOFF

Recent trends in treatment of chronic renal failure lead to the acceptance of older age groups. This, as well as hypertension, fluid overloading, and the other well-known factors of the uremic syndrome increased the demand for digitalis treatment. Either of the two substances of choice, digitoxin and digoxin, have been given preference by various authors (Doherty, 1973; Kramer, 1977; Larbig et al., 1974; Lukas, 1972; Ohnhaus, 1974; Peters et al., 1976; Storstein, 1973). This paper presents the results of a study of patients with terminal renal failure undergoing intermittent maintenance hemodialysis, who have been treated with digitoxin or digoxin. Concerning the results in patients treated with digitoxin, it is well-established that there is no correlation between renal function and serum concentration of digitoxin using a standardized maintenance dosage of the drug (Finkelstein, 1975; Lukas, 1972; Peters et al., 1976; Smith, 1970; Storstein, 1973, 1974).

Serum digitoxin levels in 51 patients with end-stage renal failure were measured by radioimmunoassay (Peters 1976; 1977) (Table 25.1). All patients received a loading dose of 1.2-1.5 mg and were subjected to at least 6 weeks of treatment with a daily maintanance dose of 0.1 mg. The serum samples were taken 24 h after the last drug ingestion and in hemodialysis patients immediatly before starting hemodialysis. Dialysis was performed three times a week for 6-10 h. Statistical breakdown of the results shows that there is a significant difference ($p < 0.05$) between the digitoxin serum levels of the 51 patients with end-stage renal failure and the group of 29 patients with heart failure and normal renal function. On the other hand, no statistically significnat difference was found between the 29 patients with heart failure and the 27 patients on dialysis treatment.

The percentage of protein bound digitoxin and its metabolites was analyzed by ultracentrifugation (Peters, 1977). In 13 patients with end-stage renal failure, the protein bound digitoxin fraction is significantly lower than in patients with heart failure (Table 25.2). On the other hand, with regard to protein bound digitoxin, there is no difference between the hemodialysis and heart failure groups. It must be noticed that the group with end-stage renal failure not yet requiring hemodialysis shows the lowest protein bound fraction of digitoxin. In individual cases with marked uremic symptoms, normal values for plasma albumin coincided with a low protein bound digitoxin fraction down to 91.6% (Peters, 1977).

317

Table 25.1. Serum digitoxin in patients with heart failure and end-stage renal failure

Diagnosis	Patients No.	Serum digit digitoxin	Total protein g/100 ml	Serum creatinine mg/100 ml
Heart failure no renal failure	29	26.5 ± 7.3	6.7 ± 0.8	< 1.2
End-stage renal failure	51	23.2 ± 7.8	6.3 ± 0.9	1.6 − 16.0
No HD	21	23.0 ± 6.4	6.4 ± 1.0	6.6 ± 4.7
HD treated	27	24.6 ± 7.9	6.5 ± 0.7	> 10.0
Nephr. S	3	11.2 ± 5.2	4.8 ± 1.0	2.5 − 12.5

Maintanance dosis: 0.1 mg digitoxin p.d. ($\overline{x}$ ± s, range resp.); HD = hemodialysis).

Table 25.2. Serum digitoxin, protein binding, and total protein in patients with end-stage renal failure

Diagnosis	Patients No.	Serum digitoxin ng/ml	Protein binding %	Total protein g/100 ml
Heart failure no renal failure	10	25.1 ± 9.3	96.9 ± 0.5	6.5 ± 0.5
End-stage renal failure	13	20.0 ± 6.3	95.3 ± 1.8	6.0 ± 1.2
No HD	8	18.4 ± 6.5	94.7 ± 2.0	5.8 ± 1.4
HD treated	5	22.5 ± 5.8	96.2 ± 0.9	6.4 ± 0.3

HD = hemodialysis.

It must be stressed that variations in intestinal absorption do not occur since it can be shown that the plasma levels of digitoxin after an oral dose of 0.5 mg digitoxin are the same for the five controls and the five patients with end-stage renal failure (Figure 25.1). The area under the curve was not significantly different (63.4 ± 8.4 renal failure group, 72.8 ± 12.9 controls, p > 0.10). Similar results were obtained by Storstein and by Finkelstein (Finkelstein, 1975; Storstein, 1973, 1974). There is no interference in cases where simultaneous therapy with aludrox was necessary.

In digoxin, it is well-established that there exists a linear correlation between renal digoxin elimination and the glomerular filtration rate (Doherty, et al., 1967; Grosse-Brockhoff et al., 1973; Kramer, 1977; Larbig et al., 1974; Marcus et al., 1966; Ohnhaus et al., 1974; Risler et al., 1974; Smith, 1975). The optimal dose required can, therefore, be calculated in every degree of renal failure. Using the nomogram published by Ohnhaus et al. (Ohnhaus et al., 1974), we found the digoxin serum levels, which are shown on Table 25.3. These digoxin serum levels were measured by radioimmunoassay (Grosse-Brockhoff et al., 1973; Smith, 1975).

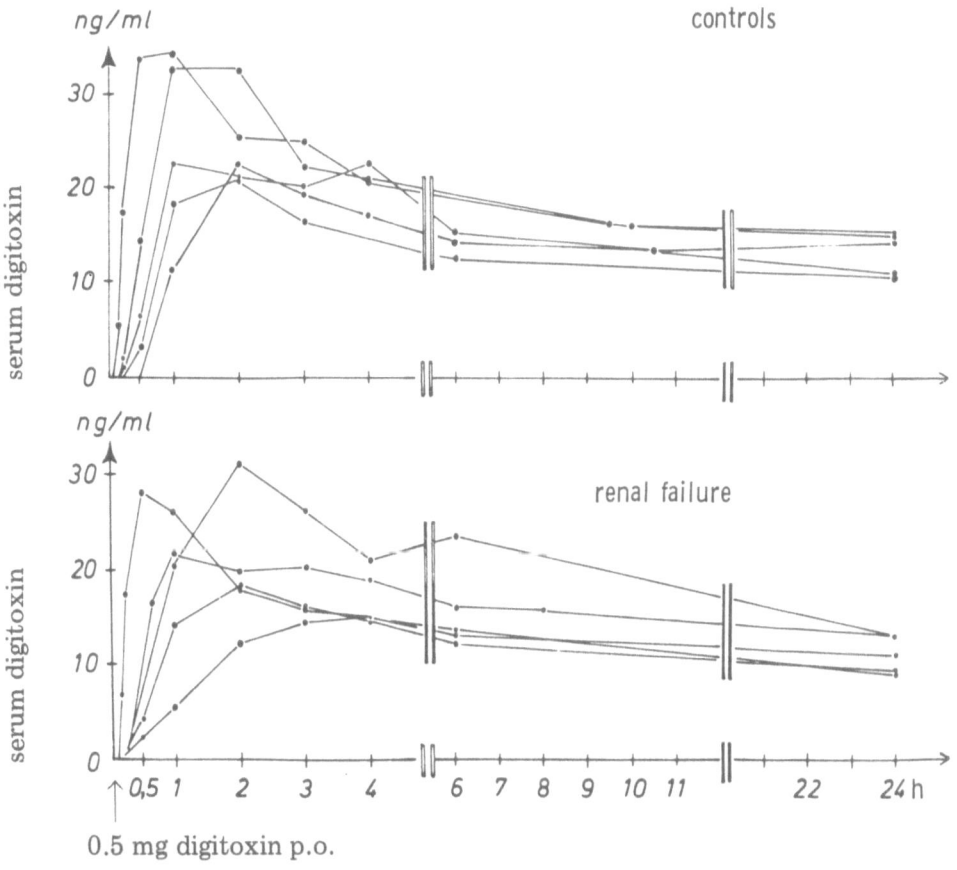

0.5 mg digitoxin p.o.

Fig. 25.1

Table 25.3. Serum digoxin in patients with end-stage renal failure und hemodialysis (HD) treatment, with reduced renal function, without HD treatment, and with heart failure (no impairment of renal function) serving as controls

Diagnosis	Patients No.	β-acetyl-digoxin mg p.d.	Serum digoxin ng/ml	Creatinine clearance ml/min
End-stage renal failure HD treated	26	0.1	1.4 ± 0.6	< 6
Red. renal function and renal failure no HD treatment	19	0.1 – 0.3	1.2 ± 0.3	5 – 65
Heart failure normal renal function	82	0.4	1.4 ± 0.4	s. creatinin mg/100 ml < 1.2

In comparison with the normal control group, the serum digoxin levels in the various stages of renal failure proved to be within satisfactory therapeutic ranges. The protein-bound percentage of serum digoxin was measured at 17% by using the same method as mentioned before for digitoxin. In normal subjects, we found a protein binding of 22% with our method.

We did not study the intestinal absorption of digoxin. The results published by Finkelstein (Finkelstein, 1975) showed that there is no variation in bioavailability. It must be mentioned that Brown at al. (Brown and Juhl, 1976) presented evidence suggesting that antacids interfere with digoxin absorption. On the other hand, we found no difference in serum digoxin levels in the control group and renal failure group, whether the patients received aludrox or not. Studies by Vöhringer et al. (Vöhringer, 1976) show that antacids do not interfere with digoxin absorption in men.

To answer the question whether it would be advantageous to treat patients with end-stage renal failure with either digitoxin or digoxin, we examined the same group of 15 patients on intermittent maintanance hemodialysis treated consecutivly with both substances. Table 25.4 shows some data of these patients. The treatment phase with digitoxin has been explained before. The changeover to digoxin was achieved in two ways: either through substitution of the maintanance dose of 0.1 mg of digitoxin by 0.1 mg of β-acetyl-digoxin or by first administering a loading dose of 0.4 mg three times and then a daily maintanance dose of 0.1 mg β-acetyl-digoxin after having dicontinued digitoxin treatment for 3 weeks. All digoxin levels were measured after at least 2 months of uninterrupted treatment. The results are shown in Table 25.5. As one can see, in digitoxin treatment as well as in the digoxin phase, therapeutic levels of both substances are present. Even so, the variation coefficient in the digitoxin group is smaller than in the digoxin group. There was no evidence of digitalis intoxication in any patient. A further point of interest is the half-life of the two drugs. Our results are shown in Table 25.6. The half-life was assessed by measuring the digitalis levels for 2-11 days after cessation of maintenance treatment. As Storstein, we also found the digitoxin half-life shortened in patients with renal failure. The surprising fact that the digoxin half-life was more prolonged than estimated and measured by other authors (Doherty et al., 1967; Larbig et al., 1974; Ohnhaus et al., 1974) needs further investigation.

Table 25.4

No.	Creat. clear.	Age	B. weight	S. protein
15	< 6ml/min	42.1 ± 9.5 years	66.5 ± 8.8 Kg	6.64 ± 0.8 g/100 ml

Hemodialysis 3 × weekly 6-10h.

Table 25.5

Treatment	Maintanance dosis mg p.d.	Serum concentr. ng/ml $\overline{x}$ ±s	No.
Digitoxin	0.1	22.8 ± 8.1	15[a]
β-acetyl-digoxin	0.1	1.1 ± 0.6	15[a]

[a] Same patients.

Summary

Patients with end-stage renal failure and on hemodialysis can be treated success-fully with a maintanance dose of 0.1 mg p.d. digitoxin as well as digoxin. There is no convincing evidence available to justify preference for either drug.

References

Brown, D.D., Juhl, R.P.: Decreased bioavailability of digoxin due to antacids and kaolin-pectin N. Engl. J. Med. 295, 1034 (1976)

Doherty, J.E.: Digitalis glycosides. Ann. Intern. Med. 79, 229 (1973)

Doherty, J.E., Flanigan, J., Perkins, H.W., Ackerman, G.L.: Studies with tritiated digoxin in anephric human subjects. Circulation 35, 298 (1967)

Finkelstein, F.O., Goffinet, J.A., Hendler, E.D., Lindenbaum, J.: Pharmacokin-etics of digoxin and digitoxin in patients undergoing hemodialysis. Am. J. Med. 58, 525 (1975)

Table 25.6. Biologic half-life of digitoxin and digoxin

Diagnosis	No.	Digitoxin days $\overline{x}$ ± s	No.	Digoxin days $\overline{x}$ ± s
Normal renal function $C_{cr} > 90$ ml/min	8	7.6 ± 1.6	2	2.0 ± 0.1
End-stage renal failure $C_{cr} <$ ml/min	4	5.7 ± 0.9	3	12 ± 2.2

Grosse-Brockhoff, F., Hengels, K.J., Fritsch, W.-P. Grabensee, B., Hausamen, T.-U.: Serumdigoxin-Spiegel und Nierenfunktion. Dtsch. Med. Wochenschr. 98, 1 (1973)

Jeliffe, R.W., Buell, J., Kalaba, R., Sridhar, R., Rockwell, R., Wagner, J.G.: An improved method of digitoxin therapy. Ann Intern. Med. 72, 453 (1970)

Kramer, P.: Digitalis pharmacokinetics and therapy with respect to impaired renal function Klin. Wochenschr. 55, 1 (1977)

Kramer, P., Quellhorst, E., Horenkamp, J., Scheler, F.: Dialysance und prozentuale Elimination verschiedener Herzglykoside während der Haemodialyse und Peritonealdialyse. Klin. Wochenschr. 50, 609 (1972)

Larbig, D., Haasis, R., Bundschu, H.D., Buckesfeld, R.G., Lankisch, P.G., Ilg, R., Girndt, J.: Radioimmunochemische Bestimmung von Digoxin und Digoxinderivaten im Serum und Urin bei normaler und eingeschränkter Nierenfunktion. Verh. Dtsch. Ges. Inn. Med. 80, (1974)

Lukas, D.S.: Of toads and flowers. Circulation 46, 1 (1972)

Marcus, F.I., Peterson, A., Salel, A., Scully, J., Kapadia, G.G.: The metabolism of tritiated digoxin in renal insufficiency in dogs and man. J. Pharmacol. Exp. Ther. 152, 372 (1966)

Ohnhaus, E.E., Spring, P., Dettli, L.: Eliminationskinetik und Dosierung von Digoxin bei Patienten mit Niereninsuffizienz Dtsch. Med. Wochenschr. 99, 1797 (1974)

Peters, U., Fritsch, W.-P., Grabensee, B., Hausamen, T.-U., Grosse-Brockhoff, F.: Serum-Digitoxinspiegel bei terminaler Niereninsuffizienz. Verh. Dtsch. Ges. Inn. Med. 82 (in press) (1976)

Peters, U., Grabensee, B., Hausamen, T.-U., Fritsch, W.-P. Grosse-Brockhoff, F.: Pharmokokinetik von Digitoxin bei chronischer Niereninsuffizienz Dtsch. Med. Wochenschr. 102, 109 (1977)

Risler, T., Grabensee, B., Grosse-Brockhoff, F.: Eliminationskinetik und Dosierung von Digoxin bei Patienten mit Niereninsuffizienz. Dtsch. Med. Wochenschr. 99, 2130 (1974)

Shoeman, D.W., Azarnoff, D.L.: Serum digitoxin in uremic patients. Clin. Pharmacol. Ther. 13, 460 (1972)

Smith, T.W.: Radioimmunoassay for serum digitoxin concentration. Methodology and clinical experience. J. Pharmacol. Exp. Ther. 175, 352 (1970)

Smith, T.W.: Digitalis toxicity. Epidemiology and clinical use of serum concentration measurements. J. Med. (Basel) 58, 470 (1975)

Storstein, L.: The influence of renal function on the pharmacokinetics of digitoxin. In: Storstein, O. (ed.): Symposium on Digitalis. Oslo: 1973 (Gyldendal Norsk Forlage

Storstein, L.: Studies on digitalis. 1. Renal excretion of digitoxin and its cardioactive metabolites. Clin. Pharmacol. Ther. 16, 14 (1974)

Storstein, L.: Studies on digitalis. 2. The influence of impaired renal function on the renal excretion of digitoxin and its cardioactive metabolites. Clin. Pharmacol. Ther. 16, 25 (1974)

Vöhringer, H.F., Kuhlmann, J., Rietbrock, N.: Der Einfluß von Antacida auf die Plasmakonzentration von Digoxin beim Menschen. Dtsch. Med. Wochenschr. 101, 106 (1976)

Discussion

Storstein, Norway: I would just like to comment on your last point. Digitoxin and digoxin could be used with equal safety in renal diseases if you really know the renal function. But in a lot of patients, especially in old patients, you don't have specific data on their renal function and you don't measure it too often. Therefore, I think it would be easier to handle digitoxin in general practice or in small hospitals where they don't have elaborate measurement of creatinine, inulin, and PAH clearance.

Kramer, Göttingen: I think we all agree that the time required for disappearance of overdosage symptoms elicited by digoxin is shorter than if elicited by digitoxin. But I think we have to consider another aspect. If there is a high interpatient variation in the plasma protein binding in uremic patients — especially in patients on hemodialysis — we have to draw conclusions with respect to the therapy control by measuring the total plasma concentration. If there is a great variation in the unbound fraction in uremic patients, the total plasma concentration in the individual case will not provide sufficient information about the degree of digitalization. In other words, if we treat a patient with digitoxin, one disadvantage would be that the control of therapy by serial determinations of the plasma concentration is not as good as with the use of digoxin.

Grabensee: I agree with you, but my data refer to patients in chronic maintenance hemodialysis, and in most of these patients we see normal plasma protein concentrations. In addition, we couldn't find a significnat difference between the unbound fraction in normal and end-stage renal failure patients.

Grahame-Smith, Oxford: Recently, Dr. Aronson and I published a paper on volumes of distribution of digoxin in renal failure. This paper came out of a little experiment that we did. Normally we don't use nomograms but on this occasion we did. In treating some patients with renal failure with digoxin, we used Dettli's nomogram. We intoxicated three out of five of those patients, and when we looked into the reasons, it seemed to us that a decreased volume of distribution of digoxin was the factor which isn't included in nomograms. This doesn't seem to have been a factor in your study.

Grabensee: It's very difficult to determine the volume of distribution in all patients with renal disease. In contrast to your findings, we had low digoxin serum levels in most patients.

Marcus, Tucson: I want to commend you for your excellent study. I do want to insert a note of caution that although there is a direct correlation between creatinine clearance and digoxin clearance, there may not be such a precise correlation between digoxin clearance and digoxin half-life. There is no question that with a very marked decrease in digoxin clearance, there is a prolonged half-life of digoxin, but we have found that there are some patients who have serum creatinines of less than 3 who have a normal digoxin half-life. I think that a lack of correlation between a decrease in creatinine clearance and increase in digoxin half-life diminishes the value of nomograms that have been proposed to be used to alter digoxin dose on the basis of creatinine clearances.

Grabensee: Were your patients in acute renal failure?

Marcus: These were patients with heart failure and renal abnormalities secondary to age and their heart disease.

Belz, Koblenz: I would like to comment on the remark by Dr. Kramer about the question of the free and the protein-bound glycoside which seems to be a disadvantage of the digitoxin. I think that we are not allowed to look at the plasma proteins only. Binding to tissue proteins — we do not know much about them — must also be taken into consideration and I believe — of course I cannot prove this — that if the protein binding in plasma decreases there may be changes in the binding on the cardiac receptors which cancel each other out. This may not be a disadvantage for digitoxin in clinical therapy.

Butler, New York: I agree with you completely; we are measuring glycosides in the blood, but what is really important is the glycoside concentration at the tissue receptor level and we are not getting at that very adequately. Perhaps Dr. Grahame-Smith's approaches to the red cells may help us in that regard.

Ohnhaus, Bern: May I just make another comment on nomograms. I think a nomogram is a mean guideline for the doctor. If you look at nomograms of different investigators who correlated creatinine clearance to drug clearances, half-lives, or elimination rate constants, there are always some patients who are out of the medium range. Probably you examined just three of them. About 1 year ago, there was a paper in the Brit. J. of Clin. Pharmacol. in which doses were calculated according to nomograms of Dettli and Ohnhaus. The predicted values and the measured values were compared, and there was a correlation coefficient about 0.8. So I do think nomograms are helpful but they are just a medium guideline.

26 International Patterns of Clinical Use and Toxicity of Digitalis Glycosides: Report From the Boston Collaborative Drug Surveillance Program[1]

D. J. GREENBLATT

Clinical pharmacokinetic studies of digitalis glycosides have the ultimate objective of providing information on drug absorption, distribution, and elimination which might promote the safe and effective use of these drugs in humans. Although understanding of the pharmacokinetics of digitalis derivatives has advanced impressively in the last decade, the impact of this new knowledge upon the clinical use of digitalis glycosides is largely unknown. This is not surprising, since assessment of a drug's "safety" and "effectiveness" in clinical practice is exceedingly difficult. Furthermore, pharmacokinetic studies have been performed in many parts of the world. It is not established whether results obtained with one subject population in one nation are applicable to subjects in other nations where genetic heritages are different and where subjects are exposed to entirely different environments. To provide some preliminary insight into these problems, the present report describes a preliminary evaluation of patterns of clinical use and toxicity of digitalis glycosides based upon data collected by the Boston Collaborative Drug Surveillance Program (BCDSP).

Methods

The BCDSP monitors and quantitates clinical effects of drugs among patients admitted to medical services of 23 hospitals in seven countries (Table 26.1). (Allen and Greenblatt, 1975; Jick, 1974; Miller and Greenblatt, 1976). Trained nurse or pharmacist monitors use standardized data sheets to record information on patient characteristics, medical history, laboratory studies, and diagnoses. Data are also recorded on details of drug therapy during hospitalization, including indication for therapy, dose, route and frequency of administration, duration of therapy, and reason for termination of treatment. When an adverse drug reaction (defined as any undesired or unintended drug effect) is suspected, the monitor records a detailed description of the event including its severity, consequences, and any palliative measures taken. The treating physician

---

1 From the Clinical Pharmacology Unit, Massachusetts General Hospital, Boston; and the Boston Collaborative Drug Surveillance Program, Boston University Medical Center, Waltham and Boston, MA, U.S.A.

Table 26.1. Hospitals currently or previously participating in the Boston
Collaborative Drug Surveillance Program

United States
  Boston, Massachusetts:
    Massachusetts General Hospital
    Boston University Medical Center
    Peter Bent Brigham Hospital
    Boston City Hospital
    Lemuel Shattuck Hospital
    Boston Veterans Administration Hospital
  Providence, Rhode Island:
    Roger Williams General Hospital
  Syracuse, New York:
    State University of New York — Upstate Medical Center
  Tucson, Arizona:
    University of Arizona Medical Center
  Richmond, Virginia:
    Medical College of Virginia Hospital
  Stanford, California:
    Stanford University Hospital

Canada
  London, Ontario:
    St. Joseph's Hospital

New Zealand
  Auckland:
    Auckland Hospital
  Lower Hutt:
    Hutt Hospital

Israel
  Jerusalem:
    Hadassah-Hebrew University Hospital
  Tel-Aviv:
    Beilinson Hospital
    Asaf Harofe Government Hospital
  Haifa:
    Rambam University Hospital
  Tiberias:
    Poriah Hospital

Germany
  Berlin:
    Klinikum Steglitz der Freien Universität Berlin

Scotland
  Glasgow:
    Western Infirmary
    Stobhill General Hospital

Italy
  Milan:
    Ospedale di Circolo

---

renders a judgement on the likelihood that the drug in question was responsible for the untoward event. A second judgement is later rendered by a clinical pharmacologist who reviews the case.

All data are coded and stored on magnetic tape for subsequent analysis.

Results

More than 33,000 patients have been monitored since the program began in 1966 (Table 26.2). Most of the data were obtained from American hospitals.

Table 26.2. Cross-national patterns of digitalis use

Country	Year of first monitoring	Total number of patients monitored	Per cent of patients	
			Receiving any digitalis glycoside	Receiving digoxin
United States	1966	18110	24.6	23.5
Canada	1969	2228	17.6	17.2
Israel	1969	5324	19.8	17.0
New Zealand	1971	2540	26.5	25.8
Scotland	1973	2580	17.0	16.9
Italy	1974	602	43.4	30.6
Germany	1972	1760	53.6	47.5

Extent of Digitalis Use

The per cent of monitored patients treated with any digitalis glycoside ranged from 17%-27% in the United States, Canada, Israel, New Zealand, and Scotland (Table 26.2). Digoxin accounted for nearly all of the glycoside use in these nations. The proportion of monitored patients receiving digitalis was higher in Italy (43%) and Germany (54%); in these two nations, a considerably higher proportion of patients received glycosides other than digoxin (Table 26.2). The per cent of digitalis-treated patients monitored by the BCDSP did not change substantially from year to year in any of the seven nations.

Among all monitored patients receiving digoxin, a high percentage (46%) had a primary (first) diagnosis consistent with cardiovascular disease. With the exception of Germany, where 31% of digoxin recipients had cardiovascular disease, the frequency was similar among nations, ranging from 41%-62%. A majority (61%) of monitored digoxin recipients had been taking a digitalis glycoside prior to admission. Again, the variation among nations in this characteristic (40%-68% of digoxin recipients) was relatively small.

Adverse Reactions to Digoxin

Adverse reactions to digoxin were divided into three categories. Cardiac toxicity included digoxin-attributed arrhythmias, conduction disturbances, or a combination of the two. Gastrointestinal (GI) manifestations included some combination of anorexia, nausea, vomiting, diarrhea, or abdominal discomfort. "Other" designated digoxin-attributed adverse reactions which could not be categorized as cardiac or GI. We included only those adverse reactions which both attending physician and the clinical pharmacologist judged were probably or definitely due to digoxin.

Table 26.3 shows the frequency of digoxin-attributed adverse reactions among patients monitored from 1970 to the present. With the exception of Italy, from which a relatively small amount of data were available, the frequencies of cardiac toxicity attributed to digoxin were similar, ranging from 2.2% (Germany and Israel) to 6.2% (Canada). The frequency of reported gastrointestinal toxicity was higher in New Zealand, Scotland, and Italy than in the United States, Canada, Israel, and Germany.

Factors Influencing the Frequency of Adverse Reactions

One possible source of nation-to-nation variations in adverse reaction rates could be "confounding," or unequal distributions of characteristics of patient and/or therapy which are known to predispose to toxicity. Table 26.4 lists such characteristics which are available for analysis by the BCDSP. While there are differences among nations in the distribution of these factors, they do not appear to be large enough to fully explain some of the exceptional differences in adverse reaction rates. In Israel, for example, a relatively low proportion of digoxin recipients were seriously ill, as judged by the proportion of elderly patients, those who died, and those with long hospitalizations; this might have contributed to the relatively low frequency of digoxin-attributed adverse reactions in that nation. However, no obvious explanation based on confounding is evident for the relatively high frequency of gastrointestinal toxicity in New Zealand and Scotland, or for the high frequency of all adverse reactions to digoxin in Italy.

329

Table 26.3. Adverse reactions to digoxin among patients monitored since 1970

Country	Number of patients receiving digoxin	Per cent of patients with adverse reaction to digoxin[a]		
		Cardiac	GI	Other
United States	2659	5.2	2.5	2.8
Canada	292	6.2	2.7	3.1
Israel	847	2.2	1.3	0.5
New Zealand	655	2.3	12.8	0.6
Scotland	437	6.6	12.1	1.1
Italy	184	13.0	21.7	10.3
Germany	836	2.2	4.2	0.6

[a] See text for explanation of manifestations of toxicity.

Table 26.4. Potential sources of confounding: factors that might influence the frequency of adverse reactions

Age
Sex
Body weight
Renal function (admission blood urea nitrogen
    concentration)
Survival
Duration of hospitalization
Diagnosis
Digitalis use prior to admission
Digoxin dose
Route of digoxin administration
Coadministration of other drugs

Discussion

The BCDSP monitors clinical drug effects among hospitalized medical patients in certain wards in selected hospitals. The findings, therefore, do not necessarily apply to all patients in a given nation nor to patients in other therapeutic settings. The results from a small number of patients in a single Italian hospital, for example, must be interpreted with caution until considerably more data are available.

Overall, the frequency of adverse reactions to digoxin among patients monitored by the BCDSP was reasonably similar from nation to nation. Nonetheless, there were a few striking differences. Gastrointestinal adverse reactions were reported more often from New Zealand, Scotland, and Italy, and the overall rate of toxicity was higher in Italy. Since confounding does not appear to account for these variations, other explanations must be sought. The problem is exceedingly complex and requires in-depth evaluation of the entire data base.

Acknowledgements

The Boston Collaborative Drug Surveillance Program is supported by United States Public Health Service Contract GM-4-2148 from the National Institute of General Medical Sciences (NIGMS) and in part by grants from the United States Food and Drug Administration, the Hadassah Medical Organization, the Kupat-Holim, Auckland Hospital, New Zealand, the Israeli Ministry of Health, the Canadian Food and Drug Directorate, the Roger Williams General Hospital (Brown University NIGMS grant No. GM-165-38-02), the Scottish Home and Health Department, and Hoffmann-LaRoche, Inc.

Dr. Greenblatt is supported in part by grant MH-12279 from the United States Public Health Service.

References

Allen, M.D., Greenblatt, D.J.: Role of nurse and pharmacist monitors in the Boston Collaborative Drug Surveillance Program. Drug Intel. Clin. Pharmacol. 9, 648-654 (1975)

Jick, H.: Drugs--remarkably nontoxic. N. Engl. J. Med. 291, 824-828 (1974)

Miller, R.R., Greenblatt, D.J. (eds.): Drug Effects in Hospitalized Patients: Experiences of the Boston Collaborative Drug Surveillance Program, 1966-1975. New York: John Wiley and Sons 1976

Discussion

Dengler, Bonn: Just to start the discussion, we are aware that we have this very high frequency of digitalis use, and it is mostly due to the following facts: first, our surgeons sometimes insist on preoperative digitalization without a clear-cut indication. Second, we have a number of conditions which are treated with digitalis not in internal medicine, not in general practice, but for instance in neurology and ophthalmology. I think that in a cardiology department there wouldn't be too much difference in our country -- the high figure comes from outside this area.

Greenblatt: I should mention that these are all hospitalized medical patients on your medical ward in Berlin, so people that are hospitalized specifically for eye disorders or on surgical wards would not be included.

Follath, Basel: We have recently conducted a prospective study on the incidence of digitalis toxicity. During a 6-month period, 260 digitalized patients were followed. On admission, 80% were already on digoxin. Using the same criteria as Beller et al. (1971) in their prospective study at Boston City Hospital, we found that 19% of the patients were intoxicated. This is a much higher percentage than mentioned in Dr. Greenblatt's paper, but corresponds to the results of Beller et al. In a similar investigation in Australia, the incidence of digitalis intoxication in general medical patients was also 15%. Another explication of the divergence could be the higher mean age (73 years) in our patients.

It seems that overall drug surveillance programs based on physicians' reports and evaluation by monitoring nurses — as the Boston Collaborative study — will miss a considerable percentage of patients who may be identified by a more specific approach.

Greenblatt: They are not necessarily missed; it's just that they did not fulfill the definition of an adverse drug reaction, being an unintended drug effect that usually requires the clinician to do something about it.

Follath: So you would admit that the actual incidence of intoxication is higher than your figure?

Greenblatt: Again it depends on how you define it; I think that this is a pretty realistic number, because it's unlikely that people would miss clinically important digitalis toxicity.

Baligadoo, Paris: I should like to add to this review some information concerning the frequency of digitoxin toxicity. We have conducted in a Parisian hospital a study on 3000 patients all on a maintenance therapy on digitoxin. I would like to stress that this study dealt with outpatients and not with inpatients as do the majority of studies concerning the frequency of toxicity of cardiac glycosides. I think we should always make a distinction between inpatients and outpatients when judging toxicity. Depending on the particular recruitment of a unit (diagnostic laboratory, general medical ward, coronary care unit), a smaller or greater percentage of inpatients are hospitalized because of an acute disease which may in itself mimic digitalis toxicity or render the patient more prone to manifest toxicity. In that study, we observed a 3% incidence of toxicity with digitoxin. The diagnosis of toxicity was not based on the appearance of "specific" signs of toxicity but only on a highly probable causal relationship between the appearance of a sign and the administration of digitoxin.

We had previously shown that in cases of digitoxin toxicity a distinction could be made on the bases of daily dose, serum concentration, and clinical appearance between early signs of toxicity (first-degree av-block and/or isolated ventricular premature beats) and other more severe signs of toxicity. With that distinction made, we observed the following: early toxicity: 2.1%, severe toxicity (with 11%

mortality): 0.9%. This distinction between early and severe toxicity is evidently a rough one, but it permits us to compare our results more accurately with those of others and to state that with the doses used a patient on digitoxin maintenance therapy has a 3% risk of developing toxicity which is severe in one of three toxic patients. One of ten patients with severe toxicity dies as a result of toxicity. All of the patients with early toxicity in this study survived.

Oliver, St. Louis: May I just ask Dr. Baligadoo over what time period were the patients at risk? It seems to make a difference whether you follow someone for a short interval or over a period of months or years.

Baligadoo: These patients were followed on average for about 2 years.

Dengler: I'd like to come back to the difference in the incidence of gastrointestinal toxicity, and you promised to comment upon it. I think it was in two countries that this incidence was unexpectedly high. Did they use particular oral preparations?

Greenblatt: We saw a high incidence in Scotland and New Zealand, and in neither case was it apparently related to use of a special oral digoxin preparation. In New Zealand, it was partly related to the high use of intramuscular digoxin which was a confounding factor accounting for the high incidence of GI toxicity. In Scotland, they were not heavy users of intramuscular digoxin, so that couldn't have accounted for it. I have no explanation for the GI toxicity in Scotland.

Shaw: I think one of the fascinating things about these figures is that it tells us as much about the countries as about the drugs. My own experience has been that in Scotland physicians quite readily attribute nausea to digitalis. If you stop the drug the nausea may go away, but perhaps it was due to some other cause and was going to go away anyway. So I think perhaps in that instance it may reflect the thinking of the physicians.

Greenblatt: In general, though, we find fewer cross-national differences among house doctors than there are among drugs. For most drugs we don't find this kind of difference.

Oliver: I don't recall your mentioning interaction between diuretics and digitalis. Did that simply not tumble out of your statistics?

Greenblatt: It did not tumble out because I didn't look for it (and I was hoping that nobody would ask me). This is very complicated, and anybody doing a definitive study on digoxin would also have to assess the effect of diuretics.

Nyberg, Sweden: You mentioned initially that most of these adverse reactions were innocent.

Greenblatt: The majority of adverse reactions were not life-threatening.

Nyberg: The recent book about the progress of your program, appearing last year, gives a rate of life-threatening intoxications of, if I remember correctly, 2.1%. Do you have any corresponding figure for the present material? Was there any relation to the higher average dose level in some countries?

Greenblatt: My impression was that in general the frequency of life-threatening toxicity relative to all digitalis toxicity was relatively small in all nations.

Nyberg: And there was no connection with the high dosages in some countries, for instance?

Greenblatt: No, not that I saw.

Reference

Baligadoo et al.: Coeur Med. Interne 15, 2, 249 (1976)

27 Pharmacokinetic and Clinical Effects During the Predistribution Phase of Digoxin Treatment

P. REISSELL, V. MANNINEN, and O. LOKKI

Pharmacokinetic studies with digoxin have shown that its distribution is rapid and corresponds to an open two-compartment model (Nyberg et al., 1974). Brock and Christensen (1974) have suggested that there might be a saturation of the receptor sites during maintenance therapy. Whether this postulate is merely an interesting excercise in theoretic pharmacokinetics or does, in fact, have practical implications in the clinical use of digoxin remains to be elucidated.

In this study, we present data which show that in healthy volunteers during maintenance digoxin a saturation of the digoxin receptor sites is achieved with higher doses. Other data demonstrate that during maintenance digoxin therapy, a high proportion of elderly cardiac patients may experience transient cardiac arrhythmias following administration of the normal maintenance doses.

Materials and Methods

Two groups of six healthy volunteers were subjected to the pharmacokinetic studies of digoxin. In the first study, single doses of first 0.25 mg and later 1.0 mg of digoxin, with an interval of at least 7 days, were injected intravenously in 20 ml saline at constant rate over 20 min. In the second study, 0.25 mg and later 0.50 mg of digoxin were injected intravenously in 10 ml saline over 5 min for a 10-day period at each dose level. The washout period between the first and second dose was at least 7 days. Steady-state serum digoxin concentrations were determined on days 8-11, and the mean of this was used as the base line steady-state concentration.

In the clinical experiments, ten elderly cardiac patients were continuously monitored for the detection of cardiac arrhythmias during 8 h after ingestion of their normal maintenance doses of digoxin in the fasting state. The Lanoxin (Burroughs Wellcome, United Kingdom) brand of digoxin tablets, with a dissolution of 95% in 1 h, was used. All subjects had normal levels of serum creatinine and electrolytes. Serum concentrations of digoxin were determined by radioimmunoassay (Ojala et al., 1972). Calculation of the rate of digoxin disappearance (b) from blood was made using the following equations:

1. for ½-1 h $\quad b_{1/2} = \log (x (\tfrac{1}{2}h)) - \log (x (1h))/0.5$
2. for 1-2 h $\quad b_1 = \log (x (1h)) - \log (x (2h))$
3. for ½-4h $\quad b_{1/2\text{-}4} h = \log (x (\tfrac{1}{2}h)) - \log (x (4h))/3.5$

Results

Single-Dose Studies

No significant difference in the disappearance of digoxin from the blood can be seen between the administrations of large (1.0 mg) or smaller (0.25 mg) doses (Fig. 27.1). By analyzing the initial phase of distribution, there were no significant time-dependent variances. The disappearance of digoxin approximates to the function $x(t) = ce^{-bt}$. It is also of interest to note that the shape of the serum digoxin curve obtained by applying the three-way analysis of variance has the same uniformity in both serum curves and that there is no significant variation between individuals.

Maintenance Studies

In Figure 27.2 the serum curves, as well as the steady-state serum digoxin levels, are shown. Disappearance rates of digoxin are given in Table 27.1. Digoxin dis-

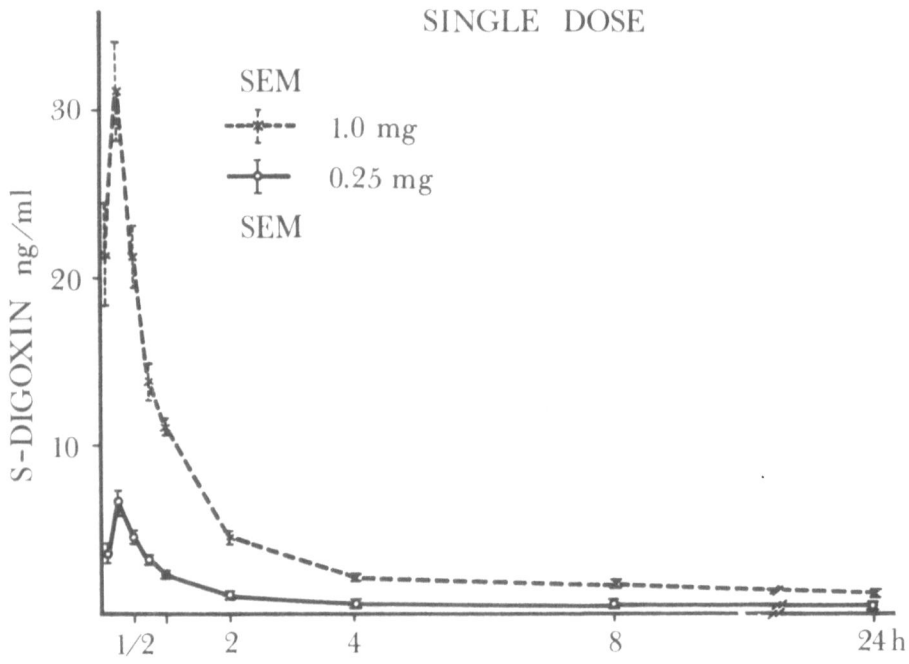

Fig. 27.1. Serum digoxin concentrations in six healthy volunteers after 20 min constant rate intravenous infusion of two different digoxin doses. Mean values and SEM are given. Values for $b_{1/2}$, b_1, and $b_{1/2-4}$ are 0.613, 0.327, and 0.229 for a dose of 0.25 mg and 0.559, 0.401, and 0.252 for a 1.0 mg dose. The disappearance rate of digoxin did not thus differ according to the dosage

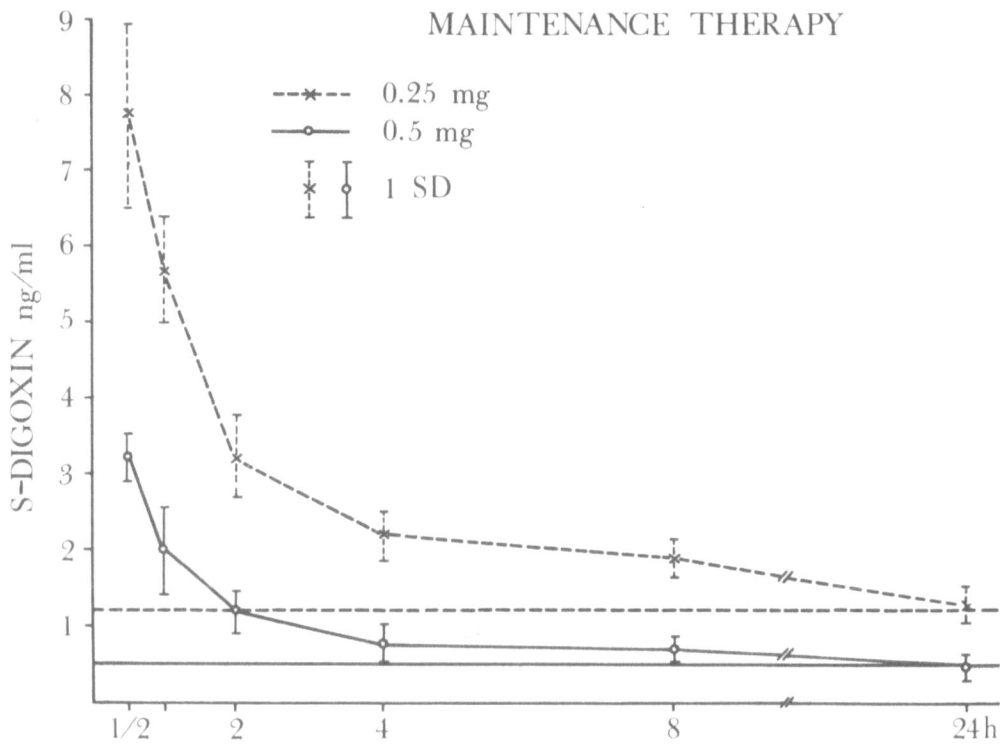

Fig. 27.2. Serum digoxin concentrations in six healthy volunteers on day 10 of the maintenance therapy with either 0.25 mg or 0.50 mg digoxin given intravenously. Steady-state concentrations (bottom lines) are calculated from values on days 8-11

appearance following the smaller dose (0.25 mg) behaved as in single-dose studies. The larger dose leads to a faster initial disappearance. This change in the disappearance rate is short, and 30 min later there were no significant differences. The relatively higher serum concentration at ½ h and 1 h, which coincide with the accelerated disappearance, favors the idea of a saturation in the reseptor sites. Three-way analysis of variance shows again that the shape of the serum curve displays no significant differences between individuals (Table 27.2). The subjective feeling of the volunteers remained good throughout the study and no complaints attributable to digoxin were noted.

Clinical Studies

The patient's characteristics and results are summarized in Table 27.3. In half of the subjects, transient arrhythmias were recorded 2-5 h after administration of digoxin. In two of these, there were episodes of ventricular extrasystoles, in two others supraventricular extrasystoles, and in one prolongation of PQ time,

Table 27.1. The disappearance rate (b) of digoxin from blood on day 10 of the maintenance therapy

Subject	Dose 0.25 mg			Dose 0.5 mg		
	$b_{1/2}$	b_1	$b_{1/2\text{-}4}$	$b_{1/2}$	b_1	$b_{1/2\text{-}4}$
LO	0.136	0.223	0.121	0.366	0.196	0.144
TH	0.224	0.240	0.167	0.258	0.336	0.155
LMJ	0.309	0.238	0.165	0.494	0.222	0.184
APJ	0.268	0.280	0.157	0.866	0.176	0.232
JR	0.340	0.284	0.182	0.420	0.206	0.211
AR	0.336	0.231	0.150	0.224	0.217	0.189
Mean	0.269	0.249	0.157	0.438	0.225	0.182

The $b_{1/2}$ of the 0.5 mg dose is significantly greater compared with the $b_{1/2}$ of the 0.25 mg dose, while the b_1 and $b_{1/2\text{-}4}$ are equal after the different dosages.

Table 27.2. Three-way variance analysis of the serum digoxin concentration curve on day 10 of the maintenance therapy

	N	
	Degrees of freedom	Variance
S_i	4	3.1348[a]
S_j	1	3.0533[a]
S_{ij}	4	0.0235
S_k	5	0.1244[b]
S_{ik}	20	0.0235
S_{jk}	5	0.0683[c]
S_{ijk}	20	0.0236

Data = log of S digoxin, i = 30, 60, 120, 240, and 1440 min, k = 6 persons, and j = 0.50-0.25 mg.

[a] Highly significant.
[b] Significant.
[c] Almost significant.

Table 27.3. Clinical data and serum digoxin concentrations in ten patients monitored for detection of cardiac arrhythmias during 8 h after intake of digoxin tablets in the fasting state

Patient	Age and sex	Digoxin dose (mg)	Serum digoxin (ng/ml) Stationary	Peak	Rhythm disturbance Type and time of occurrence
1	71 F	0.375	1.2	3.4	Nil
2	79 F	0.25	1.0	2.1	Nil
3	75 F	0.125	0.7	1.7	Nil
4	65 M	0.375	0.7	3.2	Nil
5	60 M	0.25	0.8	2.7	Nil
6	76 F	0.375	1.2	3.8	VES[a] at 3-5 h
7	76 F	0.375	1.5	4.0	SVES[b] at 3-5 h
8	60 F	0.375	1.4	3.9	Prolongation of PQ time at 3-5 h
9	69 F	0.25	1.5	3.4	SVES at 2-5 h
10	72 M	0.50	1.6	3.6	VES at 2-5 h

By permission from Manninen et al. 1976.

[a] VES ventricular extrasystoles.
[b] SVES supraventricular extrasystoles.

from 0.15 s to 0.24 s. In patients with arrhythmias, higher steady-state digoxin concentrations were found than in patients without arrhythmias, even though serum concentrations in all instances remained below 2.0 ng/ml.

Discussion

The present results show that during maintenance therapy with larger intravenous doses of digoxin, saturation of digoxin sites during the initial distribution can be demonstrated. The phenomenon is rapidly corrected and after 1 h, the disappearance rate from blood is similar with low and high doses. Doherty et al. (1967) have shown that the distribution of digoxin in the body is wide and that it can be found in almost every tissue, although in different concentrations. The theoretic maximal uptake volume has been calculated by several authors, most recently by Koup and his co-workers (1975), and it seems to be large enough to accept the quantity of digoxin we have used in this study. We have also demonstrated that in cadavers resulting from high suicidal doses of digoxin — exceeding the normal therapeutic dose by 100 times — the digoxin concentration in heart muscle is very high (Reissell et al., 1975). So it seems that there is, in fact, a real variable uptake capacity for digoxin. One question is whether this short-lived phenomenon relates to the restricted binding sites at subcellular level. Elimination of digoxin from the body might also play a role, though we were not able to separate this from other pharmacokinetic parameters in our experimental set up.

In applying the pharmacokinetic data to the clinical use of digoxin, serum digoxin levels, myocardial digoxin concentrations, and sensitivity of the individual subjects must be considered. There is increasing evidence that serum and myocardial digoxin concentrations are related (see, e.g., Härtel et al., 1976 for a review) although direct conclusions about the correlation between these concentrations and the clinical effects of digoxin cannot be drawn yet. We may speculate that during maintenance therapy, saturation of nonspecific binding sites might encourage accumulation of digoxin on the active sites in the heart, i.e., a switch of digoxin from the passive or noncardiac sites to the active sites.

It is quite clear from this study and from past clinical experience that normal healthy people tolerate digoxin well. The same applies to patients with atrial fibrillation. This variation in individual sensitivity to digoxin must be of great importance and is not a constant factor, but varies according to changes in electrolytes, oxygen tension in blood and tissues, hormonal balance (particularly catecholamines), etc. If the healthy volunteers in this study represent the highly resistent type in terms of sensitivity, the elderly cardiac patients with transient arrhythmias represent the opposite pole. We have seen that five out of ten patients on maintenance digoxin therapy, monitored after doses of digoxin tablets with excellent bioavailability, experienced disturbances of cardiac rhythm 2-5 h after the intake of digoxin.

Such a study with cardiac patients is not comprehensive, however, and obviously invites further investigations. In confirmation of our observations, Belz and his associates (1974) have demonstrated that glycoside effects on the electrocardiogram show maxima at 2-4 h after intravenous injections of digoxin and proscillaridin. The present results lead us to believe that digoxin ought to be administered with caution to elderly sensitive patients, even with normal stationary levels of serum digoxin. Administration of digoxin either in divided daily doses or with a meal (thereby slowing down the rate of absorption, White et al., 1971) is suggested in sensitive subjects.

References

Belz, G.G., Rudofsky, G., Lossnitzer, K., Wolf, G., Stauch, M.: Plasmaspiegel und Elektrokardiogramm nach intravenöser Applikation von Proscillaridin und Digoxin. Z. Kardiol. 63, 201 (1974)

Brock, A., Christensen, E.: On the elimination of digoxin from serum after intravenous injections. Acta Pharmacol. Toxicol. (Kbh.) 34, 205 (1974)

Doherty, J.E., Perkins, W.H., Flanigan, W.J.: The distribution and concentration of tritiated digoxin in human tissues. Ann. Intern. Med. 66, 116 (1967)

Härtel, G., Kyllönen, K., Merikallio, E., Ojala, K., Manninen, V., Reissell, P.: Human serum and myocardium digoxin. Clin. Pharmacol. Ther. 19, 153 (1976)

Koup, J.R., Greenblatt, D.J., Jusko, W.J., Smith, T.W., Koch-Weser, J.: Pharmacokinetics of digoxin in normal subjects after intravenous bolus and infusion doses. J. Pharmacokinet. Biopharm. 3, 181 (1975)

Manninen, V., Reissell, P., Paukkala, E.: Transient cardiac arrhythmias after single daily maintenance doses of digoxin. Clin. Pharmacol. Ther. 20, 266 (1976)

Nyberg, L., Andersson, K.-E., Bertler, Å.: Bioavailability of digoxin from tablets. II. Radioimmunoassay and disposition pharmacokinetics of digoxin after intravenous administration. Acta Pharm. Suec. 11, 459 (1974)

Ojala, K., Karjalainen, J., Reissell, P.: Radioimmunoassay of digoxin. Lancet 1972: 150

Reissell, P., Alha, A., Karjalainen, J., Nieminen, R., Ojala, K.: Digoxin intoxication determined post mortem. Abstr. Sixth Int. Congr. Pharmacol. Helsinki 1975

White, R.J., Chamberlain, D.A., Howard, M., Smith, T.W.: Plasma concentrations of digoxin after oral administration in the fasting and postprandial state. Br. Med. J. 1971 1, 380

Discussion

Oliver: Perhaps I could just begin the questions by asking if you could tell me the time of your peak concentration. At what time did that occur?

Reissell: It's at 1 h.

Greenblatt: I think you have to be exceedingly careful about drawing conclusions, especially mathematical conclusions, about drug distribution following oral administration. Depending on how the absorption rate constant compares to α, you may or may not see the distribution phase. If α is much greater than the absorption rate constant, you just don't see the distribution phase at all. On the other hand, if the reverse is true, you may see a very pronounced distribution phase. So I think that after oral administration, much of what you are seeing might be confounded by differences in absorption rate. If you really wanted to study dose-dependent drug distribution, then it clearly should be done with intravenous administration.

Reissell: That's what we have done in the first part of our study.

Greenblatt: Then I misinterpreted the graph, because it looked like the level was going up. These were individuals on maintenance therapy?

Reissell: Intravenous maintenance therapy.

Dengler: But I still have an objection very similar to that of Dr. Greenblatt. I think it's a kind of peculiar pharmacokinetics if you subdivide a curve arbitrarily into ½ h and 1 h and 1-4 h and compare single-dose administration with superimposed i.v. injections in an already digitalized patient.

Reissell: The intravenous studies were originally designed for the comparison of different dosages of digoxin on the suitability as reference solution to the tablet bioavailability — the comparison was calculated not by conventional pharmacokinetic methods but by mathematical calculations of the disappearance rate from blood at different periods of time. We do not consider these time periods as strictly the α-phase, but the results certainly suggest that the difference in the disappearance rates includes also the α-phase.

Dengler: This brings me back to the true message, and I think this is your observation of arrhythmias following the digoxin administration. They occurred in your experiments after 2-5 h. As I am responsible for this title of your presentation I want to excuse myself, but I thought we should discuss whether the achievement of a high digoxin level after oral or intravenous administration bears the risk of precipitating more extrasystoles. I would like to suggest that we should discuss this particular point which seems very important to me and neglect for a moment the pharmacokinetic situation.

Oliver: For what period of time were the patients observed?

Reissell: They were monitored continuously from the beginning of the test to 6-8 h. I think what we found actually for the transient arrhythmias is fitting very well to the observations by Dr. Belz who said that the effect of digitalis comes about 2 h after the administration.

Grahame-Smith: I am truly and completely lost. This morning, Dr. Johnson was talking about dogs. They have hearts and he showed that as far as the acetylstrophantin test was concerned, it didn't really matter very much what kind of profile the plasma level time curve had (which I found rather surprising), and in your studies, it seems that there are transient and fairly early arrhythmias occurring, possibly dependent upon the early predistribution phase. Now it seems to me that somehow or other we have got to put those two things together. I think it is important because of the question I asked yesterday "what is the meaning of the plasma level time curve in terms of the pharmacodynamic action of digitalis? " This is crucial to the understanding of how the drug works.

Reissell: We are still going on with this problem and trying to monitor the patients — several patients — to see if we can confirm our own results. But what fascinates me is exactly what you are saying about the timing of the appearing and the disappearing of these arrhythmias.

Shaw: I can't understand why you didn't do control recordings on a separate day. I think it's very important in elderly people like this who very commonly have arrhythmias on these prolonged recordings.

Oliver: And arrhythmias are certainly time dependent, even in patients who are not on digitalis. There are certain patterns to the day; events at certain times can provoke arrhythmias.

Reissell: I think this reflects more the sensitivity of the patient to digitalis. I think we had to find the patients who are sensitive to digitalis, they might be 1% or 20% of all patients.

Shaw: Without the control reading you can't say that.

Reissell: Of course, the appropriate control is needed.

Johnson: I'd like to comment on the point raised by Dr. Grahame-Smith. I think these results of Pentti Reissell's show absence of temporal relationship between the peak plasma levels and cardiotoxicity. They saw evidence of cardiotoxicity 3-5 h after administration of the last tablet; whereas peak plasma levels occurred at about 1 h. So I think there is no disagreement on that point.

I don't think that you can say anything from this experiment relevant to the nature of the plasma profile, because there was no comparison with any other type of profile. This experiment simply shows that an oral preparation which happens to produce a high peak plasma level may later be associated with evidence of cardiotoxicity. That simply reflects that the major cardiac effects of digoxin are delayed. That wouldn't be too surprising; maximal inotropic and chronotropic effects develop something like 3-8 h after an oral dose of digoxin. I don't think that this experiment could by its design say anything at all in relation to the plasma concentration profile.

Lukas: I have a question for Dr. Johnson relative to his data. He tested sensitivity to acetylstrophantidin at a time when the concentration curve was flat; I wonder whether he has data on acetylstrophantidin sensitivity at the peaks of these curves.

Johnson: We did acetylstrophantidin sensitivity testing at the time of peak concentration after giving an alcoholic solution of digoxin by esophageal tube to dogs. Sensitivity was lower at this time than at either 3 or 6 h after digoxin administration.

Smith: It has been shown in animal studies that peak myocardial levels are achieved no more than about 30 min or so after an intravenous injection of digoxin. Although the total myocardial concentration reaches a peak or really a plateau after only about that time, it's only well after that plateau is achieved that one sees the peak incidence of apparent toxicity.

Jogestrand, Stockholm: Dr. Reissell, can you tell us something about the quantity of the arrhythmia during these registrations?

Reissell: They were numbered more than 10 per min.

Oliver: Were there any repetitive ventricular beats, two in a row, three or more in a row (ventricular tachycardia), or that sort of thing?

Reissell: No.

Dengler: I think there is still some misunderstanding. You answered that these figures applied to i.v. injections, but as I understood these clinical studies are done with tablets. Am I right?

Reissell: Yes. I am trying to interpret two different studies. One with healthy people where we can see the saturation mechanism in the heart, and still they didn't have any clinical signs of digitalis intoxication, and the elderly people who are apparently sensitive to digitalis.

Dengler: Well, but then I come to the next point which is very interesting for us. The consequence of your interpretation would be that giving i.v. injections would be almost forbidden.

Reissell: Very hard to have an opinion on it at present.

Nyberg: I wish to comment on your findings from the two-compartment open model. Reuning and associates found a relationship between the amount of digoxin calculated to be in the peripheral compartment and a clinical effect, in their case the shortening of the left ventricular ejection time. We have simulated the time course in the peripheral compartment after administration of a rapidly absorbed tablet. After a single dose, there is a maximum somewhere between 6 and 7 h. During maintenance dose treatment, the maximum occurs earlier, presumably at about 5 h. This time course might be compatible with your observations.

Smith: There probably are many peripheral "compartments," and pharmacokineticists try not to attach unrealistic significance to the models they use. The time course of digoxin uptake by the heart is known to plateau, in dog studies, at about 30 min. I wouldn't really know how to interpret cardiac effects in terms of theoretic calculation that take into account the uptake of the glycoside by all the tissues, most of which are much less well perfused than the heart. I would think that what we are really interested in, primarily, would be the kinetics of uptake by the heart, and not by this theoretic second compartment we talk about.

Erdmann: I think what we are all talking about now is digitalis concentrations in serum and in the heart, but actually the concentration in the heart is not the same everywhere. It is different at different sites or places. For instance, if you inject a cardiac glycoside into a guinea pig, then after let's say 10-30 min or so you will have the peak concentration in the heart. If you take the membranes and isolate them, you will not have filled all available specific binding sites with cardiac glycosides. You have not inhibited the ATPase totally, either. Now, if you take isolated membranes and do binding experiments with them and you do it in a solution, which permits very good binding then after let's say 40-50 min, you have peak specific binding. If you perform the same binding experiment in the serum, however, you need hours until equilibrium is established. It takes a much longer time. What I want to point out with this experimental design is: it is not the heart we should look for, but we should look for the actual pharmacologically important sites where the drug acts, and I think those obey completely different kinetics or pharmacodynamics than the total heart, where we are measuring mostly unspecific binding of cardiac glycosides.

Smith: I would agree with that entirely. What I meant was that the effect at the "receptor" in the heart may or may not correlate with values derived from the shape of a plasma curve of drug going into a number of other organs and tissues.

28 Digitalis Intoxication: Clinical and Experimental Work[1]

P. F. BINNION

The appearance of various disorders of cardiac rhythms and conduction and non-specific symptoms in patients receiving digitalis is a common clinical problem. Practically all the disorders of cardiac rhythm and conduction that are known have been seen in patients taking digitalis preparations. A causal relationship is sometimes highly suggestive and numerous papers have been published on this topic (Rodensky and Wasserman, 1961); Irons and Orgain, 1966; Chung, 1967; Fisch and Knoebel, 1970), but it must be remembered that much of this work was done before estimation of blood digitalis levels became an easily obtainable clinical tool. When methods became available for measuring nanogram quantities of digoxin and digitoxin in blood from patients, the first papers used the clinical criteria for digitalis-induced arrhythmias as the basis for their investigations and found a good correlation between toxic signs and symptoms and the blood glycoside level (Grahame-Smith & Everest, 1969); Beller et al., 1971; White et al., 1970; Smith & Haber, 1970; Evered & Chapman, 1971). This lead to the idea that a plasma digoxin level exceeding 2-3 ng/ml was a toxic level, but in view of the difficulty defining digitalis toxicity, this approach was a biased one, and the errors intrinsic in these studies has been commented upon (Fogelman et al., 1970; Binnion, 1972; Binnion, 1973). By taking a series of 323 sequential patients and relating plasma digoxin levels to various arrhythmias, the only relationship which would be established was a possible one between paroxysmal atrial tachycardia with av-block (Binnion, 1973) and later work cast suspicion even on this association (Storstein & Rasmussen, 1974)

In various cases of massive digitalis overdose with obvious poisoning, extreme bradycardia, av-block, and asystole were the dominant rhythm changes (Lely & Van Enter, 1970; Asplund et al., 1971; Citrin et al., 1972; Citrin et al., 1973; Reza et al., 1974; Rumack et al., 1974) although atrial dysrhythmias were mentioned in one paper (Bertler et al., 1973). There was little relationship between the findings in these papers and the results of the earlier clinical papers on the radioimmunoassay method used by others.

I have always maintained that on both theoretic and experimental grounds there is, at best, only a weak association between serum digitalis concentration and

---

1 Supported by funds from the American Heart Association (grant no. 71-1091) and with funds contributed by the Pennsylvania Heart Association in 1971 and 1976.

digitalis toxicity. Much of the investigative work has been criticized in a recent article (Ingelfinger & Goldman, 1976) and most of the subsequent correspondence related to this article supports this view (various authors, 1976).

Myocardial Levels in Man
Human Myocardial Digoxin Concentrations

Up to now the discussion has centred on blood glycoside levels, but it is the concentration in the heart which determines the arrhythmia. Measurements of the digoxin concentration in the heart have been measured under various experimental conditions in animals (and will be reviewed in the section on "factors affecting digitalis intoxication"), and various investigators have determined the levels in the human myocardium. The first study used tritiated digoxin and showed a myocardial level about 30 times higher than the serum concentration in two patients (Doherty et al., 1967). With the advent of new assay techniques, it was possible to measure myocardial levels in fragments of human heart removed at cardiac surgery, the first values being obtained in the atrial appendage of patients undergoing mitral valvotomy (mean atrial digoxin concentration of 219 ng/g wet wt with a range of 34-648 and SEM ± 42) (Binnion et al., 1969). There was no evidence of abnormal arrhythmias before or after operation, so this would appear to be a "nontoxic" concentration, and the variability could have been due to the varying amount of fibrosis expected in atrial tissue affected by prior rheumatic disease. More accurate work on the same line has been done since that time (Carroll et al., 1973), and the results are summarized in Table 28.1. There is greater affinity of human myocardial muscle for digoxin compared with skeletal muscle (mean myocardial/plasma ratio = 67.7, mean skeletal muscle/plasma ratio = 15.9) (Coltart et al., 1972). Taking the concensus of various investigators gives a human atrial digoxin concentration in nontoxic patients about 34-77 ng/g and papillary muscle of 78-95 ng/g, but there is a great range in values obtained as was noted in the earliest paper (Binnion et al., 1969) where the ^{86}Rb uptake biologic assay technique was used before refinement which produced higher values than the radioimmunoassay method used later by others. There is an even greater range in the myocardial/plasma digoxin ratios which I consider to imply that blood levels can have only a poor relationship to any toxic manifestations of digitalis (which supports the earlier statements in this paper).

In a more controlled setting, albeit with anesthetized animals, many factors have now been found to influence the uptake of digitalis glycosides by the myocardium (Table 28.2 which will cast further doubt on finding a reasonable relationship between blood levels and adverse electrophysiologic effects.

Factors Affecting Digitalis Intoxication

Although digitalis causes arrhythmias, there are many other factors involved (Table 28.2), and it is these other factors which preclude a close association be-

Table 28.1. Human myocardial digoxin concentrations (ng/g wet wt of tissue)

Authors	Tissue site	Tissue level range	Mean	Mean Myocardial/serum ratio (range)
Binnion et al., 1969 (N = 16)	Left atrium	34-648	219	100:1
Coltart et al., 1972 (N = 8)	Left ventricular papillary muscle	15.5-132	77.7	67.7:1 (39:1-155:1)
Carroll et al., 1973 (N = 27)	Right atrium	30-175	76.5	70:1 (25:1-128:1)
Güllner et al., 1974 (N = 12)	Right atrium	14.0-86.6	34.3	23.9 (17.7-29.1)
Carruthers, et al., 1975 (N = 32)	Atria papillary muscle	2.3-130.2	50.9 94.8	45.3:1 (2.8:1-124:1) 70.6:1 (39.3:1-114:1)

N = No. of patients studied.

Table 28.2. Factors affecting digitalis intoxication

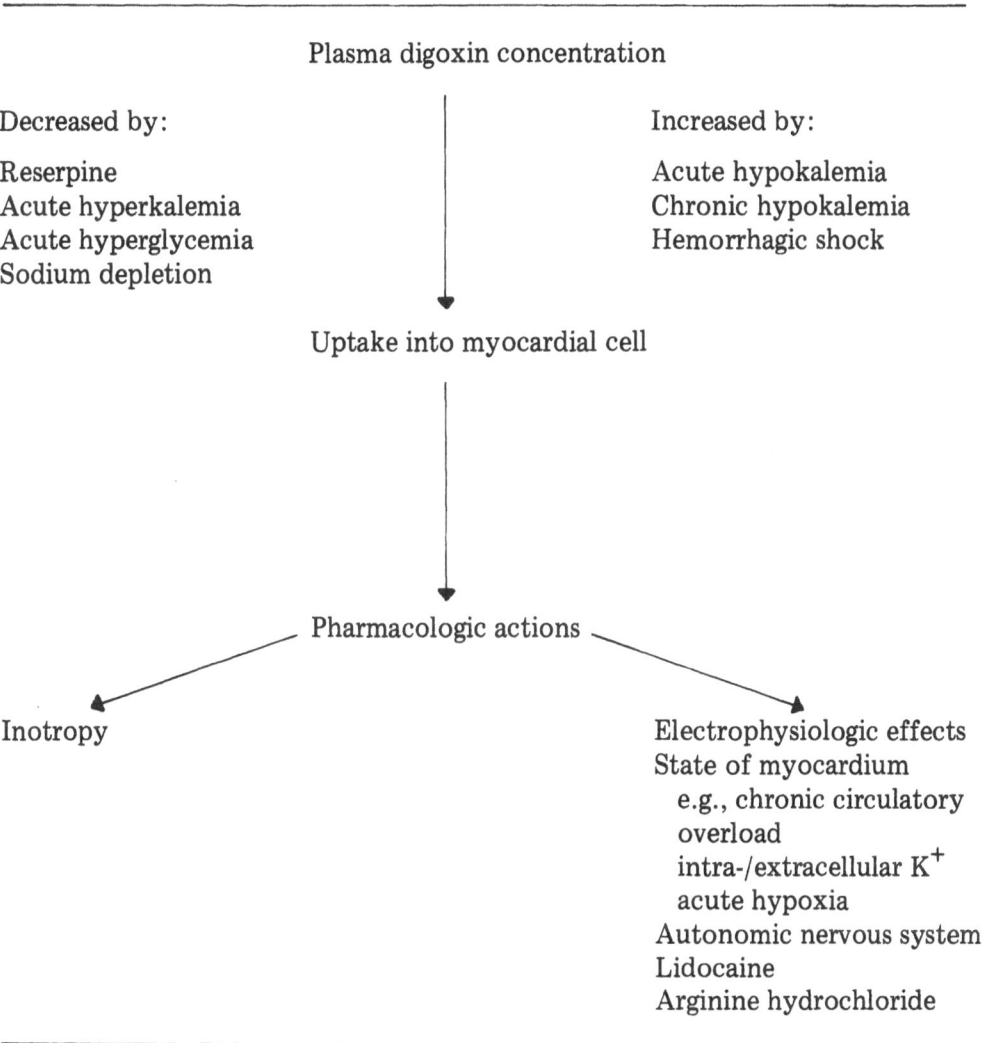

tween plasma levels and the electrophysiologic actions of digitalis. Most recent experimental work on this topic has used tritiated digoxin, and myocardial levels have been measured. Sodium depletion depresses ^{3}H-digoxin binding to the canine myocardium (Harrison and Wakim, 1969) as does hyperkalemia (Ebert et al., 1963; Marcus et al., 1969; Morgan & Binnion, 1970; Prindle et al., 1971), while hypokalemia tends to increase the uptake of digoxin by the myocardium (Cohn et al., 1967; Binnion & Morgan, 1971; Prindle et al., 1971). However, these experiments are more useful in the study of the cardiac cell capacity to take up digoxin and theories related to how this occurs (Morgan & Binnion, 1970) and are not directly related to the production of arrhythmias.

Other factors demonstrated to alter myocardial digoxin uptake are acute hypoxia which reduces the amount of glycoside needed to cause toxic arrhythmias (Harrison et al., 1968; Williams et al., 1968; Beller & Smith, 1975) in contrast to acute hypercapnia and chronic hypoxia where no reduction in ouabain dosage is needed to produce toxic arrhythmias (Halloran & Douwing, 1972; Beller et al., 1975). Hemorrhagic shock increases plasma and myocardial digoxin levels possibly due to a reduced peripheral blood flow (and hence peripheral digoxin delivery and uptake) (Lloyd & Taylor, 1975). Occlusion of a major coronary artery reduces myocardial digoxin uptake which also remains abnormally low when reperfusion is permitted later (Beller et al., 1975). Another factor of importance is chronic circulatory overload which can reduce the tolerance to a cardiac glycoside (Cope et al., 1973). Heart rate is a critical determinant of early increases in ventricular automaticity during ouabain administration (Vassale et al., 1963; Wittenberg et al., 1972). Both hypothermia and the β-blocking agent pronethalol significantly increase the threshold toxic dose of ouabain needed to produce a ventricular arrhythmia, but without cardiac concentrations we cannot speculate on the mechanism for this (El-Fiky & Katzung, 1969). Reserpine also protects the myocardium against lethal arrhythmias due to digitalis (Erlij & Mendez, 1964) possibly partially by reducing the myocardial uptake of glycoside (Marcus et al., 1968). However, sympathectomy also protects against lethal digoxin arrhythmias (Erlij & Mendez, 1964), most likely by altering the electrophysiologic responsiveness of the myocardial cells. Other substances can reverse experimentally induced ouabain arrhythmias, such as lidocaine, arginine hydrochloride, and glucagon (Alberti et al., 1971; Allen et al., 1971; Einzig et al., 1971), although the mechanisms are probably different. Hence, there are an enormous number of factors which can affect the induction of arrhythmias by digitalis glycoside, and little can be gleaned from further innumeration. It is obviously necessary to study the induction of these arrhythmias under conditions in which plasma and myocardial concentrations can be measured for, as mentioned previously, it must be the glycoside in the myocardium which ultimately causes the arrhythmia.

Experimental Work on Myocardial Glycoside Levels

Using the anesthetized dog, plasma and myocardial digoxin levels can be measured in various dysrhythmic states produced by glycoside infusion such as av-dissociation, ventricular tachycardia, and cardiac arrest. This will give us a more specific insight into the mechanisms of action of digoxin on the cardiac electrophysiologic process in the absence of myocardial disease. Table 28.3 gives a synopsis of results obtained in experiments of similar design done in our laboratory, some as yet incomplete, and left ventricular digoxin concentrations are tabulated. As might be expected, the greater the concentration in both plasma and heart, the more serious is the arrhythmia in the control animals although the difference in ventricular glycoside levels between animals in av-dissociation and those without any pumping action is relatively small. There is no relationship between these concentrations and those found in patients on chronic therapy. Human myocardial levels after death have been reported as 245 ± 33 ng/g wet wt (mean ± SEM)

Table 28.3. Myocardial digoxin concentrations

Rhythm at endpoint	Intervention	Plasma digoxin conc. at induction of arrhythmia (ng/ml)	Digoxin conc. (ng/g wet wt)		Calculated $\bar{x}$ rate of myocardial digoxin uptake	
			Atria	LV	Atria	LV
Av-dissociation		114	436	632	37	387
	Acute hypokalemia	91.4	398	663	48	521
	Chronic hypokalemia	135	373	591	35	364
	Acute hyperglycemia	150	257	494	24	307
Ventricular tachycardia		125	528	759	55	430
	Acute hypokalemia	108	483	728	52	521
	Acute hyperglycemia	170	330	540	26	300
Cardiac arrest		(N = 5)	202	889	25	286
	Pretreated with propranolol	(N = 6)	157	663	23	265
	Glucose-insulin infusion	(N = 3)	134	1005	–	–

Andersson et al., 1975) and over 201 ng/g (Jelliffe and Stevenson, 1969) which again are much less than we found for the dog and are probably accounted for by the different experimental design. Hence, the dog experiments are apparently only useful for comparison between themselves and delineating factors which alter myocardial uptake and sensitivity to cardiac glycosides.

Changes in extracellular potassium concentration produced either acutely or chronically do not reduce the myocardial digoxin concentration needed to produce av-dissociation, and this is also noted when ventricular tachycardia is the endpoint for the infusion (Table 28.3). Acute elevation of blood glucose appears to interfere with the myocardial uptake of digoxin into both atria and left ventricle (and this is supported numerically by the figures for the mean calculated rate of digoxin uptake). The rate of uptake of digoxin is increased by acute hypokalemia even though ventricular tachycardia occurs at the same myocardial level as in the control group, suggesting that a threshold level is required to induce the abnormal depolarization of the Purkinje cells in the left ventricle (Kastor et al., 1971). A certain threshold level appears to be needed for the induction of av-dissociation (as for ventricular tachycardia) with the exception of acute hypoglycemia where a lower level is recorded. The exception raises the question that the threshold level for arrhythmias is not necessarily constant, but the reasons for this are unclear at present. This could be due to a change in the intracellular distribution of digoxin, for this is the fundamental cause of the arrhythmia, and there is no work on this under these experimental conditions. It is likely that the digoxin bound to the microsomes is most important in the genesis of arrhythmias, for this is where the inotropic response appears to be generated (Dutta et al., 1968; Kim et al., 1972; Goldmann et al., 1973), but direct information is lacking.

Further doubt is cast on the concept of a fixed threshold level required to produce an arrhythmia when the results of the cardiac arrest experiments are studied (Table 28.3).

Conclusion

If there is no fixed threshold of myocardial digoxin concentration which will produce a certain arrhythmia, then we can hardly expect a close correlation between blood digoxin concentrations in man and the presence of certain arrhythmias. This has now been confirmed by others in human experiments.

References

Alberti, K.G.M.M., Shahriari, A.A., Levine, H.D., Lauler, D.P.: Reversal of ouab-
    ain-induced arrhythmias in the dog by intravenous arginine hydrochloride.
    Cardiovasc. Res. 5, 226-235 (1971)
Allen, J.D., Shanks, R.G., Zaidi, S.A.: Effects of lignocaine and propranolol
    on experimental cardiac arrhythmias. Br. J. Pharmacol. 42, 1-12 (1971)
Andersson, K.E., Bertler, Å., Wettrell, G.: Post-mortem distribution and tissue

concentrations of digoxin in infants and adults. Acta Paediatr. Scand. 64, 497-504 (1975)

Asplund, J., Edhag, O., Mogensen, L., Nyquist, O., Orinius, E., Sjögren, A.: Four cases of massive digitalis poisoning. Acta Med. Scand. 189, 293-297 (1971)

Beller, G.A., Smith T.W.: Digitalis toxicity during acute hypoxia in intact conscious dogs. J. Pharmacol. Exp. Ther. 193, 963-968 (1975)

Beller, G.A., Smith, T.W., Abelmann, W.H., Haber, E., Hood, W.B.: Digitalis intoxication. N. Engl. J. Med. 284, 989-997 (1971)

Beller, G.A., Giamber, S.R., Saltz, S.B., Smith, T.W.: Cardiac and respiratory effects of digitalis during chronic hypoxia in intact conscious dogs. Am. J. Physiol. 229, 270-271 (1975)

Beller, G.A., Smith, T.W., Hood, W.B.: Effects of ischemia and coronary reperfusion on myocardial digoxin uptake. Am. J. Cardiol. 36, 902-907 (1975)

Bertler, A., Gustafson, A., Redfors, A.: Massive digoxin intoxication. Acta Med. Scand. 194, 245-249 (1973)

Binnion, P.F.: The plasma-digoxin controversy. Lancet 1972/I, 535-536

Binnion, P.F.: Plasma Digoxin Levels and Electrocardiographic Changes in Man. Symposium on Digitalis. Storstein, O. (ed.) Oslo, Norway: Gyldendal Norsk Forlag 1973, pp. 366-379

Binnion, P.F., Morgan, L.M.: Effect of acute hypokalaemia on ^{3}H-digoxin metabolism. Cardiovasc. Res. 5, 431-435 (1971)

Binnion, P.F., Morgan, L.M., Stevenson, H.M., Fletcher, E.: Plasma and myocardial digoxin concentrations in patients on oral therapy. Br. Heart J. 31, 636-640 (1969)

Carroll, P.R., Gelbart, A., O'Rourke, M.F., Shortus, J.: Digoxin concentrations in the serum and myocardium of digitalized patients. Aust. N.Z.J. Med. 3, 400-403 (1973)

Carruthers, S.G., Cleland, J., Kelly, J.G., Lyons, S.M., McDevitt, D.G.: Plasma and tissue digoxin concentrations in patients undergoing cardiopulmonary bypass. Br. Heart J. 37, 313-320 (1975)

Chung, K.K.: Digitalis-induced cardiac arrhythmias. Am. Heart J. 79, 845-848 (1970)

Citrin, D., Stevenson, I.H., O'Malley, K.O.: Massive digoxin overdose: observations on hyperkalaemia and plasma digoxin levels. Scot. Med. J. 17, 275-277 (1972)

Citrin, D.L., O'Malley, K., Hillis, W.S.: Cardiac standstill due to digoxin poisoning successfully treated with atrial pacing. Br. Med. J. 1973/II, 526-527

Cohn, K.E., Kleiger, R.E., Harrison, D.C.: Influence of potassium depletion on myocardial concentration of tritiated digoxin. Circ. Res. 20, 473-476 (1967)

Coltart, J., Howard, M., Chamberlain, D.: Myocardial and skeletal muscle concentrations of digoxin in patients on long-term therapy. Br. Med. J. 1972/II 318-319

Cope, G.D., Hopkins, B.E., Taylor, R.R.: Effect of chronic circulatory volume overload on digitalis intoxication. Cardiovasc. Res. 7, 638-641 (1973)

Doherty, J.E., Perkins, W.H., Flanigan, W.J.: The distribution and concentration of tritiated digoxin in human tissues. Ann. Intern. Med. 66, 116-124 (1967)

Dutta, S., Goswami, S., Lindower, J.O., Marks, B.H.: Subcellular distribution
of digoxin-H^3 in isolated guinea pig and rat hearts. J. Pharmacol. Exp. Ther.
159, 324-334 (1968)

Ebert, P.A., Greenfield, L.J., Austen, W.G.: The effect of increased serum potassium on the digoxin content of the canine heart. Bull. Johns Hopkins Hosp.
112, 151-154 (1963)

Einzig, S., Todd, E.P., Nicoloff, D.M., Lucas, R.V.: Glucagon in prevention and
abolition of ouabain-induced ventricular tachycardia in normokalemic and
hypokalemic dogs. Circ. Res. 29, 88-95 (1971)

El-Fiky, S.B.I., Katzung, B.G.: Effects of hypothermia and pronethalol on
ionic correlates of ouabain arrhythmias in dogs. Circ. Res. 24, 43-50 (1969)

Erlij, D., Mendez, R.: The modification of digitalis intoxication by excluding
adrenergic influences on the heart. J. Pharmacol. Exp. Ther. 144, 97-103
(1964)

Evered, D.C., Chapman, C.: Plasma digoxin concentrations and digoxin toxicity in hospital patients. Br. Heart J. 33, 540-545 (1971)

Fisch, C., Knoebel, S.B.: Recognition and therapy of digitalis toxicity. Prog.
Cardiovasc. Dis. 13, 71-96, 1970

Fogelman, A.M., La Mont, J.T., Finkelstein, S., Rado, E., Pearce, M.L.: Fallibility of plasma-digoxin in differentiating toxic from non-toxic patients.
Lancet 1971/II, 727-729

Goldman, R.H., Coltart, D.J., Friedman, J.P., Nola, G.T., Berke, D.K., Schweizer,
E., Harrison, D.C.: The inotropic effects of digoxin in hyperkalemia. Circulation 48, 830-838 (1973)

Grahame-Smith, D.G., Everest, M.S.: Measurement of digoxin in plasma and
its use in diagnosis of digoxin intoxication. Br. Med. J. 1969/I, 286-289

Güllner, H.G., Stinson, E.B., Harrison, D.C., Kalman, S.M.: Correlation of serum
concentrations with heart concentration of digoxin in human subjects.
Circulation 50, 653-655 (1974)

Halloran, K.H., Downing, S.E.: Inotropic and toxic responses to acetylstrophanthidin in young animals; relationship of hypercapnia and beta adrenergic
blockage. J. Pharmacol. Exp. Ther. 183, 146-153 (1972)

Harrison, C.E., Wakim, W.G.: Depression of digoxin-^{3}H binding to myocardium
by sodium depletion in dogs. Am. J. Cardiol. 23, 117-118 (1969)

Harrison, D.C., Robinson, M.D., Kleiger, R.E.: Role of hypoxia in digitalis toxicity. Am. J. Med. Sc. 256, 352-359 (1968)

Ingelfinger, J.A., Goldman, P.: The serum digitalis concentration does it diagnose
digitalis toxicity? N. Engl. J. Med. 294, 867-870 (1976)

Irons, G.V., Orgain, E.S.: Digitalis-induced arrhythmias and their management.
Prog. Cardiovasc. Dis. 8, 539-569 (1966)

Jelliffe, R.W., Stephenson, R.G.: A fluorometric determination of myocardial
digoxin at autopsy, with indentification of digitalis leaf, digitoxin, and gitoxin. Am. J. Clin. Pathol. 51, 347-357, 1969

Kastor, J.A., Spear, J.F., Moore, E.N.: Origin of digitalis-induced monofocal
tachycardia from left ventricular Purkinje tissue. Circulation 44, Supp. II,
84 (1971)

Kim, N.D., Bailey, L.E., Dresel, P.E.: Correlation of the subcellular distribution of digoxin with the positive inotropic effect. J. Pharmacol. Exp. Ther. 181, 377-385 (1972)

Lely, A.H., Van Enter, C.H.J.: Large-scale digitoxin intoxication. Br. Med. J. 1970/III, 737-740

Lloyd, B.L., Taylor, R.R.: Augmentation of myocardial digoxin concentration in hemorrhagic shock. Circulation 51, 718-722 (1975)

Marcus, F.I., Pavlovich, J., Lullin, M., Kapadia, G.: The effect of reserpine on the metabolism of tritiated digoxin in the dog and in man. J. Pharmacol. Exp. Ther. 159, 314-323 (1968)

Marcus, F.I., Kapadia, G.G., Goldsmith, C.: Alteration of the body distribution of tritiated digoxin by acute hyperkalemia in the dog. J. Pharmacol. Exp. Ther. 165, 136-148 (1969)

Morgan, L.M., Binnion, P.F.: The distribution of ^{3}H-digoxin in normal and acutely hyperkalaemic dogs. Cardiovasc. Res. 4, 235-241 (1970)

Prindle, K.H., Skelton, C.L., Epstein, S.E., Marcus, F.I.: Influence of extracellular potassium concentration on myocardial uptake and inotropic effect of tritiated digoxin. Circ. Res. 28, 337-345 (1971)

Reza, M.J., Kovick, R.B., Shine, K.I., Pearce, M.L.: Massive intravenous digoxin overdosage. N. Engl. J. Med. 291, 777-778 (1974)

Rodensky, P.L., Wasserman, F.: Observations on digitalis intoxication. Arch. Intern. Med. 108, 171-188 (1961)

Rumack, B.H., Wolfe, R.R., Gilfrich, H.: Phenytoin (diphenylhydantoin) treatment of massive digoxin overdosage. Br. Heart J. 36, 405-408 (1974)

Smith, T.W., Haber, E.: Digoxin intoxication: the relationship of clinical presentation to serum digoxin concentration. J. Clin. Invest. 49, 2377-2386 (1970)

Storstein, O., Rasmussen, K.: Digitalis and atrial tachycardia with block. Br. Heart J. 36, 171-176 (1974)

Vassalle, M., Greenspan, K., Hoffman, B.F.: An analysis of arrhythmias induced by ouabain in intact dogs. Circ. Res. 13, 132-148 (1963)

White, R.J., Chamberlain, D.A., Howard, M., Smith, T.W.: Measurement of plasma digoxin by radioimmunoassay. Proc. R. Soc. Med. 63, 703 (1970)

Williams, J.F., Boyd, D.L., Border, J.F.: Effect of acute hypoxia and hypercapnia acidosis on the development of acetylstrophanthidin-induced arrhythmias. J. Clin. Invest. 47, 1885-1894 (1968)

Wittenberg, S.M., Gandel, P., Hogan, P.M., Kreuzer, W., Klocke, F.J.: Relationship of heart rate to ventricular automaticity in dogs during ouabain administration. Circ. Res. 30, 167-176 (1972)

Discussion

Grahame-Smith: Can you define what you mean by "sensitivity to digoxin?" I'll tell you why I ask. I may be wrong, but I don't look upon hypokalemia or hyperkalemia or normokalemia really as determining sensitivity to digoxin, and I look upon the plasma potassium level as determining how much digoxin binds to the myocardium.

Binnion: I would agree with you that you must either use less digoxin or have less digoxin in the tissue to say you've got increased sensitivity. One or the other will do, I think. Either a quicker rate of uptake with less digoxin being infused or else less digoxin in the final tissue, the microsome, or whatever it is, that would constitute increased sensitivity.

Grahame-Smith: But even the rate of uptake may not be the thing to measure, because I can imagine less going in at the same rate or more going in at the same rate.

Binnion: I agree with you, I mean, I can find more things going wrong with my own experiments, but there is only Dr. Marcus to compare my results with.

Lukas: Dr. Bernhard Marks has made the point from data obtained in his studies that we are not looking at the effects of glycosides on a single tissue; there is the myocardium and then there is the His-Purkinje system. I think that one should be examining uptake of glycoside by the His-Purkinje system and the pacemaker tissues when talking about cardiac toxicity.

Binnion: I agree, but how do you do it?

Lukas: Well, that's a problem. One could study uptake of glycosides in the His-Purkinje system by the complicated techniques that Dr. Marks has used. Nevertheless, it does appear that we really are in the midst of a large deficiency in our knowledge of the localization of the cardiac glycosides at their sites of action.

Marcus: Dr. Robert Goldman from Standford has recently published data that show that dogs made chronically hypokalemic by a potassium-deficient diet are more sensitive to digoxin than normokalemic dogs. His data are in disagreement with your results.

Binnion: I am aware of the disagreement.

Markus: I think it is of interest that during chronic hypokalemia, one certainly observes low serum potassiums and low skeletal muscle potassium concentrations, but it is questionable whether there is any decrease in the myocardial concentration of potassium. A possible mechanism for the observed sensitivity to digoxin in hypokalemia may not be related to decreased myocardial concentration of digoxin, but may be due to an increased binding affinity of digoxin to the receptor sites.

Binnion: But what's the situation in the patient? Maybe we didn't make the dogs hypokalemic enough, I mean not over a long enough period of time. The patient's myocardium may have less potassium in it than the dog's does after this period of time that we use, and this is a possibility, of course, that could be proven.

Marcus: The main points is that there probably is an increased sensitivity during hypokalemia, at least insofar as can be determined experimentally.

Erdmann: As I pointed out earlier today, we have measured $(Na^+ + K^+)$-ATPase activities and ouabain binding sites in chronic hypokalemia. We have done this in guinea pigs which had been kept on a potassium-deficient test diet. From these animals, we have isolated myocardial cell membranes, and we have measured ATPase activity and specific ouabain binding sites, both were increased. Furthermore, we performed an experiment demonstrating what I stated earlier, that the glycoside concentration in the myocardium — that means total tissue concentration — does not necessarily mean much. We have used guinea pigs and injected a certain amount of radioactively labeled digoxin and after equilibration, that is after 50 min, we have measured the radioactivity per gram wet weight in the myocardium. In the next guinea pig, we have diluted the labeled digoxin with unlabeled digoxin and injected that. We got the same amount of radioactivity per gram wet weight. And we went on diluting the radioactively labeled digoxin with increasing doses of unlabeled digoxin, still we measured the same amount of radioactivity in the myocardium although the animals had died because of the high digoxin doses. This result means that we have measured only unspecific binding of digoxin to the heart as the amount of unspecific binding sites is too large to detect the specific ones. But only the specific binding sites related to the pharmacologic effects are of interest. Therefore, I think the glycoside concentration "in the total heart" seems to be rather irrelevant.

Binnion: Lüllmann did something on that. He did a mathematical evaluation of the literature and came to the conclusion that about 90%-95% of all the digoxin in the myocardium was not specifically bound. That really makes the whole subject absolutely impossible. It's getting hard now to devise an experiment that solves the problem when you have so much nonspecific binding.

29 Digitalis Intoxication: Specificity of Clinical and Electrocardiographic Signs

W. Doering and E. König

The high frequency of digitalis intoxication is well documented in medical literature (for literature, see Smith, 1975). The introduction of serum concentration measurement has been of great benefit in digitalis therapy, and where it is applied, the intoxication rate has been substantially reduced (Koch-Weser and al., 1974). However, in most German hospitals, the radioimmunoassay has not as yet been introduced, and even where digoxin is measured, the physician often has to wait for one or more days for the test results. Therefore, we looked for another practical way to reduce the intoxication rate. The three main causes for the high frequency of digitalis intoxication are:

1. Pharmacologic properties of cardiac glycosides in combination with small therapeutic range
2. Determination of best individual dosage
3. Nonspecificity of intoxication symptoms

The first point is a matter of pharmacologic research to find safer glycosides. As for point 2, there is as yet no straightforward method to determine the optimal dose for an individual patient without the risk of intoxication. We thus concentrated on point 3, the nonspecificity of intoxication signs. This holds true for digitalis-induced arrhythmias (Castellanos et al., 1969; Mason et al., 1971), but extracardiac symptoms are of even less diagnostic value (Hillestad et al. 1973). Patients receiving digitalis usually belong to the old age group who suffer from several illnesses and who are already on different kinds of medicine. All of these factors may contribute to the development of intoxication-like symptoms which are so common among older polymorbid patients.

Consequently, we performed a study to assess the predictive value of certain risk factors and of the cardiac and extracardiac signs in digitalis intoxication. Our goal was to design a questionnaire with a digitalis-intoxication score which would allow for a more accurate bedside diagnosis and which would also make the physician more aware of the risk factors and thus help to prevent digitalis intoxication (Ogilvie and Ruedy, 1972).

In a group of over 1000 patients, we compared the prevalence of arrhythmias, symptoms, and risk factors in toxic and nontoxic patients. The diagnosis of digitalis intoxication was promarily based on serial ECG tracings and for the extracardiac symptoms also on the serum digoxin concentrations (SDC). Like many other research groups (for literature, see Smith, 1975), we were able to show that the SDC values differentiate quite clearly between nontoxic patients and patients with digitalis-induced arrhythmias (Doering et al. in press). Furthermore, we were able to verify that it also diffentiates distinctly between patients with digitalis-induced arrhythmias and patients under digitalis with rhythm disturbances of other origin (Doering et al., in press). From the arrhythmias observed in both groups, we learned that the prolongation of the PQ interval and premature ventricular beats, which are the most common arrhythmias encountered in digitalis intoxication, occur equally often in patients with rhythm disorders of other origin (Doering and König, in press). Their diagnostic value is, therefore, limited while arrhythmias like paroxysmal atrial tachycardia (PAT) with block, ventricular bigeminy, nonparoxysmal nodal tachycardia, and the second degree atrioventricular block of the Wenckebach type were significantly more prevalent in the toxic group (Doering and König, in press).

As already mentioned, the true origin of the extracardiac intoxication-like symptoms is rather difficult to elicit because these symptoms could stem from other accompanying illnesses, other drugs administered, etc., and they will often vanish when the general state of health of a patient improves whether digitalis is withheld for a couple of days or not. In a previous paper (Doering et al., in press), we were able to demonstrate the difficulty in assessing the true origin of intoxication-like symptoms. According to the physicians' initial diagnosis based on extracardiac symptoms, the patients were classified as probably intoxicated or nonintoxicated. Comparing the SDC values, we found a complete overlap of these two groups. Of the probably intoxicated patients, a considerable number had very low or even unmeasurable digoxin concentrations. So these results represent very clearly the physician's diagnostic dilemma in patients taking digitalis and suffering from extracardiac intoxication-like symptoms.

The relationship between extracardiac symptoms and SDC levels becomes evident when dividing the patients into small groups according to different digoxin concentration ranges and calculating the percentage of probably intoxicated patients per concentration range (Fig. 29.1). From SDC values of about 2.0 ng/ml on, there is a rising percentage of patients with extracardiac symptoms with rising digoxin concentrations — as to be expected in dose-related effects. In the lower concentration ranges, there is a constant 20% portion of the patients for whom the origin of the symptoms is to be sought elsewhere. This concentration-related rise of extracardiac symptoms can also be demonstrated in patients with digitalis-induced arrhythmias (Doering et al., in press). According to their prevalence in patients with normal and elevated SDC values, the various extracardiac symptoms were of lower predictive value than the rhythm disturbances. Only visual symptoms were somewhat more pathognomonic of digitalis intoxication (Doering et al., in press).

Compared to nontoxic patients, the toxic patients were of significantly higher mean age, lower body weight, they had higher creatinine concentrations, and were on a higher mean maintenance dose (Doering et al., in press). However, these risk factors did not score very high in the toxicity questionnaire which

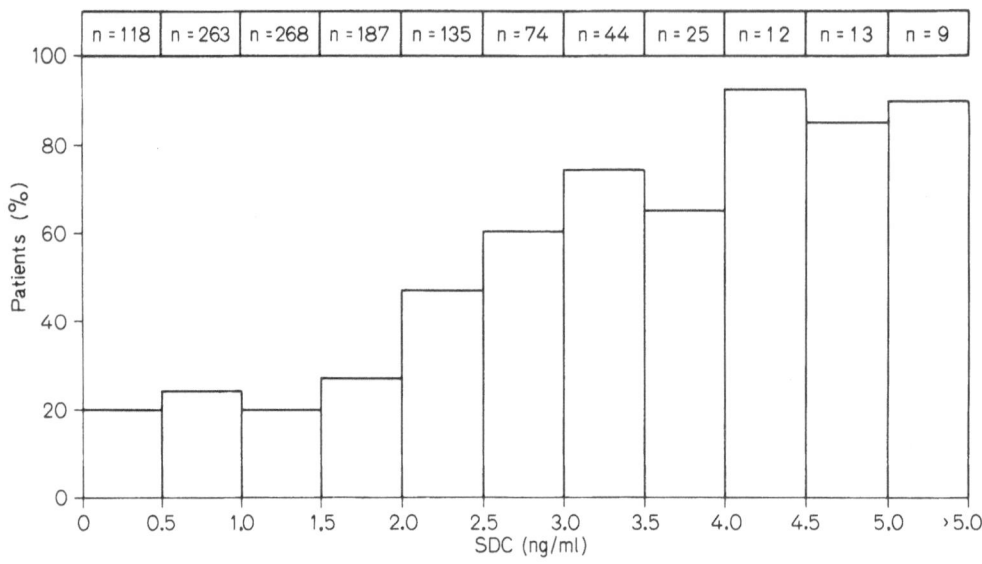

Fig. 29.1. Percentage prevalence of patients with extracardiac signs of digitalis intoxication per concentration range. Total number of patients n = 1148

also included the judgement of the physician as to whether the arrhythmia and/ or the symptoms were digitalis induced or not.

By using the statistical method of "odds ratio", we calculated the "relative risk" of a patient being intoxicated when he demonstrated one or more of intoxication-like signs. In a prospective study, the intoxication score was then applied to 96 patients under digoxin or β-methyl-digoxin. In all patients with extracardiac intoxication-like symptoms and/or arrhythmias, the glycoside was withheld until a final diagnosis of intoxication or nonintoxication was established.

Patients' complaints and 12 lead ECG tracings were documented daily while the digoxin concentration was measured every second day. For various reasons, a final diagnosis of the origin of the arrhythmia and/or of the extracardiac symptoms could not be established for 11 patients in each respective group. These were patients with pacemakers, changing patterns of arrhythmias, intercurrent severe illenesses, coma, or patients who died. In some of these patients (n = 10), either the arrhythmia or the extracardiac symptoms could not be validated initially, and therefore no total score could be calculated (patients with predominant pacemaker rhythm or somnolent patients).

Figure 29.2 shows the correlation between total score, SDC values, and final diagnosis. Nontoxic patients without any intoxication-like symptoms and signs (control group) are marked as squares, patients where no final diagnosis could be established as triangles. Only 6 (18.2%) of the 33 toxic patients had SDC values below 2.0 ng/ml or total score values below 8.0. From the 43 nontoxic patients, 4 (9.3%) had total scores of 8.0 and higher and only 2 (4.7%) nontoxic

360

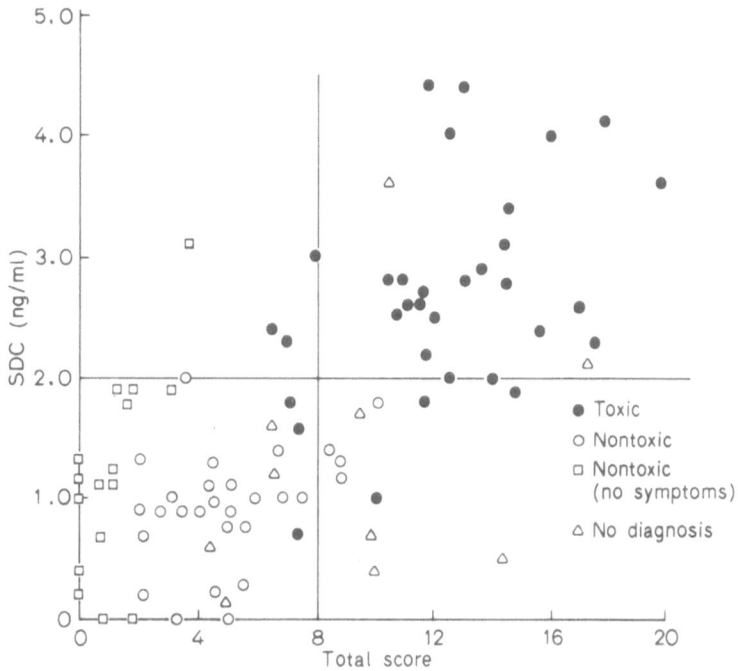

Fig. 29.2. Correlation between SDC and total score

patients had SDC values of 2.0 ng/ml or more. The respective chi-square values
are significant with p < 0.001. Of the 43 nontoxic patients, the mean total
score is 3.61 ± 2.68, the mean SDC 1.03 ± 0.64 ng/ml compared to a total score
of 12.30 ± 3.39 and a mean SDC of 2.67 ± 0.88 ng/ml for the 33 toxic patients
(p < 0.001). As seen from Figure 29.2 there is not only close agreement between
final diagnosis and score results but also between toxic and nontoxic SDC and
score values, even for most of those patients where a final diagnosis could not
be established. The linear correlation between SDC and score values, however,
is not very close with a correlation coefficient of 0.54. On the one hand, this
is due to a wide range of variation of individual reaction toward the same toxic
concentration and on the other hand, to the incidence of intoxication-like signs
in nontoxic patients. The most essential point, however, is that SDC and score
values permit a sound prediction of the final diagnosis, of the two the SDC value
being somewhat more accurate.

Taking only one category of criteria of toxicity, the correlation coefficient becomes somewhat better with 0.61. Figure 29.3 includes only the patients with
arrhythmias classified according to the final diagnosis of the origin of the arrhythmia. For patients with extracardiac symptoms, the coefficient of correlation is 0.64. As already mentioned, the relationship between the physicians'
preliminary diagnosis based on extracardiac intoxication-like symptoms and the

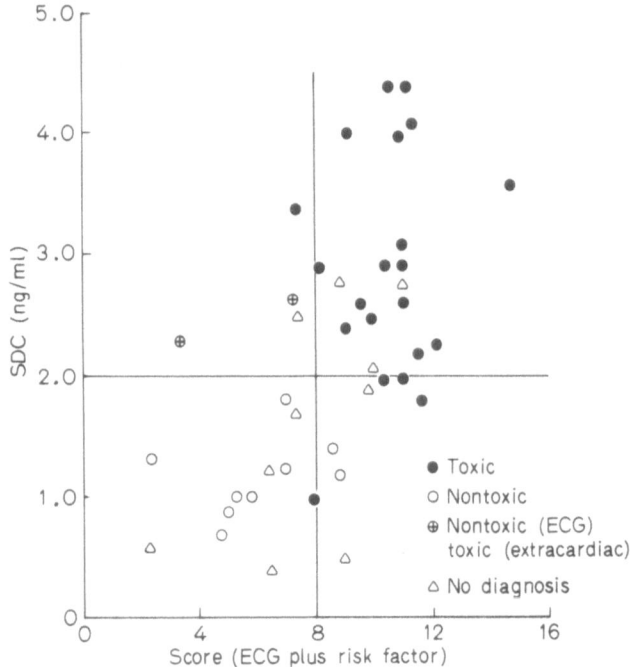

Fig. 29.3. Correlation between SDC and ECG score (arrhythmetic pat. only)

SDC values is rather poor. Using a similar form of presentation (Figure 29.4), we compared the score results for extracardiac symptoms with the final diagnosis and found a considerably smaller overlap between toxic and nontoxic patients.

We therefore consider this intoxication score as a useful means for a preliminary diagnosis especially in the large number of patients suffering from extracardiac intoxication-like symptoms. Yet, for the severely ill patients with rhythm distirbances and intoxication-like symptoms, this preliminary diagnosis should if possible be ascertained quickly by digoxin concentration measurement.

References

Castellanos, A., Jr., Ghafour, A.A., Soffer, A.: Digitalis-induced arrhythmias: Recognition and therapy. Cardiovasc. Clin. I/3, 108-123 (1969)

Doering, W., König, E.: Digitalisintoxikation: Ursachen, Diagnose, Prophylaxe. Dtsch. Med. Wochenschr. (in press)

Doering, W., König, E., Sturm, W.: Digitalisintoxikation: Wertigkeit klinischer und elektrokardiographischer Befunde im Vergleich zur Digoxinkonzentration im Serum. Z. Kardiol. (in press)

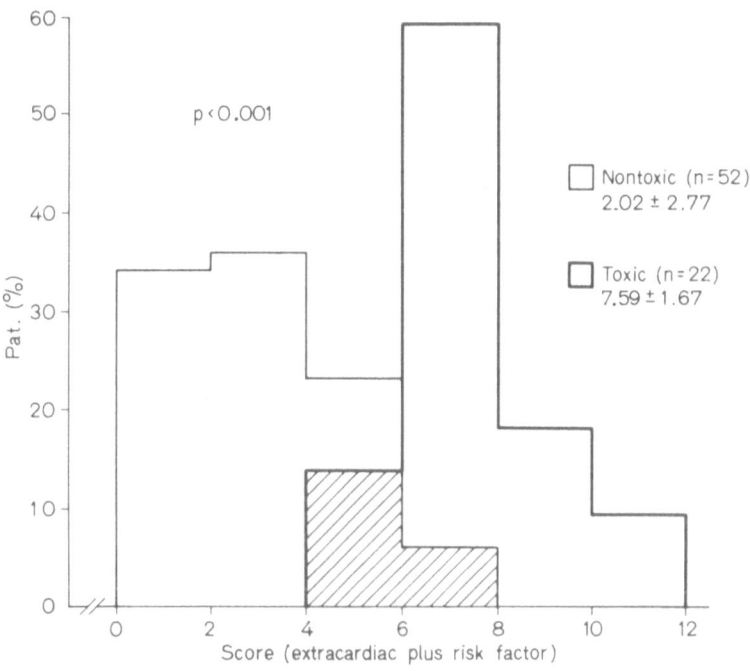

Fig. 29.4. Extracardiac score in toxic and nontoxic pat.

Hillestad, L., Hansteen, V., Hatle, L., Storstein, L., Storstein, O.: Digitalis
    intoxication: Preliminary data from a prospective study. In: Symposium
    on digitalis . 1973 pp. 281-286
Koch-Weser, J., Duhme, D.W., Greenblatt, D.J.: Influence of serum digoxin
    concentration measurements on frequency of digitoxicity. Clin. Pharmacol.
    Ther. 16, 286 (1974)
Mason, D.T., Zelis, R., Lee, G., Hughes, J.D., Spann, J.F., Amsterdam, E.A.:
    Current concepts and treatment of digitalis toxicity. Am. J. Cardiol. 27,
    546-557 (1971)
Ogilvie, R.I., Ruedy, J.: An educational program in digitalis therapy. J. Am.
    Med. Assoc. 222, 50-55 (1972)
Smith, T.W.: Digitalis toxicity: Epidemiology and clinical use of serum concen-
tration measurements. Am. J. Med. 58, 470-476 (1975)

Discussion

Storstein, Norway: I would like to make a comment on your paper. We did a
prospective study on digitoxin intoxication in 650 patients on digitoxin maintenance therapy. A clinician looked at the patients when they first were admitted
to hospital. If symptoms or signs of digitoxin intoxication were found during

the first evaluation of the patients, they were reassessed and a final diagnosis was made after 6 days of drug discontinuance. Of these, 5.8% resulted in a definite diagnosis of intoxication, and almost twice as many patients had signs or symptoms of digitalis toxicity, but these were not found to be due to digitalis on the second evaluation. We tried to see if any of the symptoms or signs were more specific of digitalis intoxication than other symptoms and signs. The comparison between the toxic and the suspected toxic patients showed that no single arrhythmia occurred significantly more often in the toxic group than in the suspected toxic group, which was very disappointing. The same holds true for the extracardiac symptoms. I think this very briefly illustrates the difficulties in diagnosing digitalis intoxication. Even when doing prospective study, one is not always sure that all the patients adhering to the criteria really were toxic.

Doering: I certainly agree with you that it sometimes may be extremely difficult to come to a final conclusion whether there was an intoxication or not. But in contrast to your results, we did find that some rhythm disturbances were more prevalent in digitalis intoxication, and this has been the experience of other investigators, too. I cannot explain the discrepancy between your results and ours, I am sure it is not due to the use of either digitoxin or digoxin.

Oliver: Dr. Doering, what were the final criteria that you used in deciding toxicity?

Doering: Patients were classified as intoxicated if their rhythm disturbances and/or extracardiac symptoms disappeared when digoxin was withheld.

Schneider, Berlin: Dr. Doering, we found a similar overlap of glycoside serum concentrations in the toxic and nontoxic patients as you did, but this overlap was much smaller if patients with thyroid dysfunction were excluded. Did you exclude these patients, too?

Doering: The setting of this study was quite different from yours. We got the serum samples with a sheet from the physician in which he stated whether he considered this patient to be intoxicated or not and whether the diagnosis of toxicity was based on extracardiac or on cardiac signs or on both. We wanted to find out how many patients with digitalis intoxication are diagnosed properly when first seen by a clinician. As other authors, we found that many digitalized patients with extracardiac symptoms are suspected to be intoxicated while, in fact, their symptoms are of other origin.

Baligadoo: I agree with Dr. Storstein that there is no electrocardiographic sign that is really specific of digitalis toxicity. However, the results presented here should be interpreted as failure of classic statistical methods to show a significant difference in the frequency of certain arrhythmias in toxic and nontoxic patients. Statistical bias may be introduced in this kind of study through the selection of patients as the arrhythmias presented by the nontoxic patients depend evidently on the underlying cardiac disease.

In a study that we conducted at Tenon Hospital, we found the association of first-degree av-block and ventricular premature beats commonly as a sign of early digitoxin toxicity, this association being more frequent than in patients with more florid toxicity. I agree evidently that these arrhythmias are also seen in nontoxic patients, but I would suggest that failure to find statistically significant difference in the frequency of these arrhythmias in your toxic and nontoxic patients may be due to the types of patients studied. In our study, we included only cases with valvular disease and ischemic heart disease outside the period of acute infarction and we found that first-degree av-block and ventricular premature beats occur more frequently in toxic patients but with serum concentrations intermediate between that seen in normal patients and patients with severe toxicity.

Doering: What I wanted to show is that these two most common arrhythmias encountered in digitalis intoxication, first-degree av-block and ventricular premature beats, are as often seen in patients with arrhythmias of other origin. So the occurrence of these arrhythmias are not very helpful in the diagnosis of digitalis intoxication. From our results, we concluded that there are certain arrhythmias which are more common in digitalis intoxication than in arrhythmic patients under digitalis maintenance therapy but with arrhythmias not due to the cardiac glycoside. The probability that a patient really is intoxicated rises if he shows certain dysrhythmias like nodal tachycardia, for example. Of course there are no specific rhythm disorders in digitalis intoxication.

Baligadoo: I agree with you that there are certain arrhythmias which are more common in digitalis toxicity and which should awake the suspicion of the clinician. However, and here I disagree with you, we should not lose our vigilance in the presence of certain arrhythmias which you find to occur equally well in your nontoxic patients. I feel that if we do not think of toxicity in the presence of first-degree av-block and ventricular premature beats in digitalized patients — as your results would suggest — we shall only diagnose cases of severe toxicity.

In our experience with digitoxin — your experience with digoxin may be different — daily dose seems to be the most discriminant factor in the separation of patients into toxic and nontoxic groups. A number of physicians in our unit feel that when one knows the case history and the daily dose, clinical judgement is as valuable as a serum concentration in making the diagnosis. I would like to know your opinion about that.

Doering: This means that you have very compliant patients. As other studies have shown, about 40% of in-patients do not take their medicine properly, and if you evaluate outpatients, this percentage is even higher. In our experience, outpatients' serum levels are about one-third lower than inpatients' serum levels, both groups being on the same daily maintenance dose.

Larbig: I would like to make a comment on the problem of how to identify whether a disturbance of rhythm is due to digitalis or not. It is sometimes quite helpful to look at the ST segment, because if you notice, for instance in second-degree av-block, the typical descension of the ST segment, you can be quite sure that you are dealing with digitalis intoxication. This sign may be valuable, especially when the ST segment is normal in patients before digitalization.

Doering: We studied the prevalence of typical ST segment changes and indeed found a significant difference between patients with digitalis-induced arrhythmias and patients with arrhythmias of other origin.

30 Treatment of Digitalis Intoxication

H. JAHRMÄRKER

This survey should be restricted to the unwanted cardiac effects of glycosides, because side-effects from the CNS and gastrointestinal tract are more a problem of differential diagnosis than of therapy. There are three principal ways to treat glycoside intoxication:
1. Eliminate the substance from the body
2. Displace the substance at the receptor side
3. Counteract the unwanted cardiac effects by drugs and other treatment

I avoid talking about the immediate stop of glycoside administration, which is obligatory in any case of suspected serious glycoside intoxication. It depends on the clinical state if and when to restart digitalis treatment, usually at a lower dosage. It might be justified to maintain a fairly high digitalis blood level in some cases, close monitoring provided.

Elimination of Glycosides From the Body

The first principal way of therapy is to enhance the elimination of the glycosides. This is especially important after ingestion of very large amounts of a digitalis glycoside. These patients took the drug mostly with suicidal intention. They differ from the conventional patients with a digitalis intoxication in several respects. They show high digitalis blood concentrations up to 20-fold the therapeutic level, predominantly conduction blockade (rarely tachycard arrhythmias since we are dealing with a primarily normal heart), and development of hyperkalemia (Smith and Willerson, 1971; Smith et al., 1976).

Gastric lavage may be useful followed by application of cholestyramine and charcoal. At this very early phase, these maneuvers are indicated following oral ingestion of all glycosides. Later on, cholestyramine is effective in digitoxin poisoning only (Caldwell and Greenberger, 1971) due to its substantial enterohepatic circulation. In case there is a high glycoside concentration in the blood, elimination of some percent can be achieved by hemodialysis (Kramer et al., 1972), somewhat better with charcoal hemoperfusion (Carvallo et al., 1976; Pritchard et al., 1976), and possibly with hemofiltration. The absolute amounts of glycoside eliminated by these methods are very limited, and the therapeutic success after ingestion of great amounts of glycosides remains doubtful.

In the usual cases of digitalis intoxication, i.e., glycoside-dependent arrhythmias associated with normal or slightly elevated blood levels, the enhancement of elimination procedures is practically of no clinical relevance at present. In these everyday cases the underlying heart disease is essential for the pathogenesis of the arrhythmias. Very promising are experimental studies and the first clinical results with Fab fragments of glycoside-specific antibodies with high affinity.

Displacement of Glycosides at the Receptor Site

Displacement at the receptor — Na, K-dependent membrane ATPase — can be achieved by potassium and by phenytoin. Both substances have in addition to the displacing effect a direct antiarrhythmic activity, independently if there is glycoside action or not. Phenytoin is difficult to handle due to its longer serum half-life. Thus, potassium treatment in general is the first choice in cases of hypo- and normokalemia. Confirming former clinical experience, the affinity of the receptor is high in hypokalemia and lower in the presence of normal or high potassium concentrations. According to the experiments of Erdmann et al. (1976) with human heart membrane ATPase preparations, this potassium dependency is a matter of glycoside association which is increased in a hypokalemic medium. The dissociation of the glycoside from membrane ATPase proceeds much slower than association and is not dependent on the external potassium concentration. The slow time course of dissociation was also shown by normalization of electric activity (Anderson et al., 1976) which in turn corresponds to the mechanical activity.

One could conclude that prevention of digitalis toxicity by prophylactic administration of potassium is more effective than potassium treatment afterwards. This is in agreement with experimental and clinical observations (Williams et al., 1966; Zelis et al., 1970, Goldsmith et al., 1969; Prindle et al., 1969, Allen and Schwartz, 1971). The empiric effectivity of potassium in glycoside-dependent arrhythmias might be partially due to dimished steady-state binding and partially due to the direct electrophysiologic effects of an increased extracellular potassium concentration. The same applies to phenytoin therapy.

Counteraction of Glycoside-Dependent Arrhythmias by Antiarrhythmic Therapy

Searching for a rational basis for the antiarrhythmic therapy in digitalis intoxication we have to consider:
1. The complicated electrophysiologic effects of toxic doses of cardiac glycosides on the heart.
2. The different physiologic behavior of normal and diseased cardiac structures which might react to drugs differently. This makes the predicting of drug effects difficult.

Glycoside-dependent tachycard arrhythmias result either from impulse formation (automaticity) or from reentry mechanisms or from both. Summarizing the evidence accumulated by Rosen et al. (1975), one can conclude that higher doses of glycosides decrease the conduction within the specific system by lowering the resting membrane potential as well as decreasing the fast upstroke velocity and duration of the action potential.

Conduction delay and shortening of the refractory period facilitate reentry. Purkinje fibers may develop two possibly different phenomena which may occur alone or in combination and which increase the excitability. They can show increased automaticity which is facilitated by low potassium concentrations and by cardiac damage. The other possibility consists in delayed afterdepolarizations occurring at normal potassium concentrations. They have a higher incidence at fast rates or during premature depolarizations and show, when reaching the threshold, a changing conduction velocity. They may correspond to repetitive ventricular response (Lown, 1968; Hagemeijer and Lown, 1970). Delayed afterdepolarizations are also observed following β-receptor stimulation (Cranefield and Wit, 1974). Verapamil decreases the magnitude of digitalis-induced delayed afterdepolarizations (Ferrier and Mow, 1973; Rosen et al., 1974) and also counteracts the effects of digitalis on automaticity (Rosen et al., 1974), suggesting that calcium current (slow response) is responsible at least in part for these phenomena.

I addition, I would like to stress some clinical evidence (Jahrmärker et al., 1974; Theisen and Jahrmärker, 1975; Theisen et al., 1975) supporting the possibility of reentry phenomena by our own work. In severe glycoside intoxication, TU abnormalities in the electrocardiogram are a common finding, indicating an abnormal behavior of the repolarization in different parts of the myocardium. This is important since it proves an electric inhomogeneity within the myocardium. Local prolonged depolarization and delayed conduction may induce an echo beat or even lead ro reentry tachycardia following a regular or premature impulse.

When choosing the way of treatment in digitalis-dependent arrhythmias, we have to consider the possibility if not probability of reentry phenomena. I admit that this is a simplification, but as long as no other information is available, I would like to recommend in potential dangerous ventricular tachyarrhythmias and also in supraventricular tachycardias with block due to digitalis therapy that such antiarrhythmic drugs which shorten the action potential and the effective refractory period in addition to enhancing the conduction velocity be preferred. Thereby, the electric homogeneity of the myocardium can be improved and the impulse formation suppressed. By increasing the conduction velocity, an important prerequisite for a reentry mechanism is abolished. Therefore, lidocain and phenytoin are the drugs of first choice. Both are known to be effective against digitalis-induced premature beats and tachyarrhythmias. The efficacy of both drugs is dependent on the extracellular potassium concentration. Their antiarrhythmic activity can be improved by simultaneous administration of potassium which is recommended in hypo- and normokalemia. For infusion therapy, lidocain is more suitable. Due to its shorter serum half-time, it is easier to achieve a constant blood level. In resistant cases, verapamil should be tried. Propranolol as a typical adrenergic blocking agent is often effective since an increased adrenergic drive is often an important supporting factor in the pathogenesis of glycoside-dependent tachyarrhythmias (Waxman et al., 1971), but its use is very limited in patients with heart failure.

Other antiarrhythmic agents, for example quinidine, might also — in addition to the suppression of starting extrasystoles — interrupt reentry mechanisms by further slowing or blocking the conduction. At the same time, however, they increase electric inhomogeneity and in this way might favor reentry mechanisms. Thus, in my personal opinion, drugs of the quinidine type are the second and only experimental choice in the treatment of digitalis-induced arrhythmias.

Electric treatment is gaining increasing importance in digitalis-dependent arrhythmias. Defibrillation is indicated as an emergency treatment only in ventricular fibrillation. It is well-known that electric instability is enhanced after electroshock for digitalis-induced tachyarrhythmias. Simultaneous administration of potassium and lidocain or DPH is advisable under such circumstances. Considering that in many forms of glycoside-induced arrhythmias reentry phenomena might be in operation, stimulation procedures (overdriving or single or repetitive intracardiac pacemaker stimuli) might be effective in cases of tachyarrhythmias to bridge the first hours and deserve further trial. In glycoside dependent-bradyarrhythmias — av-block II and III and atrial fibrillation with slow ventricular response, administration of atropine is the first choice and may sometimes, by repeated administration, bridge the situation. Infusion of isoproterenol should be avoided whenever possible as one cannot predict whether it first will increase the heart rate or lead to ectopia. In atropine-resistant cases, the use of provisional pacemakers is the method of choice.

In conclusion, I would like to add the ceterum censeo: prevention of glycoside intoxication should be our first goal and can be achieved to a large extent by taking into account all factors which are known to lower glycoside tolerance.

References

Allen, J.C., Schwartz, A.: Further therapeutic implications of potassium-digitalis interaction with the transport enzyme Na, K-ATPase. Circulation 44, Suppl. 2, 134 (1971)
Anderson, G.J., Bailey, J.C., Reiser, J., Freeman, A.: Electrophysiological observations on the digitalis-potassium interaction in canine Purkinje fibers. Circ. Res. 39, 717 (1976)
Caldwell, J.H., Greenberger, N.J.: Interruption of enterohepatic circulation of digitoxin by cholestyramine. I. Protection against lethal digitoxin intoxication. J. Clin. Invest. 50, 2626 (1971)
Carvallo, A., Ramirez, B., Honig, H., Knepschield, I., Schreiner, G.E., Gelfand, M.C.: Treatment of digitalis intoxication by charcoal hemoperfusion (CHP). Trans. Am. Soc. Artif. Intern. Organs 22, 718 (1976)

Cranefield, P.F., Wit, A.L.: Sustained rhythmicity in cardiac fibers with slow response activity triggered by propagated action potentials. Circulation 49-50, Suppl. III, 97 (1974)

Erdmann, E., Presek, P., Swozil, R.: Über den Einfluß von Kalium auf die Bindung von Strophanthin an menschliche Herzmuskelzellmembranen. Klin. Wochenschr. 54, 383 (1976)

Ferrier, G.R., Moe, G.K.: Effect of calcium on acetylstrophanthidin induced transient depolarizations in canine cardiac tissues. Circ. Res. 33, 508 (1973)

Goldsmith, C., Kapadia, G.G., Nimmo, L., Murphy, C., Moran, H., Marcus, F.I.: Correlation of digitalis intoxication with myocardial concentration of tritiated digoxin in hypokalemic and normokalemic dogs. Circulation 39-40, Suppl. III, 92 (1969)

Hagemeijer, F., Lown, B.: Effect of heart rate on electrically induced repetitive ventricular responses in the digitalized dog. Circ. Res. 23, 233 (1970)

Jahrmärker, H., Theisen, K.: Kammerflattern und Kammerflimmern. In: Herzrhythmusstörungen. II. Wiener Symposium, Stuttgart 1974

Kramer, P., Quellhart, E., Hosenkamp, J., Scheler, F.: Dialysance und prozentuale Elimination verschiedener Herzglykoside während der Hämo- und Peritonealdialyse. Klin. Wochenschr. 50, 609 (1972)

Lown, B.: Electrical stimulation to estimate the degree of digitalization. Am. J. Cardiol. 23, 251 (1968)

Prindle, K.H., Skelton, C.L., Epstein, S.E., Marcus, F.I.: Influence of extracellular potassium concentration on myocardial uptake and inotropic effect of tritiated digoxin. Circulation 39-40, Suppl. III, 165 (1969)

Prichard, S., Chirito, E., Chang, T., Sniderman, A.D.: Microencapsulated charcoal hemoperfusion: a possible therapeutic adjunct in digoxin toxicity. Clin. Res. 24, 409 A (1976)

Rosen, M.R., Wit, A.L., Hoffmann, B.F.: Electrophysiology and pharmacology of cardiac arrhythmias. IV. Cardiac antiarrhythmic and toxic effects of digitalis. Am. Heart J. 89, 391 (1975 a)

Rosen, M.R., Wit, A.L., Hoffmann, B.F.: Electrophysiology and pharmacology of cardiac arrhythmias. VI. Cardiac effects of Verapamil. Am. Heart J. 89, 665 (1975 b)

Smith, T.W., Haber, E., Yeatman, L., Butler, V.P., Jr.: Reversal of advanced digoxin intoxication with Fab-fragments of digoxin-specific antibodies. N. Engl. J. Med. 294, 797 (1976)

Smith, T.W., Willerson, J.T.: Suicidal and accidental digoxin ingestion. Report of five cases with serum level correlations. Circulation 44, 29 (1971)

Theisen, K., Jahrmärker, H.: Re-entry Mechanismus ventrikulärer Tachykardien bei inhomogener Repolarisation. Unter besonderer Berücksichtigung des Jervell- und Lange-Nielsen-Syndroms sowie ähnlicher Zustände und ihrer Therapie. Dtsch. Med. Wochenschr. 100, 1141 (1975)

Theisen, K., Haider, M., Jahrmärker, H.: Untersuchungen ventrikulärer Tachykardien durch Re-entry bei inhomogener Repolarisation. Dtsch. Med. Wochenschr. 100, 1099 (1975)

Waxmann, M.B., Chan, H.K., Heimbecker, R.O.: Influence of variations in sympathetic drive on digitalis tolerance. Clin. Res. 19, 763 (1971)

Williams, J.F., Klocke, F.J., Braunwald, E.: Studies on digitalis. 13. Comparison of the effects of potassium on the inotropic and arrhythmia-producing actions of Ouabain. J. Clin. Invest. <u>45</u>, 346 (1966)

Zelis, R., Mason, D.T., Spann, J.F., Braunwald, E.: Effects of ventricular stimulation and potassium administration on digitalis-induced arrhythmias. Am. J. Cardiol. <u>25</u>, 428 (1970)

Discussion

Belz, Koblenz: From the standpoint of the electrophysiologic observation, the application of procainnamide seems not to be useful because there might be an increased risk of reentry. On the other hand, I have to say from my clinical experience that we were successful in many kinds of tachycardiac arrhythmias (extrasystolies, bigemini, ventricular tachycardia) using procainamide. I think the advantage of this drug is that you can apply it by intramuscular route or also by peroral route. So I would suggest we should not absolutely forget this drug.

Jahrmärker: In the case of digitalis intoxication, I prefer to avoid antiarrhythmic drugs which increase the refractory period and possibly cause an inhomogeneous repolarization which facilitates reentry. But I agree that in reentry you can be successful both with an antiarrhythmic agent which accelerates conduction and with drugs which dealy conduction. In the latter case, however, you favor inhomogeneity. These considerations are based on observations in Jervell syndrome and in symptomatic forms of TU abnormalities.

Oliver: Dr. Jahrmärker, I wonder if you or anyone else might choose to comment on the use of potassium as a treatment for digitalis intoxication, particularly in patients who might be hypokalemic. What is your view about the efficacy of giving potassium?

Jahrmärker: Our goal is to reach a potassium value in the upper normal range, which is effective in diminishing digitalis-induced ectopy.

Larbig: You said pacemaker treatment is indicated when critical bradycardia ensues. What is your definition of critical bradycardia?

Jahrmärker: Critical heart rate means bradycardia with impending shock. It is necessary to monitor such a patient closely, otherwise the pacemaker might be indicated even earlier. Extrasystoles might be favored by bradycardia which suggests pacemaker application.

Schaumann: What do you think about a low dose of a β-blocker, one which does not have a quinidine-like action? I'm asking that because it's known that particularly the danger of ventricular tachycardia is potentiated by the sympathetic tone. I also would like to ask: what about vitamin E? Hochrein claims that he successfully treated digitalis intoxication with large doses of vitamin E.

Jahrmärker: The effect of β-blocking agents in glycoside-induced extrasystoles and ventricular tachycardia is good and better than in arrhythmias of other cause. But β-blockade is limited by induction of heart failure, conduction delay, and bradycardia. As to vitamin E, I don't think that it is important.

Oliver: I think whether or not β-blockade would seem appropriate might indeed depend upon the type of toxicity one is treating. Clearly a tachycardia with a rapid ventricular response might behave one way whereas a rapid atrial rate with a high degree of av-block is really quite another circumstance. Would you not agree with that?

Jahrmärker: I certainly agree.

Hombach, Köln: Dr. Jahrmärker, have you any clinical experience in treatment of digitalis intoxication with a potassium-saving diuretic such as amiloride or triamteren?

Jahrmärker: We have no data on a direct antiarrhythmic action of these substances . We use potassium-saving diuretics to keep potassium high.

Belz, Koblenz: Can't you say anything about magnesium? There is some evidence from experimental procedures that it is possible to prevent digitalis intoxication by magnesium ions. Another question refers to heart failure in digitalis intoxication. We only spoke about the arrhythmias yet, but there are experimental and also clinical observations indicating that an overdosage of digitalis may also induce another cardiac failure not due to arrhythmias.

Jahrmärker: A long time ago, it was already shown that magnesium is effective against digitalis ectopy. Today, however, we can handle digitalis intoxication in a better way. There are only very few patients who have low magnesium concentrations if you exclude patients (alcoholics) with myocardiopathy. Some authors prefer to give potassium together with magnesium. Concerning the question if heart failure might be increased due to intoxication, this is a clinical impression and might happen in advanced severe cardiac failure. But it is difficult to prove that impression because intoxication is connected with complex electrolyte changes and arrhythmias which might increase heart failure. Extreme doses of digitalis indeed impair contraction, as we know from animal experiments.

31 Biologic Effects of Specific Antibodies in Reversing the Pharmacologic and Toxic Effects of Digoxin[1]

V. P. BUTLER, JR.[2], T. W. SMITH[3], D. H. SCHMIDT, and E. HABER

By virtue of their ability to bind the cardiac glycoside, digoxin, with high specificity and affinity (Butler and Chen, 1967; Smith et al., 1970), antidigoxin antibodies are capable (Table 31.1) of acting as specific antagonists of digoxin, both in vitro and in vivo (Butler, 1970; Butler et al., 1973; 1974; Smith, 1974; Smith et al., 1977; Butler et al., 1977b). In vitro, antibodies to digoxin are capable of preventing the uptake of digoxin by rat renal cortical slices (Watson and Butler, 1972) and by human erythrocytes (Watson and Butler, 1972; Gardner et al., 1973). In inhibiting digoxin uptake by human red blood cells, digoxin-specific antibodies prevent the glycoside from exerting a pharmacologic effect on these cells in that, after a brief incubation with antidigoxin antibodies, digoxin is unable to inhibit the influx of potassium (Watson and Butler, 1972; Gardner et al., 1973) or of rubidium (Curd et al., 1971) into erythrocytes; antibodies to proscillaridin (also a cardiac glycoside) exert a similar effect on rubidium uptake (Belz et al., 1973). Antibodies to digoxin and to ouabain, another cardiac glycoside, have been shown to be capable of preventing the corresponding cardiac glycosides from exerting their positive inotropic effects on isolated cat papillary muscle strips (Skelton et al., 1971; Gold and Smith, 1974). Antibodies to digoxin (Smith, 1974), ouabain (Smith, 1972), and to proscillaridin (Kleeberg and Belz, 1974), respectively, prevent these cardiac glycosides from exerting their in vitro inhibitory effect on the catalytic activity of isolated $(Na^+ + K^+)$-ATPase preparations.

Rabbits that have been immunized with digoxin-protein conjugates and whose sera contain antidigoxin antibodies are protected from the toxic cardiac effects of a lethal dose of digoxin. This was demonstrated in a study in which a single intravenous dose of digoxin (0.5 mg/kg body weight) produced serious cardiac rhythm disturbances and, in all of 15 nonimmunized control rabbits studied, death within 1-2 h. In contrast, ten digoxin-immunized rabbits showed no significant abnormalities during 2 h of electrocardiographic monitoring following a single intravenous dose of 0.6 mg digoxin per kg body weight (Schmidt and Butler, 1971a). Antibodies to ouabain have also been shown to confer protection

1 Supported in part by grants from the United States Public Health Service (HL 10608; HL 18003) and the New York Heart Association.
2 Recipient of an Irma T. Hirschl Career Scientist Award.
3 Established Investigator of the American Heart Association.

Table 31.1. Biologic properties of digoxin-specific antibodies

1. Prevention of uptake of digoxin by cells in vitro
    Rat renal cortical cells
    Human erythrocytes
2. Prevention of pharmacologic effects of digoxin in vitro
    Prevention of inhibitory effect of digoxin on cation influx in human
        erythrocytes
    Prevention of digoxin-induced inhibition of myocardial ($Na^+ + K^+$)-ATPase
    Prevention of positive inotropic effect of digoxin on isolated myocardial
        preparations
3. Prevention of digoxin intoxication in digoxin-immunized rabbits
4. Removal of digoxin from cells in vitro
    Rat renal cortical cells
    Human erythrocytes
5. Reversal of pharmacologic and toxic effects of digoxin in vitro
    Reversal of inhibitory effect of digoxin on cation influx in human
        erythrocytes
    Reversal of digoxin-induced inhibition of myocardial ($Na^+ + K^+$)-ATPase
    Reversal of positive inotropic and toxic electrophysiologic effects of
        digoxin on isolated myocardial preparations
6. Reversal of established digoxin intoxication in nonimmunized dogs
7. Alteration of digoxin metabolism in rabbits and dogs
    Increased serum concentrations
    Decreased urinary excretion
    Prolongation of serum $t_{1/2}$

in rabbits against the toxic effects of this cardiac glycoside (Ciofalo and Ashe, 1971).

Antidigoxin antibodies have also been shown to be capable of removing digoxin rapidly from rat renal cortical slices (Watson and Butler, 1972) and from human erythrocytes (Watson and Butler, 1972; Gardner et al., 1973) in vitro. It was originally thought that the rapid removal of digoxin from the red cells was almost complete (Watson and Butler, 1972), but later studies revealed that the rapid removal of digoxin is restricted to that fraction of the digoxin which had been taken across the cell membrane into the erythrocyte. For example, in the experiment illustrated in Figure 31.1, the concentration of intracellular digoxin (defined as that fraction of the total cellular digoxin which is not membrane-bound after cell lysis) was decreased from 23.2 pmol/ml cells to 0.2 pmol/ml cells within 6 min after the addition of antidigoxin serum, while antiserum to an antigen unrelated to digoxin had no significant effect. Analysis of the data suggests that the antibodies remove the intracellular digoxin by lowering the effective extracellular concentration of free glycoside, since repetitive washing of the cells produces a similar effect on intracellular, but not on membrane-bound digoxin. Membrane-bound digoxin is also

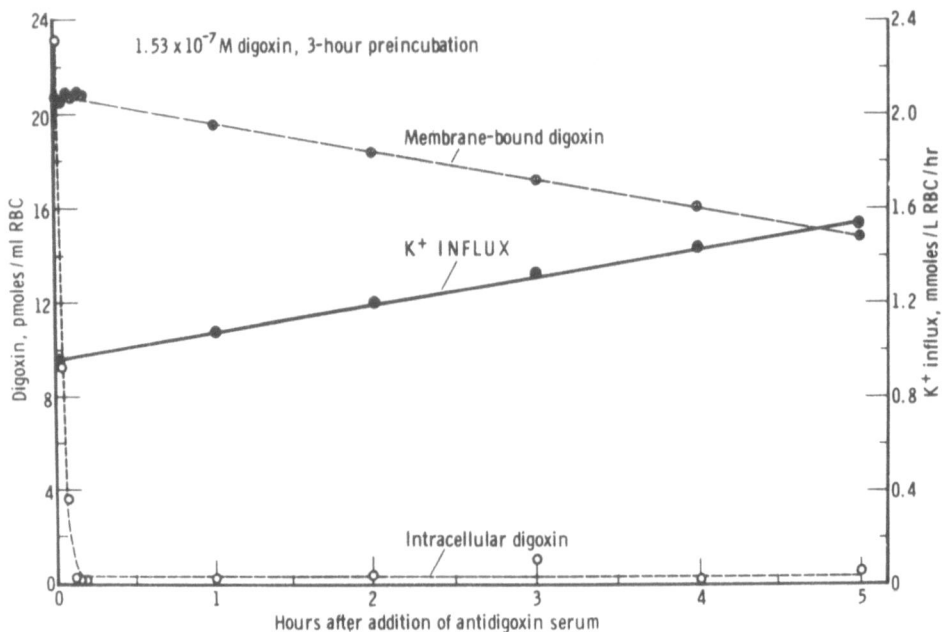

Fig. 31.1. Effect of antidigoxin serum on loss of erythrocyte digoxin and restoration of potassium influx. Human erythrocytes were incubated for three hours at 37°C in the presence of 1.53×10^{-7}M digoxin-^{3}H. Aliquots were removed for determination of total cellular digoxin, the amount of membrane-bound digoxin, and potassium influx just before and at various times after the addition, at zero time, of sheep antidigoxin serum. Membrane-bound digoxin is depicted as scored circles (⊕). Intracellular digoxin (o) was calculated as total cellular digoxin minus membrane-bound digoxin. Potassium influx (o) was determined over a 20-minute period with ^{42}K and a final K$^+$ concentration of 15.3 millimolar; potassium influx in control red cells not treated with digoxin was 2.41 mmol K$^+$/l. cells/hour. The values noted at zero time did not change significantly over the five-hour study period after the addition of control antiserum containing antibodies to an antigen structurally unrelated to digoxin. (Reproduced with permission from the Annals of the New York Academy of Sciences (Butler et al., 1974))

removed from human erythrocytes by antidigoxin antibodies, but at a much slower rate; removal is only partial after 5 h, the longest period studied (Fig. 31.1). Since in the presence of excess ouabain (10^{-3}M), membrane-bound ^{3}H-digoxin decreases at a rate very similar to its rate of decrease in the presence of antibody, it has been postulated that digoxin-specific antibodies bind this fraction of the red cell digoxin in the extracellular space after dissociation from membrane binding sites, and that the mechanism by which antibodies decrease membrane digoxin concentrations is by preventing reassociation of digoxin with these binding sites (Gardner et al., 1973). In removing digoxin from human erythrocytes, antidigoxin antibodies reverse the inhibitory effect of the glyco-

376

side on the active influx of monovalent cations, such as potassium and rubidium, into these cells (Watson and Butler, 1972; Gardner et al., 1973; Curd et al., 1971). In the experiment shown in Figure 31.1, $^{42}K^+$-influx had been decreased from 2.41 mmol/liter red cells/h in control erythrocytes to 0.93 mmol/liter red cells/h in erythrocytes which had been allowed to incubate for 3 h in the presence of 1.53×10^{-7} M digoxin. After addition of antidigoxin antibodies, progressive restoration of $^{42}K^+$-influx occured, but it was incomplete (1.54 mmol/liter red cells/h) at the termination of the experiment 5 h later. This reversal of a demonstrable effect of the glycoside on cells appeared to be correlated temporally with the removal of the membrane-bound fraction of erythrocyte digoxin (Fig. 31.1). These studies lend strong support to other experiments which suggest that there are at least two fractions of red cell digoxin but that only one of these fractions, namely the membrane-bound, contains the digoxin molecules which are responsible for the inhibitory effect of the glycoside on monovalent cation transport (Gardner et al., 1973).

Antibodies to digoxin and to other cardiac glycosides are also capable of reversing certain pharmacologic and toxic effects of these drugs on isolated cardiac preparations in vitro; the reversal of these effects of digoxin by antibody is more rapid than the reversal of the effects of digoxin on red cell cation influx by these antibodies. Digoxin-specific antibodies have been shown to be capable of reversing the toxic electrophysiologic effects of digoxin on isolated canine Purkinje fibers and on rabbit atrioventricular node preparations (Mandel et al., 1972). Digoxin-induced increases in active tension development by guinea pig atrial strips (Curd et al., 1971) and by cat papillary muscle preparations (Skelton et al., 1971) can be reversed by digoxin-specific antibodies. Antibodies to ouabain can reverse the positive inotropic effect of ouabain or of acetylstrophanthidin on isolated cat papillary muscle preparations (Gold and Smith, 1974). Antibodies to ouabain (Smith, 1972) and to digoxin (Smith, 1974) are capable of reversing the inhibitory effects of these cardiac glycosides on the catalytic activity of partially purified canine myocardial $(Na^+ + K^+)$-ATPase preparations; similarly, antibodies to proscillaridin can reverse the inhibitory effect of this glycoside on the catalytic activity of a partially purified cat brain $(Na^+ + K^+)$-ATPase preparation (Kleeberg and Belz, 1974).

Digoxin-specific antibodies are capable of reversing established digitalis intoxication when passively administered to nonimmunized, digoxin-intoxicated dogs. This property of antidigoxin antibodies was first demonstrated in a study in which 17 dogs were given large doses of digoxin (0.09 mg per kg body weight, intramuscularly, once daily for 3 days). All 17 dogs developed vomiting, weakness, lethargy and, within 1-3 h after the final dose, a toxic arrhythmia. In nine dogs, none of which received antidigoxin antibodies, the arrhythmias persisted throughout a 6-h period of continuous electrocardiographic monitoring; normal sinus rhythm was not observed at any time. Seven of the nine control dogs were dead within 24 h and all had died by 48 h (one moribund animal was sacrificed at 24 h). In contrast, in six of eight dogs given antidigoxin plasma or serum, antidigoxin antibodies reversed the toxic rhythm disturbances and restored normal sinus rhythm during the 6-h study period. In the two remaining animals given antidigoxin antibodies, serious ventricular arrhythmias were replaced by atrial tachycardia with atrioventricular block and a relatively slow ventricular rate; both dogs later reverted to normal sinus rhythm. All eight antibody-treated dogs were also promptly relieved of their gastrointestinal and other overt manifestations of digitalis toxicity (Schmidt and Butler, 1971b).

Antidigoxin antibodies exert profound effects on the pharmacokinetics of digoxin. For example, when digoxin is administered to digoxin-immunized rabbits whose sera contain digoxin-specific antibodies, these antibodies prevent renal excretion and initially produce 90-fold higher serum digoxin concentrations, principally in the form of protein-bound, inactive glycoside. For example, 12 h after a single intravenous dose of ^{3}H-digoxin (0.4 mg per kg body weight), the mean serum digoxin concentration in nine nonimmunized rabbits was 92 ng/ml, while the mean serum digoxin level in five digoxin-immunized animals was 8300 ng/ml. The mean serum half-life of digoxin was prolonged 21-fold from 3.4 days in nonimmunized animals to 72 days in the digoxin-immunized group; significant concentrations of circulating protein-bound digoxin were present in the sera of actively immunized rabbits 14 months after a single injection of the drug (Schmidt et al., 1974).

Antidigoxin antibodies also alter the pharmacokinetics of digoxin in nonimmunized dogs. A study has recently been completed of the effect of passively administered sheep antidigoxin antibodies on the pharmacokinetics of nontoxic doses of ^{3}H-digoxin (0.02 mg per kg body weight) in dogs. Antibodies, given in the form of whole antidigoxin serum, caused a 33- to 57-fold increase in serum digoxin concentrations, presumably due to the removal of digoxin from tissues by antibody. More than 90% of the serum digoxin was antibody-bound in these passively immunized dogs. Thus, as was the case in actively immunized rabbits, the urinary excretion of digoxin in passively immunized dogs became negligible and the biologic half-life of the drug was substantially prolonged (Butler et al., 1977a). Sheep antidigoxin antibodies have also been found to exert similar effects on the pharmacokinetics of digitoxin in monkeys (Ochs et al., 1976).

Potential problems connected with the possible clinical use of antidigoxin antibodies in the reversal of digoxin intoxication in man include the possibility of hypersensitivity reactions to foreign proteins and the possibility that late release of digoxin from the inactive, antibody-bound state might occur during immune degradation of the foreign protein and could conceivably result in recrudescence of toxicity, particularly if the total body burden of digoxin were large and degradation of infused antibody rapid.

Two approaches to these problems have been pursued. The first has been purification of digoxin-specific antibody to remove all extraneous protein. This has been achieved by an affinity chromatographic approach in which the cross-reacting ligand ouabain is coupled to bovine pancreatic ribonuclease and thence to the solid support bromoacetyl cellulose (Curd et al., 1971). More recently, this approach has been extended to the purification of digoxin-specific Fab fragments (Smith, 1974; Butler et al., 1977a). Fab fragments provide several advantages over intact antibody, including absence of antigenic and complement-binding determinants of the Fc fragment. Their smaller size should permit more rapid diffusion into the interstitial space and also results in relatively rapid excretion via glomerular filtration, a process known to occur with a half-life of about 4-5 h (Spiegelberg and Weigle, 1965; Waldmann and Strober, 1969).

Digoxin-specific Fab fragment reversal of established digoxin toxicity has been demonstrated in dogs given digoxin intravenously in doses sufficient to produce ventricular tachycardia (Smith, 1974; Curd et al., 1971). When administered to digoxin-treated dogs, antidigoxin Fab fragments also produce a significant increase in serum concentrations analogous to the rises observed when intact antidigoxin antibodies are administered. In contrast to dogs treated with intact antibodies, urinary excretion of digoxin in Fab-treated animals is comparable to that observed in control dogs, and hence serum digoxin concentrations fall more rapidly in Fab-treated dogs than in animals receiving intact antibodies; much of the urinary digoxin is Fab bound (Butler et al., 1977a). Recently, it has been demonstrated that sheep antidigoxin Fab fragments are capable of enhancing the urinary excretion of digitoxin in primates treated with this cardiac glycoside (Ochs et al., 1976). These findings indicate that antidigoxin Fab fragments share with intact antidigoxin antibodies the capacity to remove glycoside from tissue and that, in addition, the Fab fragments are capable of promoting the relatively prompt urinary excretion of bound digoxin, a capacity not present in the larger intact antibody molecule. Further experimental studies will be required, however, to determine the best approach to the reversal of toxic effects of digoxin with antidigoxin Fab fragments in patients who may require the maintenance of at least some digoxin effect for therapeutic purposes. Preliminary results of immunogenicity studies (Smith, Spicer and Haber, unpublished observations) indicate that purified Fab fragments of ovine digoxin-specific antibodies are weakly immunogenic compared with intact γ-globulin in both rabbit and baboon experimental models.

A patient has recently been treated with purified digoxin-specific Fab fragments with gratifying results (Smith et al., 1976). A 39-year-old man maintained on digoxin for management of atrial fibrillation ingested 90 0.25 mg digoxin tablets (22.5 mg) with suicidal intent. The initial serum digoxin concentration at the time of hospital admission was greater than 25 ng/ml. A pervenous endocardial pacemaker catheter was placed because of bradycardia and rising serum potassium concentration. During several ensuing hours of close observation, the serum potassium concentration rose steadily despite aggressive treatment with glucose and insulin, bicarbonate, and polystyrene sulfonate cation exchange resin. The heart rate continued to slow to a rate of 10 per min when the pacemaker was briefly turned off. The QRS complex progressively widened, and the threshold for pacing steadily rose. When the serum potassium concentration reached 8.7 mEq/liter, in view of the grave prognosis for massive digoxin intoxication with these manifestations (Bismuth et al., 1973), treatment with purified digoxin-specific Fab fragments was undertaken. A total of 1100 mg of Fab fragments were infused over a period of about 2 h. Within 10 min of completion of the infusion, the patient was in a stable sinus rhythm at a rate of 75 per min, and the serum potassium concentration fell rapidly back to the normal range.

The patient showed no signs of hemodynamic instability nor of immunologic side-effects.

The effects of the antidigoxin Fab fragments on digoxin pharmacokinetics in this patient were similar to the effects on digoxin pharmacokinetics previously noted in dogs (Butler et al., 1977a). Although a rapid increase in total serum digoxin concentration, from 17.6 to 223 ng/ml, occurred within 1 h after institution of the Fab infusion, the free serum digoxin concentration fell precipitously to undetectable levels (less than 1 ng/ml) during this same time interval; the free serum digoxin concentration remained low (less than 2 ng/ml) over the next 2½ days as the total (and largely Fab-bound) serum digoxin concentration, after remaining in the 210-230 ng/ml range for 12 h, progressively fell as the serum Fab concentration also decreased. Substantial renal excretion of digoxin occurred and, during the initial 6 h after the institution of Fab therapy, more than 99% of the urinary digoxin was Fab bound (Smith et al., 1976).

Further studies are planned to assess the efficacy and safety of antidigoxin Fab fragments in the treatment of digoxin intoxication in man. If, as anticipated, they prove to be effective and relatively safe for clinical use, they would constitute a useful addition to the therapeutic armamentarium of the physician.

References

Belz, G.G., Brech, W.J., Kleeberg, U.R., Rudofsky, G., Belz, G.: Characterization and specificity of proscillaridin antibodies. Naunyn Schmiedebergs Arch. Pharmakol. 279, 105 (1973)

Bismuth, C., Gaultier, M., Conso, F., Efthymiou, M.L.: Hyperkalemia in acute digitalis poisoning. Prognostic significance and therapeutic implications. Clin. Toxicol. 6, 153 (1973)

Butler, V.P., Jr.: Digoxin: Immunologic approaches to measurement and reversal of toxicity. N. Engl. J. Med. 283, 1150 (1970)

Butler, V.P., Jr., Chen. J.P.: Digoxin-specific antibodies. Proc. Natl. Acad. Sci. U.S.A. 57, 71 (1967)

Butler, V.P., Jr., Watson, J.F., Schmidt, D.H., Gardner, J.D., Mandel, W.J., Skelton, C.L.: Reversal of the pharmacological and toxic effects of cardiac glycosides by specific antibodies. Pharmacol. Rev. 25, 239 (1973)

Butler, V.P., Jr., Schmidt, D.H., Watson, J.F., Gardner, J.D.: Production and properties of digoxin-specific antibodies. Ann. N.Y. Acad. Sci. 242, 717 (1974)

Butler, V.P., Jr., Schmidt, D.H., Smith, T.W., Haber, E., Raynor, B.D., Demartini, P.: Effects of sheep antidigoxin antibodies and their Fab fragments on digoxin pharmacokinetics in dogs. J. Clin. Invest. 59, 345 (1977a)

Butler, V.P., Jr., Smith, T.W., Schmidt, D.H., Haber, E.: Immunological reversal of the effects of digoxin. Fed. Proc. 36, 2235 (1977b)

Ciofalo, F., Ashe, H.: Ouabain-induced ventricular arrhythmia in rabbit: influence of antibodies. Life Sci. 10, part I, 341 (1971)

Curd, J., Smith, T.W., Jaton, J.C., Haber, E.: The isolation of digoxin-specific antibody and its use in reversing the effects of digoxin. Proc. Natl. Acad. Sci. U.S.A. 68, 2401 (1971)

Gardner, J.D., Kiino, D.R., Swartz, T.J., Butler, V.P., Jr.: Effects of digoxin-specific antibodies on accumulation and binding of digoxin by human erythrocytes. J. Clin. Invest. 52, 1820 (1973)

Gold, H.K., Smith, T.W.: Reversal of ouabain and acetyl strophanthidin effects in normal and failing cardiac muscle by specific antibody. J. Clin. Invest. 53, 1655 (1974)

Kleeberg, U.R., Belz, G.G.: The reactivation of the proscillaridin-inhibited membrane ATPase by specific antibodies. Naunyn Schmiedebergs Arch. Pharmakol. 282, 433 (1974)

Mandel, W.J., Bigger, J.T., Jr., Butler, V.P., Jr.: The electrophysiologic effects of low and high digoxin concentrations on isolated mammalian cardiac tissue: Reversal by digoxin-specific antibody. J. Clin. Invest. 51, 1378 (1972)

Ochs, H., Haber, E., Smith, T.W.: Enhancement of digitoxin excretion by Fab fragments of specific antibodies. Circulation 54, Suppl. II-19 (1976) (Abstract)

Schmidt, D.H., Butler, V.P., Jr.: Immunological protection against digoxin toxicity. J. Clin. Invest. 50, 866 (1971a)

Schmidt, D.H., Butler, V.P., Jr.: Reversal of digoxin toxicity with specific antibodies. J. Clin. Invest. 50, 1738 (1971b)

Schmidt, D.H., Kaufman, B.M., Butler, V.P., Jr.: Persistence of hapten-antibody complexes in the circulation of immunized animals after a single intravenous injection of hapten. J. Exp. Med. 139, 278 (1974)

Skelton, C.L., Butler, V.P., Schmidt, D.H., Sonnenblick, E.H.: Immunologic reversal of the inotropic effects of digoxin. J. Clin. Invest. 50, 85a (1971) (Abstract)

Smith, T.W.: Ouabain-specific antibodies: Immunochemical properties and reversal of Na^+, K^+-activated adenosine triphosphatase inhibition. J. Clin. Invest. 51, 1583 (1972)

Smith, T.W.: Use of antibodies in the study of the mechanism of action of digitalis. Ann. N.Y. Acad. Sci. 242, 731 (1974)

Smith, T.W., Butler, V.P., Jr., Haber, E.: Characterization of antibodies of high affinity and specificity for the digitalis glycoside digoxin. Biochemistry 9, 331 (1970)

Smith, T.W., Haber, E., Yeatman, L., Butler, V.P., Jr.: Reversal of advanced digoxin intoxication with Fab fragments of digoxin-specific antibodies. N. Engl. J. Med. 294, 797 (1976)

Smith, T.W., Butler, V.P., Jr., Haber, E.: Cardiac glycoside-specific antibodies in the treatment of digitalis intoxication. In: Antibodies in Human Diagnosis and Therapy. Haber, E., Krause, R.M. (eds.) New York: Raven Press pp 365-389 (1977)

Spiegelberg, H.L., Weigle, W.O.: The catabolism of homologous and heterologous 7S gamma globulin fragments. J. Exp. Med. 121, 323 (1965)

Waldmann, T.A., Strober, W.: Metabolism of immunoglobulins. Prog. Allergy 13, 1 (1969)

Watson, J.F., Butler, V.P., Jr.: Biological acitivity of digoxin-specific antisera. J. Clin. Invest. 51, 638 (1972)

Discussion

Dengler: Dr. Butler, in the immunoassay only a part of digoxin is bound to antibodies. And this should be true in the in vivo situation. But why is then the digoxin excretion in urine as low as you showed?

Butler: Well, first of all, in those experiments employing intact antibody we gave a large molar excess of antibody: the figure ranged from an 11-fold to a 21-fold molar excess of antibody over digoxin. This excess of digoxin binding sites allows for very little free digoxin in the serum. In addition, there are the tissue digoxin binding sites. If occasionally a molecule dissociates from antibody in vivo, it can be bound by $(Na^+ + K^+)$-ATPase or other receptors which are absent in the immonoassay system. We too were surprised by the small amount of free digoxin excreted by antibody-treated dogs. The excretion was not zero, but the collection over the first 4 days after antibody administration was about 7% of the administered dose. So it was really a very small amount, and that did bother us a little bit, too.

Johnson, Chapel Hill: This is very interesting material. Of course, the major factor which would limit its use is potential immunogenicity, particularly the danger of severe anaphylaxis, and that's why I'm very interested in your comment that the Fab fragment would lack immunogenic properties. Is that certain?

Butler: The Fc portion is the species-specific part of the immunoglobulin molecule. The Fab antigen-binding part has similarities from one species to another. The Fab molecule is smaller than intact antibody molecules and is rapidly metabolized and excreted. Perhaps because of its interspecies similarities and its rapid degradation and excretion, it is significantly less immunogenic than intact antibody. For example, Dr. Hans Spiegelberg of the Scripps Clinic, La Jolla, California has tried to raise antibodies to Fab fragments in experimental animals and has had difficulties. I do think that antibodies can be raised. Dr. Smith has immunized both rabbits and monkeys, and certainly the amount of antibody that's formed is very low, but I don't think it's undetectable. If one repeatedly immunizes or if one denatures the Fab fragments, one gets some antibodies, but if undenatured material is injected, the amount of antibody formed is very small. Is that right, Dr. Smith?

Smith, Boston: That's right. If one gives repeated intravenous injections of IgG, one can usually elicit an antibody response. If one gives repeated intravenous injections of Fab fragments, one can, after several injections in most animals, detect a small, sluggish, but measurable antibody response. We haven't seen the animals show any apparent ill effects from it. Responses from Fab are generally seen only after more than one injection.

Butler: We would hope that antidigoxin Fab fragments would only be used once per patient; multiple use would almost certainly increase the chances of allergic reactions.

The other point I should have made is that appropriate skin testing should be done before administering Fab fragments. This is really the same as what people did in the old days when they used serotherapy, and so, if carefully administered, it will probably be safe. However, the considerations which Dr. Johnson brings up are very real, and this is the reason why I think that, in 99% of the patients (in 99.9% at the present time), we would subscribe to the principles that Dr. Jahrmärker outlined in the preceding lecture and would treat the patient symptomatically. Until more is known about the possible adverse effects of these Fab fragments, their use should be limited to really life-threatening situations. And this is all that we have approval for, both in the Boston hospitals and in our own institution. The use of antidigoxin Fab fragments should be reserved for the most serious situations at present.

Abshagen, Berlin: Would it be possible in order to exclude side-effects from immunologic reactions to combine hemoperfusion with the specific antibodies?

Butler: Are you talking about giving the intact antibodies? Or the Fab fragments?

Abshagen: The intact antibodies in hemoperfusion capsule.

Butler: I think you could do this. There are other methods that one could use too. If one were going to use intact antibodies, one could do plasmapheresis or one could combine it with perfusion of charcoal: that might be feasible. However, if you are referring to the extracorporeal perfusion of an immunoadsorbent-containing antibody, I doubt that it would be as effective as infused antibodies or Fab fragments. I think you do have to administer the antibody or Fab fragments to get digoxin-binding molecules close to the digoxin at receptor sites. The Fab fragments also have the advantage that they are excreted in the urine and Dr. Smith is going to give us some better data about their capacity to promote the excretion of digitoxin, evidence which we were unable to get in these studies with digoxin.

32 Reversal of Digitoxin Toxicity and Modification of Pharmacokinetics by Specific Antibodies[1]

H. R. OCHS and T. W. SMITH

Advanced digitalis toxicity unresponsive to conventional therapy continues to
be an important clinical problem (Smith and Willerson, 1971; Bismuth et al.,
1973; Lely and van Enter, 1970). The cardiac glycoside digitoxin is used in
about 16%-20% of digitalis-treated patients in the United States (National Prescription Audit) and is in more common use in some European countries such
as France, where 96% of a series of 115 patients treated for acute digitalis poisoning had taken digitoxin with a resulting morality of 22% (Bismuth et al.,
1973). Cardiac glycoside-specific antibodies or their Fab fragments have been
shown to be capable of reversing a number of pharmacologic and toxic effects
of digoxin and ouabain (Butler et al., 1973; Smith et al., 1977). Purified Fab
fragments of digoxin-specific antibodies have recently been used clinically to
reverse intractable hyperkalemia and advanced atrioventricular block following
massive suicidal digoxin ingestion (Smith et al., 1976). Due to the high mortality rate associated with overwhelming digitoxin toxicity and the need for more
effective therapy, we have undertaken studies with high affinity digitoxin-specific antibodies to determine their effects in an experimental model of lethal digitoxin toxicity. We have also extended earlier studies of Butler et al. (Butler et
al., 1977) with digoxin-specific antibodies and Fab fragments to determine
how intact antibodies and Fab fragments with high affinity for digitoxin would
influence the pharmacokinetics of digitoxin in an animal model. The latter
pharmacokinetic studies required the use of a primate species, the rhesus monkey, to provide an adequate model for digitoxin pharmacokinetics in man.

Antibody Production

To obtain antibodies with high affinity for digitoxin, digoxin was coupled to bovine
serum albumin (BSA) by periodate oxidation and Schiff's base formation and
reduction (Butler and Chen, 1967; Erlanger and Beiser, 1967). Sheep were
immunizied with BSA-digoxin in complete Freund's adjuvant and serially boosted and bled (Smith et al., 1970). Initial studies identified an animal that responded to immunization with a high titer of antibodies having high affinity

1 This work was supported in part by NHLI Award HL-18003 and NHLI Program Project Award HL-19259. Dr. Ochs was a Fellow of Deutsche Forschungsgemeinschaft.

for digitoxin. Pooled antiserum from consecutive bleedings of this animal was then used in subsequent experiments. The IgG fraction was obtained by ammonium sulfate precipitation (Campbell et al., 1963), and Fab fragments were prepared by papain digestion (Nisonoff, 1964). Undigested IgG was removed by gel filtration chromatography on Sephadex G-150. Digitoxin binding capacities of Fab fragments and IgG preparations were determined by a dextran-coated charcoal method (Herbert et al., 1965). Control (nonspecific) IgG and Fab fractions were prepared in identical fashion from sera of sheep not previously immunized with cardiac glycoside conjugates. The average intrinsic association constant (K_O) of the antibody population for digitoxin was determined by equilibrium dialysis (Smith et al., 1970). The K_O for digitoxin of the pooled antiserum used in experiments discussed in this paper, as determined by equilibrium dialysis and Scatchard analysis, was 1.4×10^{10} M^{-1}, confirming the high affinity for digitoxin of this sheep antibody population. Studies of rate constants for formation and dissociation of this antibody-digitoxin complex further document an affinity constant in the 10^{10} M^{-1} range, with rapid association and slow dissociation kinetics (Smith and Skubitz, 1975; Skubitz and Smith, 1975).

Toxicity Reversal Experiments

Experiments to determine the ability of Fab fragments of specific antibodies to reverse established, potentially lethal digitoxin intoxication were carried out in 16 mongrel dogs. Animals were anesthetized with intravenous pentobarbital (30 mg/kg) and ventilated with a Harvard respirator at 12 cycles per min with a tidal volume adjusted to the weight of the animal. Digitoxin, 0.5 mg/kg, was injected intravenously over 10 min. Ventricular tachycardia occurred in all animals; 5 min after its onset, eight control dogs were then given control Fab fragments intravenously. The remaining eight dogs received an amount of specific Fab fragments equal in molar terms to the digitoxin dose over 3 min, followed by a 30-min infusion of an additional one-third of the initial dose. Blood samples for determination of serum digitoxin concentrations were drawn at the onset of ventricular tachycardia and at hourly intervals after administration of Fab fragments. After 3 h in stable sinus rhythm, surviving dogs were allowed to breathe spontaneously and to awaken; electrocardiograms were again recorded 24 h later.

The usual pattern of digitoxin toxicity was an initial sinus bradycardia with varying degrees of atrioventricular block shortly after glycoside administration, sometimes followed by supraventricular tachycardia. Ventricular tachycardia ensued shortly after the appearance of the first ventricular premature beats, at an average time of 23.4 ± 3.8 (SEM) min after digitoxin injection in the eight control dogs. All of these animals died, with ventricular fibrillation occuring terminally in six animals and ventricular standstill in the other two. Average time of death in the eight control dogs was 101.4 ± 36.1 min after digitoxin injection.

The group of eight dogs subsequently treated with specific Fab fragments similarly developed ventricular tachycardia an average of 28 ± 3 min after digitoxin administration. In marked contrast to the control group, however, all specific Fab fragment-treated dogs survived. Conducted sinus beats reappeared in all animals in this group, an average of 18 ± 4 min after the initial dose of specific Fab fragments. Stable sinus rhythm without ventricular or supraventricular ectopic activity returned an average of 54 ± 16 min after Fab injection.

Plasma digitoxin concentrations at the onset of ventricular tachycardia in dogs that subsequently received specific Fab fragments averaged 762 ± 67 ng/ml, similar to a value of 834 ± 56 ng/ml for control dogs. The total plasma digitoxin concentration increased significantly to 2143 ± 144 ng/ml ($p < 0.0001$) during the hour after specific Fab infusion. The only control animal that died later than 1 h after onset of ventricular tachycardia showed the expected decline in plasma digitoxin concentrations from 1000 to 820 ng/ml.

This increase in plasma total digitoxin levels after Fab administration is consistent with removal of digitoxin from the tissues and sequestration in the circulation in a protein-bound, pharmacologically inactive form, analogous to the response previously documented in digoxin-treated dogs given digoxin-specific antibody (Schmidt and Butler, 1971; Curd et al., 1971).

Pharmacokinetics Studies

It was of particular interest in the course of these investigations to study the influence of specific antibodies and their Fab fragments on the pharmacokinetics of digitoxin in a suitable animal model. The elimination half-lives for digitoxin in dogs, cats, and rats are 14, 60 and 18 h, respectively, values which are considerably shorter than in humans (Okita, 1967). We therefore studied the pharmacokinetics of this glycoside in the rhesus monkey in the hope that this species would prove to have an elimination half-life for digitoxin similar to the 5-6 day values reported for man (Lukas, 1971).

In mice it had been demonstrated that rabbit Fab fragments are excreted via the kidneys with an elimination half-life of 3.6 h (Wochner et al., 1967). Therefore, in an animal model with a digitoxin elimination half-life considerably longer than for Fab fragments, we postulated that injection of specific Fab fragments would lead to enhancement of digitoxin excretion. Three male rhesus monkeys were sedated with ketamine 1 h before digitoxin administration to facilitate handling. The experiments comprised four parts. Initially, animals received 0.2 mg digitoxin intravenously over 5 min. In the subsequent three phases, each separated in time by 4-6 weeks, the same dose of digitoxin included ^{3}H-digitoxin to permit determination of serum and urine digitoxin or metabolite concentrations by direct counting of radioactivity as well as by radioimmunoassay. Blood samples in all experiments were obtained at 0.5, 1, 2, 3, 4, 6, 8, 10, 12, 24, 48, 52, 72, 76, 96, and 100 h after digitoxin administration and also on the 7th, 9th, 11th, 14th, and 21st days. The four experimental phases for each animal were:

1. Digitoxin administration followed by control (nonspecific) Fab fragments 6 h later
2. Digitoxin administration followed by specific Fab fragments 6 h later (two-fold stoichiometric excess of binding sites over digitoxin dose)
3. Digitoxin administration followed by specific IgG 6 h later (two-fold stoichiometric excess of binding sites over digitoxin dose)
4. Digitoxin administration without subsequent IgG or Fab infusion for comparison with phase 1

Spontaneously voided urine was collected during time intervals between 0-6, 6-12, 12-24, 24-48, 48-72, and 72-96 h after digitoxin administration.

Plasma digitoxin concentrations prior to specific IgG or Fab administration were determined by radioimmunoassay as previously described (Smith, 1971). For the direct determination of ^3H counts in samples, 0.2 ml of urine or serum was counted in 10 ml of the liquid scintillation medium described by Bray (Bray, 1960). Separation of antibody- or Fab fragment-bound from free digitoxin in early plasma and urine samples was accomplished by equilibrium dialysis (Smith et al., 1970).

Our initial data showed that the rhesus monkeys studied had a β (elimination) half-life of 135 h. quite similar to values previously reported for man (Lukas, 1971). Thus, the rhesus appeared to be a suitable model in which to study the influences of specific Fab fragments and intact antibody on the pharmacokinetics of digitoxin.

Administration of a twofold stoichiometric excess of Fab fragments 6 h after digitoxin infusion led to a rapid 4.3-fold increase in total plasma radioactivity in comparison to control values. Total plasma digitoxin concentrations then declined with an initial mean half-life of 4 h. Plasma concentrations of digitoxin returned to control levels found in experiments in which no specific Fab fragments were given 12-16 h after specific Fab injection. The equilibrium dialysis studies showed that the increase in plasma digitoxin levels was accompanied by greater than 99% binding of the drug to specific Fab fragments in early samples. This is further substantiated by the half-life of digitoxin elimination of 4 h initially after Fab administration, which is in accordance with the $t\frac{1}{2}$ of Fab fragments reported in the literature (Wochner et al., 1967).

Administration of a twofold stoichiometric excess of specific IgG resulted in a sharp increase in total plasma radioactivity to a mean peak value 12.9-fold above the pre-IgG infusion levels at about the 28th h of the experiment. This was followed by a gradual decline of plasma radioactivity until the 4th day, after which a more rapid fall was observed between the 4th and 9th days after specific IgG administration. Two weeks after antibody injection, mean plasma radioactivity concentrations had returned to levels comparable to those observed in control experiments. The increase in plasma digitoxin levels after IgG administration was in bound form, as demonstrated by equilibrium dialysis studies.

Mean urinary excretion of digitoxin and metabolites in the absence of specific antibody or Fab fragments totaled 11 721 ng ±2416 ng, or 6% of the dose given over 96 h, the largest amounts being excreted during the first and second 6-h collection periods. After infusion of specific Fab fragments, excretion of radioactivity increased 12.6-fold in comparison to the first 6-h period of the experiment and 14-fold over control values (from 0.6%-8% of the digitoxin dose given). This, to our knowledge, is the first demonstration of enhanced excretion of a drug by the use of an immunoglobulin fragment. These studies further document that the rhesus monkey eliminates Fab fragments in part by urinary excretion, as has been demonstrated for mice.

In marked contrast to Fab infusion, administration of intact antibodies significantly reduced the urinary digitoxin excretion rate to 37% of control during the interval between the 6th-12th h of the experiment. The serum $t\frac{1}{2}$ of homologous and heterologous γ-globulin injected into rabbits or guinea pigs has been shown to be between 4.2 and 6 days, and only very small amounts of intact IgG were excreted in the urine. The reduction in urinary excretion of digitoxin in our study was, therefore, not an unexpected observation. It is possible that an increase in urinary excretion of radioactivity took place at the time of maximal IgG degradation during days 5-9 when total plasma digitoxin levels were falling more rapidly and digitoxin was being released from the antibody binding sites.

In comparison to whole antiserum, administration of IgG preparations or Fab fragments decreases the foreign protein load with its attendant volume expansion and immunogenic hazards. The use of Fab fragments has several advantages over intact antibodies. First, Fab fragments lack the species-specific antigenic determinants of Fc fragments and are, therefore, less immunogenic, The smaller molecular size may permit more rapid diffusion to glycoside binding sites in tissue. Furthermore, Fab fragments enhance urinary excretion of digitoxin, at least in the rhesus monkey, whereas administration of IgG leads to the opposite effect and retains the potentially toxic glycoside stores in the body. On the basis of these observations, we conclude that:
1. Specific Fab fragments rapidly reverse advenced, otherwise lethal digitoxin intoxication in the dog by removal of the drug from tissue binding sites and sequestration in the extracellular space in an antibody-bound, pharmacologically inactive form.
2. Specific Fab fragments are capable of substantially accelerating urinary digitoxin excretion and reducing the plasma half-life of the drug in the rhesus monkey, which was found to have a β-elimination half-life similar to that in man.
3. Clinical trials of purified digitoxin-specific Fab fragments appear to be warranted in carefully selected cases of overwhelming, life-threatening digitoxin toxicity that fail to respond to conventional therapeutic measures.

References

Bismuth, C., Gaultier, M., Conso, F., Efthymiou, M.L.: Hyperkalemia in acute digitalis poisoning: Diagnostic significance and therapeutic implications. Clin. Toxicol. 6, 153-162 (1973)

Bray, G.A.: A simple efficient liquid scintillator for counting aqueous solutions in a liquid scintillation counter. Anal. Biochem. 1, 279-285 (1960)

Butler, V.P., Jr., Chen, J.P.: Digoxin-specific antibodies. Proc. Natl. Acad. Sci. U.S.A. 57, 71-78 (1967)

Butler, V.P., Jr., Watson, J.F., Schmidt, D.H., Gardner, J.D., Mandel, W.J., Skelton, C.L.: Reversal of pharmacological and toxic effects of cardiac glycosides by specific antibodies. Pharmacol. Rev. 25, 239-248 (1973)

Butler, V.P., Jr., Schmidt, D.H., Smith, T.W., Haber, E., Raynor, B.D.: Demartini, P.: Effects of sheep digoxin-specific antibodies and their Fab fragments on digoxin pharmacokinetics in dogs. J. Clin. Invest. 59, 345-359 (1977)

Campbell, D.H., Garvey, J.S., Cremer, N.E., Sussdorf, D.H.: Methods in Immunology. Benjamin, W.A. (ed.) New York: pp. 118-120 (1963)

Curd, J., Smith, T.W., Jaton, J.C., Haber, E.: The isolation of digoxin specific antibody and its use in reversing the effects of digoxin. Proc. Natl. Acad. Sci. U.S.A. 68, 2401-2406 (1971)

Erlanger, B.F., Beiser, S.M.: Antibodies specific for ribonucleosides and ribonucleotides and their reaction with DNA. Proc. Natl. Acad. Sci. U.S.A. 52, 68-74 (1967)

Herbert, V., Lau, K.S., Gottlieb, C.W., Bleicher, S.J.: Coated charcoal immunoassay for insulin. L. Clin. Endocrinol. Metab. 25, 1375-1384 (1965)

Lely, A., VanEnter, C.H.J.: Large-scale digitoxin intoxication. Br. Med. J. 1970/III, 727-740

Lukas, D.S.: Some aspects of the distribution and disposition of digitoxin in man. Ann. N.Y. Acad. Sci. 179, 338-361 (1971)

National Prescription Audit: IMS American Ltd., Ambler, PA

Nisonoff, A.: Enzymatic digestion of rabbit gamma globulin and antibody and chromatography of digestion products. Methods Med. Res. 10, 134-141 (1964)

Ochs, H.R., Vatner, S.F., Smith, T.W.: Reversal of the inotropic effects of digoxin by specific antibodies in the conscious. dog. Am. J.: Cardiology 39, 313 (1977)

Okita, G.T.: Species difference in duration of action of cardiac glycosides. Fed. Proc. 26, 1125-1130 (1967)

Schmidt, D.H., Butler, V.P., Jr.: Reversal of digoxin toxicity with specific antibodies. J. Clin. Invest. 50, 1738-1744 (1971)

Skubitz, K.M., Smith, T.W.: Determination of antibody-hapten association kinetics: a simplified experimental approach. J. Immunol. 114, 1369-1374 (1975)

Smith, T.W.: Radioimmunoassay for serum digitoxin concentration: Methodology and clinical experience. J. Pharmacol. Exp. Ther. 175, 352-360 (1971)

Smith, T.W., Skubitz, K.M.: Kinetics of interactions between antibodies and hapten. Biochemistry 14, 1496-1502 (1975)

Smith, T.W., Willerson, J.T.: Suicidal and accidental digoxin ingestion: Report of five cases with serum digoxin level correlations. Circulation 44, 29-36 (1971)

Smith, T.W., Butler, V.P., Jr., Haber, E.: Characterization of antibodies of high affinity and specifity for the digitalis glycoside digoxin. Biochemistry 9, 331-337 (1970)

Smith, T.W., Haber, E., Yeatman, L., Butler, V.P., Jr.: Reversal of advanced digoxin intoxication with Fab fragments of digoxin specific antibodies. N. Engl. J. Med. 294, 797-800 (1976)

Smith, T.W., Butler, V.P., Jr., Haber, E.: Digoxin-specific antibodies in the treatment of digitalis intoxication. In: The Future of Antibodies in Human Diagnosis and Therapy. Krause, R., Haber, E. (eds.) New York: Raven Press 1977

Wochner, R.D., Strober, W., Waldmann, T.A.: The role of the kidney in the catabolism of Bence Jones proteins and immunoglobulin fragments. J. Exp. Med. 26, 207-221 (1967)

Discussion

Grahame-Smith: I can see now why you have been rather keen throughout this meeting on the speed of reversibility of certain cardiac effects, because although Dr. Butler showed that the dissociation of digoxin from red cells is a rather slow process, in the experiments you have just described, both in the patient and in the dog, it is apparent that the arrhythmias are very rapidly reversible. Do you think that the positive inotropic effect is quickly reversible or do you think you are pulling out some more quickly reversible sort of effect?

Smith: No, the inotropic effect is not so rapidly reversible. In isolated papillary muscle preparations, we showed that the reversal of ouabain-induced inotropy occurs with a relatively long half-time in response to ouabain-specific antibodies. Dr. Butler and his colleagues have also studied the reversal of digoxin inotropy in the papillary muscle preparation. In experiments in collaboration with Drs. Ochs and Vatner (Ochs et al., 1977), we've shown that the half-time of antibody reversal of digoxin-induced inotropy in the intact dog is about 8 h. It's about one-third as long as in the control state. I don't believe that one can argue from these findings, however, that different receptors or compartments are involved in inotropic and arrhythmogenic effects.

Schaumann: There is an increasing discussion about the cost of treatment — therefore this is an unscientific question — what is the cost of the material you would need for a treatment of a severe life-threatening intoxication in man? Would it be possible to reduce the dose which you have used? I think Dr. Butler mentioned that it was about 10-20 times as much as you would need stoichiometrically?

Smith: The patient who was treated received just one stoichiometrically equivalent dose. We probably would not in general choose to use more than about a stoichiometrically equivalent dose of Fab fragments. It's very hard to cost account a fundamental research project of this kind. My guess would be that if this were scaled up to a pilot plant scale, the cost would not be prohibitive in terms of the potential good it could do for a patient with life-threatening toxicity.

Shaw: Do you think that the kinetics and quantities are such that in a patient with an arrhythmia, you could use the antibody as a diagnostic test for digoxin toxicity?

Smith: It's a fond hope of ours to do that. It's appealing to try to titrate the patient back into a state of nontoxicity and use that as a diagnostic maneuver. If one had in hand a preparation that was nonantigenic, then it would be an attractive proposition to use it as a "reverse" acetylstrophanthidin tolerance test.

Greeff, Düsseldorf: Is there a cross-reaction of Fab binding between digitoxin and steroid hormones?

Smith: No, These antibodies are quite comparable in specificity to the ones that we use in the immunoassay, so that one would see significant binding only at at least 1000-10,000-fold higher concentrations of steroid hormones such as progesterone and testosterone.

33 β-Methyl-Digoxin Disposition During Spironolactone Treatment

U. ABSHAGEN

Some years ago (Abshagen, 1973) we showed that the pharmacokinetics of β-methyl-digoxin in female SD rats were markedly influenced by a 3-day pretreatment with 100 mg spironolactone/kg b.i.d. After i.d. administration of ^{3}H-β-methyl-digoxin, the half-life of ^{3}H activity in blood dropped down in controls from 9.18 ± 0.6 h to 3.19 ± 0.08 h in spironolactone-pretreated animals (Fig. 33.1). Since for i.v. administration in man the dethioacetylated spironolactone metabolite with an opened γ-lactone ring, the fairly water-soluble canrenoate-potassium, is widely used, we also tested the effect of pretreatment with iso-molar amounts of this drug. Thereby, an enhanced elimination of ^{3}H activity could also be observed but the effect ($t_{1/2}$: 4.33 ± 0.55 h) was not as pronounced as after pretreatment with spironolactone. Corresponding to the elimination from blood, the biliary excretion (Fig. 33.2) of ^{3}H activity was almost quadrupled in spironolactone-pretreated rats, whereas a somewhat smaller increase could be observed after pretreatment with canrenoate-K. TLC analysis of the biliary excreted ^{3}H activity (Fig. 33.3) revealed that the 0-demethylation of β-methyl-digoxin — as evidenced by the 12.5 times increase of digoxin — as well as the splitting of glycosidic bounds — as evidenced by the 9.3 times increase of bisglycoside — were enhanced by pretreatment with spironolactone. At the same time, the conjugation reactions leading to polar metabolites were augmented — as can be seen from the low amounts of the monoglycoside which serves as predominant conjugation partner (Abshagen and Rietbrock, 1973) and the concomitant higher amounts of the resulting polar conjugates. The fact, however, that the unchanged mother compound β-methyl-digoxin was also excreted to a higher degree after pretreatment with spironolactone pointed to an additional mechanism besides induction of glycoside degredation. In this respect, an higher uptake of the glycoside into the liver could be demonstrated as a result of spironolactone pretreatment which was evidenced both by experiments with liver slices (Abshagen, 1973) and in vivo (Castle and Lage, 1972).

Alteration of distribution, enhanced metabolism, and increased biliary and fecal elimination with consequently lower blood levels resulting from pretreatment with spironolactone could also be demonstrated in experimental animals for other glycosides, especially for digitoxin, by several authors during the last 4 years (Castle and Lage, 1972, 1973 a, b; Vöhringer and Rietbrock, 1974; Wirth et al., 1974). These phenomena were regarded as the underlying mechanism for

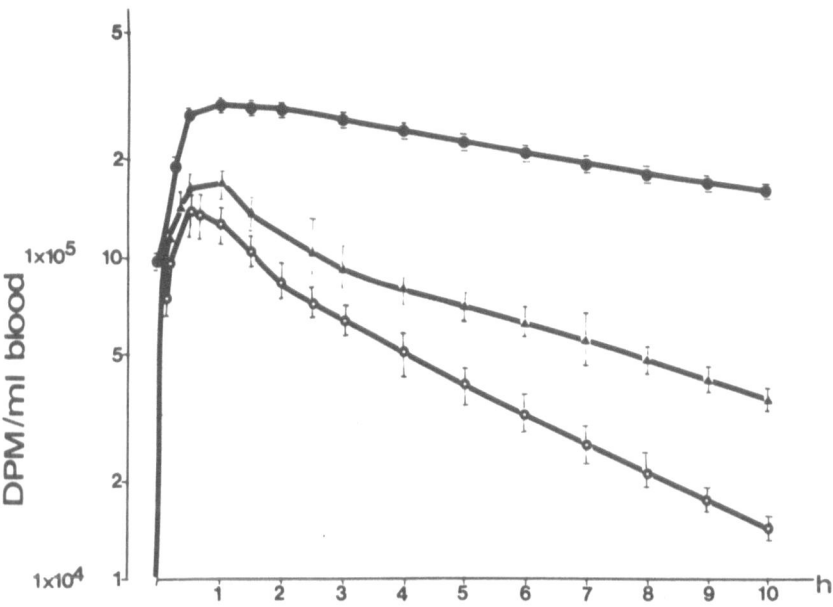

Fig. 33.1. Kinetics of ^{3}H activity in blood of biliary fistula rats after intraduodenal administration of 80 μCi ^{3}H-β-methyl-digoxin without ●——● and with pretreatment with 100 mg spironolactone ○——○ or 95 mg canrenoate-K ▲——▲ per kg body weight twice daily for 3 days. ($\overline{x} \pm s\ _{\overline{x}}$; n = 8)

the reduction of digitalis toxicity first reported in rats by Selye et al., (1969). In clinical experiments in man, however, spironolactone failed to reduce digitalis toxicity (Krämer et al., 1973 a, b). Therefore, it seemed a priori improbable that such profound alterations of digitalis metabolism as seen in rats and mice could also occur in man. Since both drugs, however, often are combined in clinical practice, this assumption had to be proved in man.

In an intrapatient trial (methodical details, see Abshagen et al., 1976 a), pharmacokinetics of β-methyl-digoxin were first studied in three persons after oral (2) and after i.v. (1) administration. The persons were treated 8 weeks later with 7 mg spironolactone/kg daily for 7 days and received a second single dose of ^{3}H-β-methyl-digoxin in the morning of the 8th day. Just before administration of the second dose of digitalis, the concentrations of the main metabolites of spironolactone in blood — canrenone and canrenoate-K — were determined in order to assure that the experimental conditions were comparable to our studies in rats (Table 33.1). In man, the concentrations of these metabolites were even distinctly higher than in rats in spite of the by far lower doses of spironolactone/ kg. This occurs as a consequence of the more than ten times longer half-lives of these substances with subsequent cumulation during the longer pretreatment period in man (Sadée, et al., 1974; Abshagen et al., 1976 b).

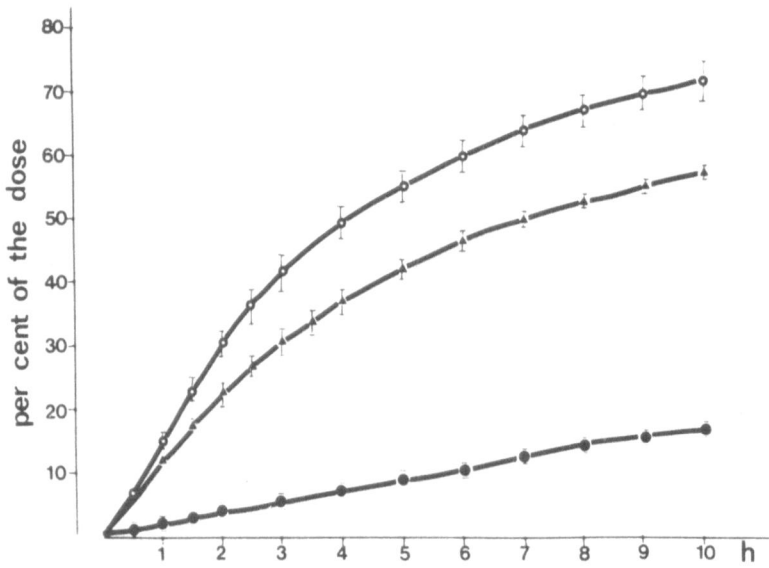

Fig. 33.2. Cumulative excretion of ^{3}H activity in bile of biliary fistula rats after intraduodenal administration of 80 μCi ^{3}H-β-methyl-digoxin without ●——● and with pretreatment with 100 mg spironolactone ○——○ or 95 mg canrenoate-K ▲——▲ per kg body weight twice daily for 3 days ($\overline{x} \pm s\ _{\overline{x}}$; n = 9)

Pretreatment of spironolactone in man resulted in a delayed invasion velocity of ^{3}H activity after oral administration of ^{3}H-β-methyl-digoxin. This leads to lower maximum concentrations which were reached later than without pretreatment (Fig. 33.4). The terminal elimination velocity, however, was unchanged in every case. Since the areas under the concentration curves in plasma, as well as the cumulative excretion in urine and feces (Fig. 33.5), were almost identical with and without pretreatment, the delayed invasion into the central compartment might not reflect an altered absorption but rather an initial higher uptake into the liver as seen in animal experiments. As it was expected from the excretion data, only insignificant alterations in the metabolic excretion pattern in urine were observed (Fig. 33.6). Slightly higher demethylation rates after pretreatment with spironolactone in V.G. and F.A. might be consistent with the initial higher uptake into the liver where demethylation takes place. These alterations, however, lie within the interindividual range of controls. Since biliary excretion of glycosides was so markedly increased in rats·after spironolactone pretreatment, we finally studied this route of elimination in a patient with biliary drainage, too, after sprionolactone pretreatment in comparison with three control patients. This investigation (Fig. 33.7) revealed that the 48-h recoveries of the label in urine as well as that in bile were not influenced by spironolactone pretreatment.

Thus, besides an initial slightly delayed invasion after oral administration, non-interaction of spironolactone with the pharmacokinetics of β-methyl-digoxin

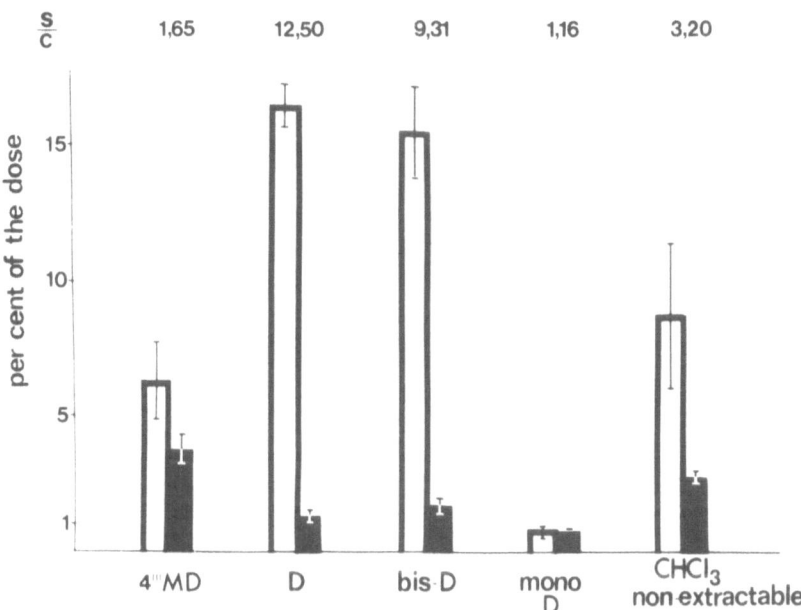

Fig. 33.3. Composition of ^3H activity in bile (0–4 h) after intraduodenal administration of 80 μCi ^3H-β-methyl-digoxin in biliary fistula rats without ■ and with pretreatment □ with 100 mg spironolactone/kg body weight twice daily for 3 days. s:c = multiplication factor after pretreatment; 4'''' MD = β-methyldigoxin; D = digoxin; bis-D = digoxigeninbisdigitoxoside; mono-D = digoxigeninmonodigitoxoside

Table 33.1. Concentration of spironolactone metabolites in plasma of rats and of man at the end of pretreatment (12 h after the last dose of spironolactone)

Species	Rat ng/ml	Man ng/ml
Canrenone	104.09 ±45.63	1190.00 ±255.15
Canrenoate-K	90.83 ±27.79	1580.00 ±152.75

and digoxin could be established. This agrees with the observation that in man spironolactone acts in contrast to its effects in experimental animals only as a weak inducer (Taylor et al., 1972), if at all (Abshagen et al., 1977). The example presented here, where profound interactions of two frequently clinically combined drugs were demonstrated in rats and where nothing of the kind occurs in man, alludes to the old saying, "man is no frog," and calls for human pharmacology.

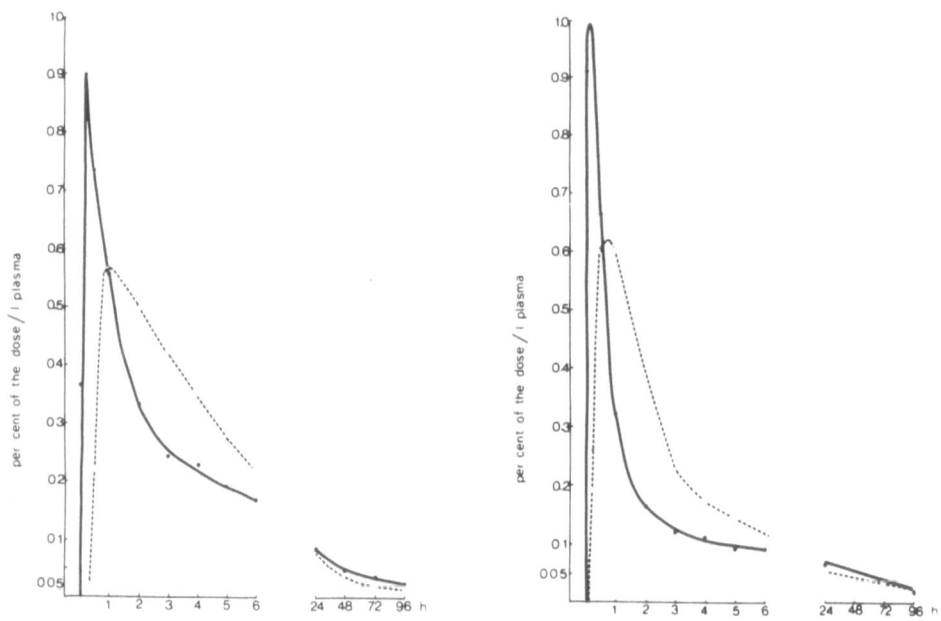

Fig. 33.4. Kinetics of ^{3}H activity in plasma of two normal persons after oral administration of 100 μCi ^{3}H-β-methyl-digoxin without —— and with — — — pretreatment with 7 mg spironolactone/kg body weight for 7 days

References

Abshagen, U.: Effects of pretreatment with spironolactone on pharmacokinetics of 4′′′-methyldigoxin in rats. Naunyn Schmiedeberg's Arch. Pharmacol. 278, 91-100 (1973)

Abshagen, U., Rietbrock, N.: Metabolism of digoxigenin, digoxigeninmono-digitoxoside and digoxigeninbisdigitoxoside in rats. Naunyn Schmiedeberg's Arch. Pharmacol. 276, 157-166 (1973)

Abshagen, U., Rennekamp, H., Kuhlmann, J.: Effects of pretreatment with spironolactone on pharmacokinetics of 4′′′-methyl-digoxin in man. Naunyn Schmiedeberg's Arch. Pharmacol. 292, 87-92 (1976 a)

Abshagen, U., Rennekamp, H., Luspinszki, G.: Pharmacokinetics of spironolactone in man. Naunyn Schmiedeberg's Arch. Pharmacol. 296, 37-45 (1976 b)

Abshagen, U., Rennekamp, H., Luspinzski, G.: Disposition kinetics of spironolactone in hepatic failure after single doses and prolonged treatment. Eur. J. Clin. Pharmacol. 11, 169-176 (1977)

Castle, M.C., Lage, G.L.: Effects of pretreatment with spironolactone, phenobarbital or β-diethylaminoethyl-diphenpylpropylacetate (SKF 525-A) on tritium levels in blood, heart and liver of rats at various times after administration of ^{3}H-digitoxin. Biochem. Pharmacol. 21, 1449-1455 (1972)

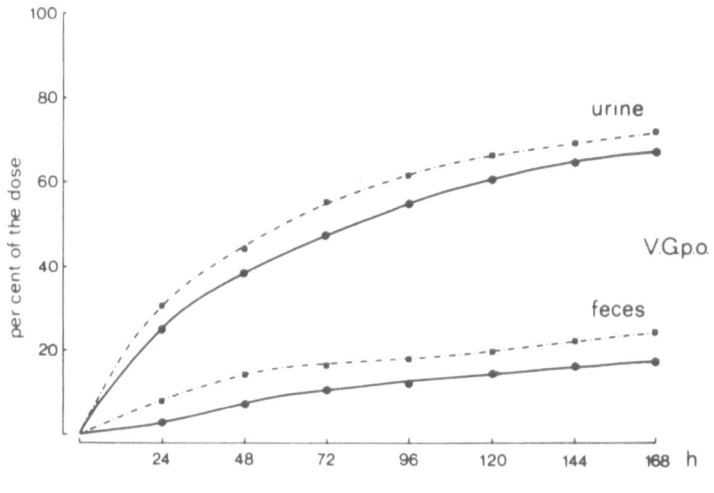

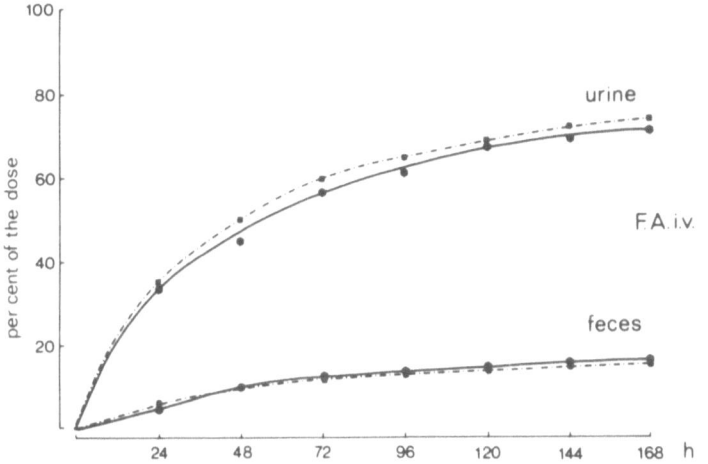

Fig. 33.5. Cumulative excretion of ^{3}H activity in urine and feces ot two normal persons after administration of 100 μCi ^{3}H-methyl-digoxin without —— and with — — — pretreatment with 7 mg spironolactone/kg body weight for 7 days

Castle, M.C., Lage, G.L.: Enhanced biliary excretion of digitoxin following spironolactone and its relation to the prevention of digitoxin toxicity. Res. Commun. Chem. Pathol. Pharmacol. 5, 99-108 (1973 a)

Castle, M.C., Lage, G.L.: ^{3}H-digitoxin and its metabolites following spironolactone pretreatment of rats. Res. Commun. Chem. Pathol. Pharmacol. 6, 601-612 (1973 b)

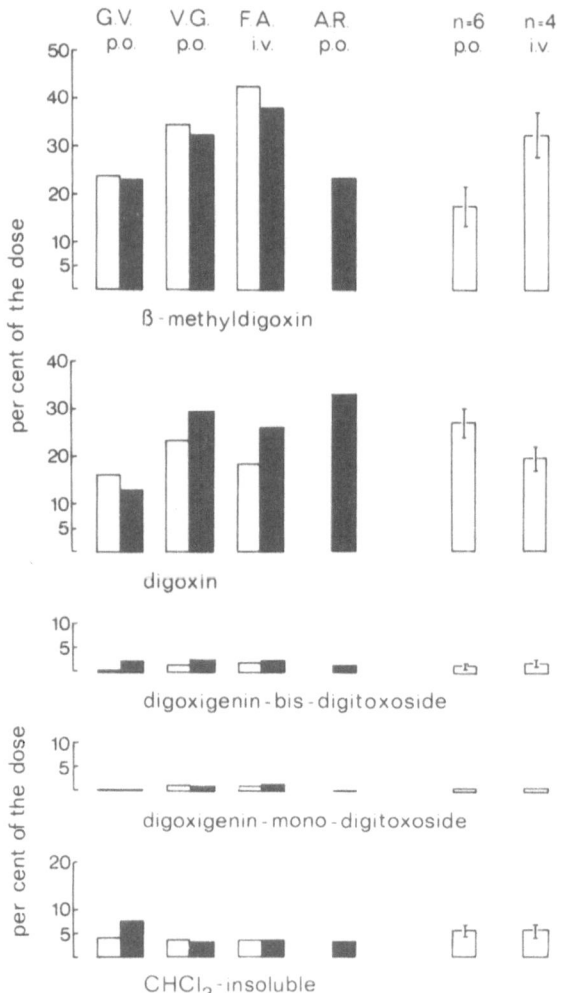

Fig. 33.6. Composition of ^{3}H activity in urine (0-7 days) after oral or intravenous administration of 100 μCi ^{3}H-β-methyl-digoxin without □ and with ■ pretreatment with 7 mg spironolactone/kg body weight for 7 days. Controls p.o. and i.v. in comparison. (From Abshagen et al., Naunyn-Schmiedebergs Arch. Pharmacol. 292.87, 1976)

Krämer, K.-D., Ghabussi, P., Hochrein, H.: Klinische Prüfung der subtoxischen Vollwirk- und Erhaltungsdosis von Digoxin unter dem Einfluß von Spironolakton. Arzneim. Forsch. (Drug Res.) 23, 508-511 (1973 a)

Krämer, K.-D., Vogt, W., Ghabussi, P., Hochrein, H.: Therapeutischer Wert des Aldosteron-Antagonisten Kalium-Canrenoat bei der Digitalisintoxikation. Med. Welt 24, 462-467 (1973 b)

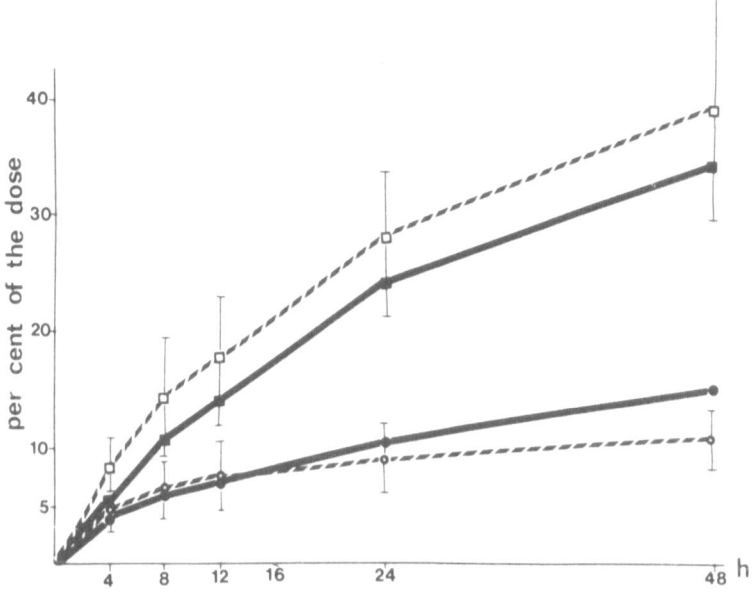

Fig. 33.7. Cumulative excretion of ^{3}H activity in urine □ ■ and bile ○ ● after oral administration of 100 μCi ^{3}H-β-methyl-digoxin in a patient with T-tube drainage after choledochetomy with previous pretreatment with 7 mg spirono-lactone/kg body weight for 7 days. Controls without pretreatment ($\overline{x} \pm s_{\overline{x}}$; n = 3) : open symbols

Sadée, W., Abshagen, U., Finn, C., Rietbrock, N.: Conversion of spironolactone to canrenone and disposition kinetics of spironolactone and canrenoate-potassium in rats. Naunyn Schmiedebergs Arch. Pharmakol. 283, 303-318 (1974)

Taylor, S.A., Rawlins, M.D., Smith, S.E.: Spironolactone — a weak enzyme inducer in man. J. Pharm. Pharmacol. 24, 578-579 (1972)

Vöhringer, H.F., Weller, L., Rietbrock, N.: Influence of Spironolactone Pre-treatment on Pharmacokinetics and Metabolism of Digitoxin in Rats. Naunyn Schmiedebergs Arch. Pharmakol. 287, 129-139 (1975)

Wirth, K.E., Frölich, J.C.: Effect of spironolactone on excretion of ^{3}H-digoxin and its metabolites in rats. Eur. J. Pharmacol. 29, 43-51, (1974)

Discussion

Preibisz, Warsaw: I have data which support your results. We did a study with healthy volunteers on a chronic digoxin treatment over 7-9 days. During the following 6 days, digoxin was continued and in addition the subjects received

399

spironolactone in a dosis about twice as high as you have given. The serum levels and urinary excretion of digoxin was not altered during the treatment with spironolactone. So our data would support your theses that we have to be careful to extrapolate the results from animal experiments to the human beings.

Abshagen: This morning Dr. Ohnhaus showed me data which have not been published yet. He measured the clearance of digoxin under a spironolactone treatment in man, and the clearance was essentially unchanged. He also determined other parameters of the metabolic capacity of the drug-metabolizing enzymes such as antipyrine N-demethylation, which was not influenced by spironolactone.

34 Digitoxin Disposition Under Rifampicin Treatment[1]

U. PETERS, T. U. HAUSAMEN, and F. GROSSE-BROCKHOFF

Introduction

Several drugs were found which influence absorption, metabolism, and excretion of digitoxin (Bazzano et al., 1970; Caldwell and Greenberger, 1971; Jeliffe and Blankenhorn, 1966; Solomon and Abrams, 1972). Substances like ion-exchange resins and charcoal interfere with absorption and enterohepatic recycling of

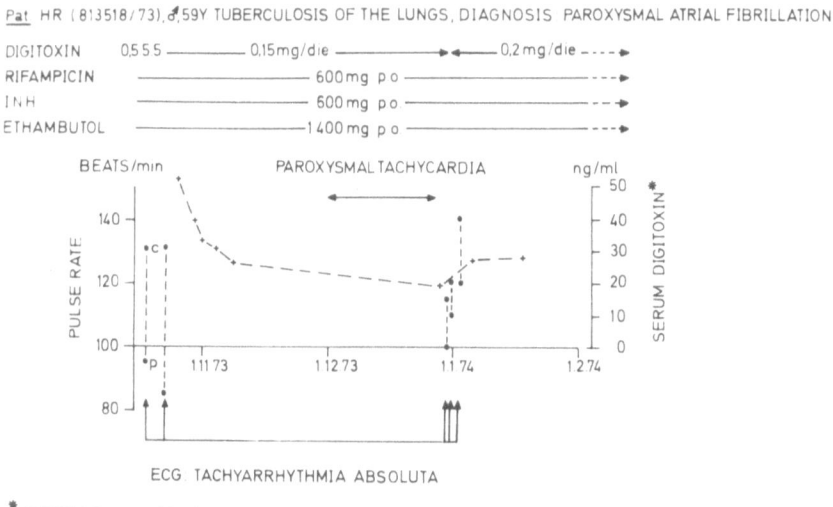

Fig. 34.1. Serum digitoxin during rifampicin therapy. In a patient (H.R. 8113518/73, 59 years) suffering from tuberculosis of the lung and paroxysmal atrial fibrillation with resulting tachyarrhythmia absoluta, digitoxin therapy initially could suppress atrial fibrillation. 4-6 weeks after continuous treatment with 600 mg per day p.o., rifampicin paroxysmal tachycardia was observed again by the patient and the reoccurrence of atrial fibrillation documented by ECG. After increase of the daily digitoxin dose t o 0,2 mg p.o., atrial fibrillation and tachycardia no longer occurred.
c.----p. Peripheral and central pulse rate 4° +----+ Digitoxin concentration in serum

1 Supported by "Deutsche Forschungsgemeinschaft (SFB 30)".

digitoxin and its metabolites. Other compounds, which are known to induce enzymes involved in drug metabolism like phenobarbital, phenytoin, and phenyl-butazone (Jeliffe and Blankenhorn, 1966; Solomon and Abrams, 1972) increase digitoxin metabolism. So far, however, there is no evidence, that these inter-actions create a major clinical problem in digitoxin therapy. The failure to control tachyarrhythmic atrial fibrillation with digitoxin in a patient receiving rifampicin, ethambutol, and isoniazid because of tuberculosis of the lungs (Fig. 34.1) led us to further investigations on the assumed interaction between these drugs and digitoxin. The results of these studies will be reported.

Patients

Included in the study were 63 inpatients (29 patients with various heart diseases and 34 patients with active and inactive tuberculous disease). None of them showed evidence of manifest heart failure or impaired liver or kidney function as judged by clinical examination, x-ray studies, and laboratory data. None of the patients received diuretics. All subjects obtained an oral loading dose of 0.6 mg digitoxin the first 2 days and 0.2 mg on day 3. The oral maintainance dose was 0.1 mg/day. Tuberculostatic treatment consisted of 5-10 mg isoniazid, 20-25 mg ethambutol and 5-10 mg rifampicin per kg body weight and day p.o. Five patients obtained rifampicin as monotherapy. Blood samples were taken from all subjects 24 h after the last application of drugs.

Methods

All methods used in this study concerning digitoxin determination, thin layer chromatography, and extraction methods of urine have been described elsewhere (Peters et al., 1974, 1976)

Statistics

For statistical analysis, the student t-test for unpaired data and the Wilcoxon test were used.

Results

Serum Digitoxin Concentrations During Tuberculostatic Treatment With Isoni-azid Ethambutol, Rifampicin, and During Monotherapy With Rifampicin

Serum digitoxin concentrations in 29 patients who obtained 0.1 mg digitoxin p.o. as maintainance dose for 8 days after the loading dose but no tuberculostatic drugs amounted to ($x \pm s$) 26.6 ± 7.3 ng/ml (Table 34.1). Twenty-one patients with tuberculous disease under therapy with isoniazid, ethambutol, and rifampicin and an equal digitoxin treatment had serum digitoxin concentrations (x ± s) of 18.4 ± 3.9 ng/ml. The difference of the mean serum digitoxin values between both groups was statistically significant (p < 0.0005). The time course of the decrease of serum digitoxin during the tuberculostatic treatment is shown in Figure 34.2. The lowest digitoxin values were reached within 2 weeks. No further decrease was observed thereafter.

Also during monotherapy with rifampicin, a decrease in serum digitoxin concentration occurred (Table 34.1), which was equal to the effect observed in patients receiving all three tuberculostatic drugs. No statistically significant difference was observed, if the patients under tuberculostatic treatment received the digitoxin orally or intravenously (Table 34.2).

Table 34.1. Serum digitoxin concentrations under tuberculostatic therapy

Treatment	n	ng/ml ($\overline{x}$ ± s)	p
No tuberculostatic treatment [a]	29	26,5 ± 7,3	
Triple tuberculostatic treatment[a]	21	18,4 ± 3,9	< 0,0005[b]
Rifampicin monotherapy[a]	5	12,8 ± 2,4	< 0,0005[b]

[a] and oral maintainance therapy with 0,1 mg digitoxin daily.
[b] Statistical significant difference to serum digitoxin concentrations of the subjects not receiving tuberculostatic drugs.

Table 34.2. Serum digitoxin after oral and intravenous administration of digitoxin in patients treated with tuberculostatics[a]

Digitoxin dosage during 3 days	Route of administration	Digitoxin serum concentration (ng/ml)	p
0.6; 0.6; 0.2	oral	27.2 ± 2.8	
0.6; 0.6; 0.2	intravenous	24.2 ± 4.2	p > 0.1

[a] Isoniazid 5 - 10 mg/kg.
    Ethambutol 20 - 25 mg/kg.
    Rifampicin 5 - 10 mg/kg.

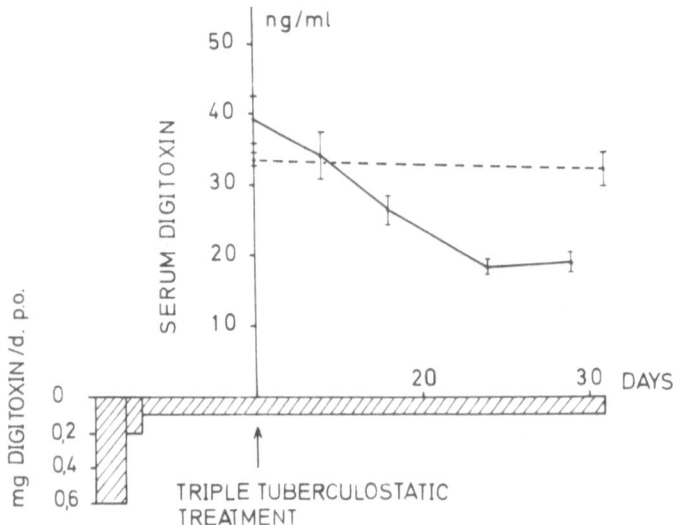

Fig. 34.2. Serum digitoxin concentration (x ± SEM) during treatment with rifampicin, isoniazid, and ethambutol and oral maintainance therapy with 0.1 mg digitoxin per day.

o ----o. Serum digitoxin in healthy volunteers (n = 4)

o——o. Serum digitoxin in patients receiving triple tuberculostatic treatment (n = 6)

Serum Half-life Time and "Digitoxin Clearance"

Serum half-life of digitoxin was determined in nine healthy subjects and in eight patients under tuberculostatic treatment. All subjects were under maintainance therapy with 0.1 mg digitoxin/day for at least 8 days. After discontinuation of digitoxin therapy, serum levels of digitoxin decreased exponentially. Serum half-life in healthy subjects was calculated with 7.6 ± 1.6 days and in the patients group with 4.5 ± 1.5 days. The difference between both groups was statistically significant (p < 0.0005). In five healthy subjects, "digitoxin clearance" was 1.2 ± 0.1 ml/min, while eight patients under tuberculostatic treatment had 2.2 ± 0.4 ml/min. The difference between both groups was statistically significant (p < 0.0005).

Protein Binding of Digitoxin

In six healthy subjects and in six patients under tuberculostatic treatment, the protein binding of digitoxin was determined. Serum protein concentration and serum albumin concentration in both groups was within the normal range. In the healthy subjects 97,3% ± 0.6% of digitoxin was bound to serum proteins, while in the patients group a value of 97,6% ± 0.5% was found. There was no statistically significant difference between both groups (p > 0.15). Equal results were obtained using equilibrium dialysis.

In three patients, the water-soluble and methylene chloride-soluble fraction of
^{3}H-digitoxin and its metabolites were measured in urine. The results are demonstrated in Figure 34.3. The ^{3}H activity in the water-soluble fraction increased
in the first patient from 19.1% ± 1.3% to 42.7% ± 5.5%, in the second patient
from 16.4% ± 2.4% to 48.0% ± 16.5%, and in the third patient from 40.8% ±
3.4% to 60.3% ± 4.4% before and after rifampicin treatment, respectively. The
increase of the water-soluble fraction during rifampicin treatment was statistically significant if compared with the pretreatment values (p < 0.0005). The
pretreatment values of water-soluble ^{3}H activity in urine of these three patients
was not significantly different from the values of nine other untreated patients,
which were found to be ($\overline{x}$ ± s) 23.9% ± 7.9%.

The amount of water-soluble ^{3}H activity was relatively constant in the urine
samples collected in the pretreatment period. In the second period of urine collection, however, two patients showed an increase of the water-soluble fraction
of ^{3}H activity during the whole collection period. Only in one patient relatively
constant values were obtained (Figure 34.3). This patient was distinguished
from the other two patients by a relatively high amount of water-soluble ^{3}H activity already in the pretreatment period.

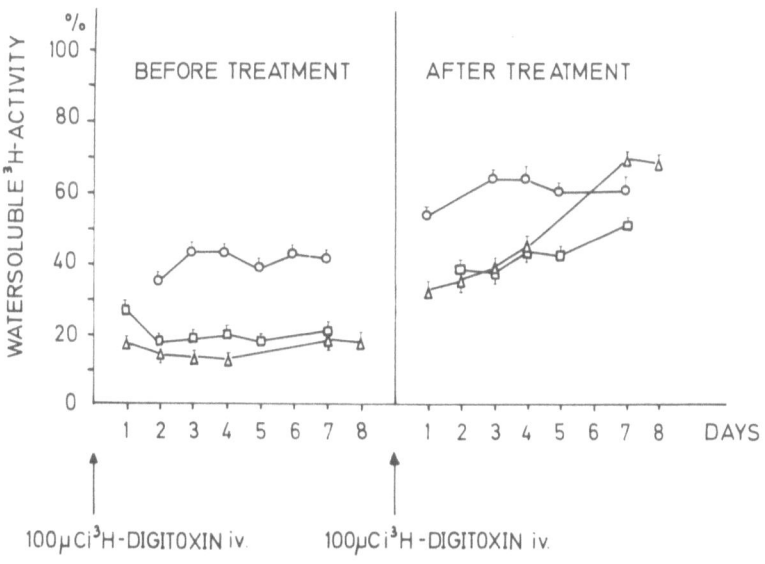

Fig. 34.3. Water-soluble ^{3}H activity (x ± SD) in urine of three patients after
intravenous application of 100 μCi ^{3}H-digitoxin before and after treatment with
rifampicin.
Note the relative constant values for all patients in the pretreatment period and the
steady increase of the water-soluble fraction in patient J.H. and A.L. during the
rifampicin treatment period
o----o patient P.K. △----△ patient J.A. □----□ patient A.L.

TLC of the methylene chloride extract from urine before and after treatment with rifampicin revealed no significant difference in the chromatograms. Main ^{3}H activity was related to digitoxin. Some ^{3}H activity could be detected in the areas of digitoxin and digitoxosides of both digoxin and digitoxin. However, the amounts of these metabolites were too small for quantitative analysis by TLC.

Discussion

These results demonstrate that under tuberculostatic therapy with rifampicin, ethambutol, and rifampicin, as well as under monotherapy with rifampicin, a significant decrease of serum digitoxin concentrations occurs. In patients receiving monotherapy with rifampicin, the fall of serum digitoxin levels was about the same as in patients treated with all three tuberculostatic drugs. It can be suggested, therefore, that the observed effect on serum digitoxin levels is mainly due to rifampicin.

Several mechanisms have to be considered for the explanation of the rifampicin effect on serum digitoxin concentrations. An inhibition of digitoxin absorption or of enterohepatic recycling of digitoxin metabolites excreted with the bile see to be unlikely. Our results demonstrate no significant difference in serum digitoxin concentrations under rifampicin therapy, if digitoxin was administered orally or intravenously. However, no investigations have been carried out to estimate excretion of digitoxin and its metabolites in the stool.

An increase of the free digitoxin fraction in blood would make available more digitoxin for ultrafiltration in renal glomeruli and thus contribute to a shortened half-life. For several drugs, changes in protein binding of digitoxin could be demonstrated. In our experiments, no change in protein binding of digitoxin could be observed. The values reported here were in the range observed by others (Kuschinsky, 1969; Lukas, 1973; Scholtan et al., 1966; Storstein, 1973).

The decrease of serum digitoxin concentration under rifampicin therapy, the shortened serum half-life of the drug, as well as the increased digitoxin clearance could be best explained by an augmented excretion due to a stimulation of digitoxin metabolism. In contrast to digoxin, digitoxin is extensively metabolized in the liver (Ashley, 1958; Doherty et al., 1971; Okita, 1964). Although many questions about digitoxin metabolism remain unanswered, two major pathways are widely accepted at present: 1. the production of genins, which are rapidly converted to cardioinactive compounds by conjugation of glucuronic or sulfuric acid and 2. the conversion of digitoxin to digoxin by 12-β-hydroxylation which occurs under normal conditions to a very small amount (Ashley, 1958; Doherty et al., 1971; Kolenda et al., 1971; Okita, 1954; Repke, 1959; Solomon and Abrams, 1972; Storstein, 1973; Talcott and Stohs, 1972). Stimulation of 12-β-hydroxylation in man and animals has been reported under phenobarbital treatment and is accompanied by a decrease of serum digitoxin concentrations and shorter serum half-life of the compound

(Jeliffe and Blankenhorn, 1966; Solomon and Abrams, 1972). Recently, it has been shown that hydroxylation of ethinylestradiol is augmented under rifampicin therapy (Bolt et al., 1974). It also has been reported that the pharmacologic half-life of cortisol is diminished under rifampicin therapy, which is accompanied by an increase of inactive conjugated metabolites in urine (Edwards et al., 1974). Our data suggest that under rifampicin treatment digitoxin metabolism is also increased. The appearance of a larger fraction of water-soluble ^{3}H activity in urine implies that the rate of conjugation of digitoxin metabolites is stimulated by rifampicin. This results in an increase of water-soluble metabolites, which can be excreted via bile and urine. However, it has to be emphasized that tritiated digitalis preparations given to subjects receiving maintainance digitalis therapy do not equilibrate equally with each body compartment of digitalis. Thus, our results must not necessarily be representative for digitalis metabolism in all body stores.

Some studies have been carried out to measure 12-β-hydroxylation products of digitoxin before and during rifampicin therapy. So far, these studies have not yet revealed conclusive results. It could be demonstrated by TLC that before and during rifampicin treatment digitoxin is the main cardioactive substance excreted with urine. The amount of 12-β-hydroxylation products was too small to allow quantitative analysis by TLC. More sensitive methods like gas chromatography with electron capture (Watson et al., 1972) have to be applied to this problem for a final answer.

References

Ashley, J.J., Brown, B.T., Okita, G.T., Wright, S.W.: The metabolites of cardiac glycosides in human urine. J. Biol. Chem. 232, 315-322 (1958)

Bazzano, G., Gray, M., Sansone-Bazzano, G.: Treatment of digitalis intoxication with a new steroid-binding resin. Clin. Res. 18, 592 (1970)

Bolt, H.M., Kappus, H., Bolt, M.: Rifampicin and oral contraception. Lancet 1280-1281

Caldwell, J.H., Greenberger, N.J.: Interruption of enterohepatic circulation of digitoxin by cholestyramine. 1. Protection against letal intoxication. J. Clin. Invest. 50, 2626-2637 (1971)

Doherty, J.E., Hall, W.H., Murphy, M.L., Beard, O.W.: New information regarding digitalis metabolism. Chest 59, 433-437 (1971)

Edwards, O.M., Courtenay-Evans, R.J., Galley, J.M., Hunter, J., Tait, A.D.: Changes in cortisol metabolism following rifampicin therapy. Lancet 1974/VII, 549-551

Jeliffe, R.W., Blankenhorn, M.H.: Effect of phenobarbital on digitoxin metabolism. Clin. Res. 14, 160 (1966)

Kolenda, K.-D., Lüllmann, H., Peters, T.: Metabolism of cardiac glycosides studied in isolated perfused guinea-pig liver. Br. J. Pharmacol. 41, 661-673 (1971)

Kuschinsky, K.: Über die Bindungseigenschaften von Plasmaproteinen für Herzglycoside. Naunyn-Schmiedeberg's Arch. Pharmakol. Exp. Pathol. 262, 388-398 (1969)

Lukas, D.S.: The pharmacokinetics and metabolism of digitalis in man. In: Storstein, O (ed.): Symposium on Digitalis. Oslo: Gyldendal Norsk Forlag 1973, pp. 84-102

Okita, G.T.: Metabolism of radioactive cardiac glycosides. Pharmacologist 6, 45 (1964)

Peters, U., Hausamen, T.U., Grosse-Brockhoff, F.: Therapie mit Digitoxin unter Kontrolle des Serum-Digitoxinspiegles. Dtsch. Med. Wochenschr. 99, 1701-1707 (1974)

Peters, U., Hausamen, T.U., Grosse-Brockhoff, F.: Einfluß von Tuberkulostatika auf die Pharmakokinetik des Digitoxins. Dtsch. Med. Wochenschr. 99, 2381-2386 (1974)

Peters, U., Grabensee, B., Hausamen, T.U., Fritsch, W.-P., Grosse-Brockhoff, F.: Pharmakokinetik von Digitoxin bei chronischer Niereninsuffizienz. Dtsch. Med. Wochenschr. 102, 109-115 (1976)

Repke, V.: Die Bis- und Monodigitoxoside des Digitoxigenins und Digoxigenins: Metaboliten des Digitoxins. Naunyn Schmiedeberg's Arch. Pharmakol. 237, 155-170 (1959)

Scholtan, W., Schlossmann, K., Rosenkranz, H.: Bestimmung der Eiweißbindung von Digitalis-Präparaten mittels der Ultrazentrifuge. Arzneim. Forsch. 16, 109-118 (1966)

Solomon, H.M., Abrams, W.B.: Interactions of digitoxin with other drugs. Am. Heart J. 83, 277-280 (1972)

Storstein, L.: The influence of renal function on the pharmacokinetics of digitoxin. In: Storstein, O. (ed.): Symposium on Digitalis, Oslo: Gyldendal Norsk Forlag 1973, pp. 158-168

Talcott, R.E., Stohs, S.J.: Interactions of digitoxigenin and digoxigenin with cytochrome P 450. Res. Commun. Chem. Pathol. Pharmacol. 4, 723-732 (1972)

Watson, E., Tramell, P., Kalman, S.M.: Identification of submicrogram amounts of digoxin, digitoxin and their metabolic products. Isolation by chromatography and preparation of derivatives for assay by electron capture detector. J. Chromatogr. 69, 157-163 (1972)

Discussion

Schaumann: Do you know whether rifampicin also increases the clearance of digoxin or methyl-digoxin?

Hausamen: We have measured digoxin serum concentrations under rifampicin therapy only in a few patients. It appears that the values in those patients are also decreased. We did not measure digoxin clearances.

Greenblatt: It seems when you study people taking both rifampicin and isoniazid, you are mixing up two opposite effects of two different drugs. Isoniazid has been shown to be a metabolic poison, and if anything we might expect that to impair the extrarenal clearance of digitoxin. Did you know there is a difference between rifampicin alone versus triple therapy?

Hausamen: We did not see any differences in digitoxin serum concentrations. The decrease of serum digitoxin was about the same under both therapeutic regimens. Under monotherapy and under triple tuberculostatic treatment, it amounted to about 50% of the pretreatment values. The same holds true for the renal clearance of digitoxin.

35 Is There a Need for New Cardiac Glycosides? For More Blood Level Determinations?

G. KAUFMANN

It is a great honor to a cardiologist in medical practice to present the last paper of the symposium to this distinguished audience. With your kind permission, I shall first deal with the question: is there a need for more digitalis blood level determinations? A positive answer primarily depends on the reliability of the method. The commercially available kits for the radioimmunoassays of digoxin and digitoxin have improved during the last years and give satisfactory results if handled by a critical laboratory. So we can concentrate on the question: what is the practical value of digitalis blood level determinations?

I tried to evaluate the usefulness of digoxin serum level determinations in medical practice. The following observations relate to outpatients. The conclusions drawn should be modified accordingly for severely ill cardiac patients in hospitals. Digoxin serum level determinations were carried out by radioimmunoassay in a private laboratory (Dr. P. Neumann, Zürich). Blood samples were taken 6-9 h after the morning dose. At that time, the therapeutic range varies from 0.8-2.0 ng/ml. Concentrations below 0.5 ng/ml are not detected. Serums of patients treated with drugs other than digitalis gave no obvious false positive response (Kaufmann and Neumann, 1977).

In 6 out of 215 determinations in patients having one or more tablets of digoxin-Sandoz (0.25 mg) daily (Beveridge et al., 1975), no digoxin was detectable (<0.5 ng/ml). Probably, the patients either did not take the prescribed drug or did not take it regularly. 3% is a low rate of nonreliability. It compares favorably to similar series of outpatient departments (Chavaz, Balant and Fabre, 1974; Chavaz et al., 1974).

In six patients and in six volunteers (not included in this series), the serum level of digoxin was determined on different days in apparently unchanged conditions. The results varied within 0.45 ng/ml or within ± 40% of the first determination. To check the usefulness of the method, some correlations were calculated. The age classes from 40-69 years had the same range of body weight, whereas patients above 69 and below 40 years of age had lower body weight. To avoid errors, the following correlations include patients aged from 40-69 years only. When I provisionally tried to predict digoxin serum levels in relation to body weight and old age, unexpectedly high values were frequently associated with some additional drugs. The drugs involved were spironolactone, amiodarone, quinidine,

410

and with less coincidence triamterene, amiloride, reserpine, and calcium antagonists. Patients who took one or more of these additional drugs were excluded.

When we look to the digoxin serum concentrations at various maintenance doses, the standard deviations are somewhat smaller than those found by other authors (Larbig and Haasis, 1975). The only significant concentration difference of digoxin is between the doses of 0.25 and 0.375 mg daily (Fig. 35.1).

The highest dose of 0.5 mg has been selected according to body weight. But when correction for body weight is made, patients with 0.5 mg digoxin daily still have unexpected low digoxin levels. To avoid a bias, this group was not included in the correlations.

The next step was to correlate body weight and digoxin serum concentration per one tablet digoxin daily. Sixty-six determinations of patients with normal serum creatinine, aged 40-69 years, and daily maintenance doses of 0.25 or 0.375 mg digoxin were evaluated. On the double logarithmic scale, there is a negative linear relationship between body weight and digoxin serum concentration. The regression coefficient calculated by the logarithms of body weight and digoxin serum concentration is -1.08. It does not differ significantly from -1 (Fig. 35.2). This confirms the expected inverse proportionality between body weight and digoxin serum level for a given maintenance dose. Many dosage rec-

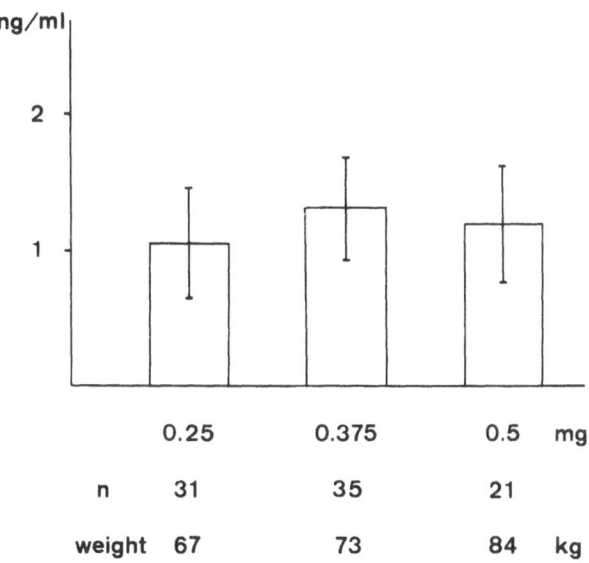

Fig. 35.1. Correlation between maintenance dose of digoxin Sandoz (tablets) and digoxin serum concentration. The absence of linear relationship is deliberate and in part due to the different body weight. Normal serum creatinine, age 40-69 years, no interfering drugs. Means and SD

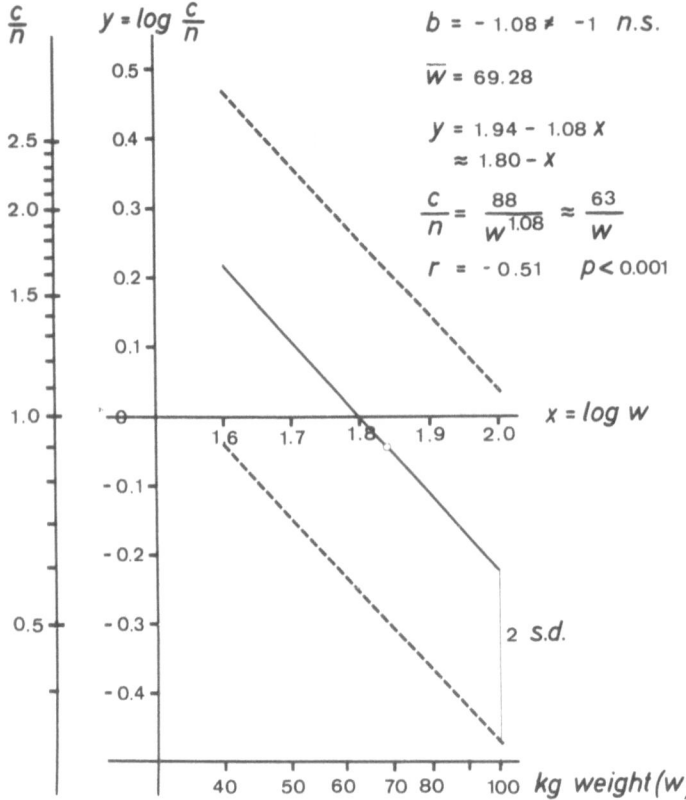

Fig. 35.2. Correlation between body weight and digoxin serum concentration (c) corrected for number of tablets (n) of 0.25 mg digoxin as maintenance dose. Almost reciprocal relationship. N = 66. Normal serum creatinine, age 40-69 years, digoxin maintenance dose 0.25 or 0.375 mg, no interfering drugs

ommendations for digoxin are based on this correlation (Aronson and Grahame-Smith, 1976; Chavaz, Balant and Fabre, 1974; Chavaz et al., 1974; Siersbaek-Nielsen et al., 1971).

According to general consensus, elderly patients need less digoxin (Ewy et al., 1969). On the other hand, several investigators were impressed by unexpectedly low serum concentrations in young volunteers. In Figure 35.3, the digoxin serum level has been corrected for one tablet digoxin daily and for a mean body weight of 69.28 kg according to the above regression equation. A total of 96 determinations of patients aged 20-90 years with normal serum creatinine was included. A loose positive correlation is obtained between age and digoxin serum level corrected for daily dose and body weight. For the means of the age decades, the linearity is strong. In the age class from 80-89 years, the mean digoxin serum concentration is roughly double that of the age class from 20-29 years. Within the normal range of serum creatinine, the creatinine clearance has been shown to

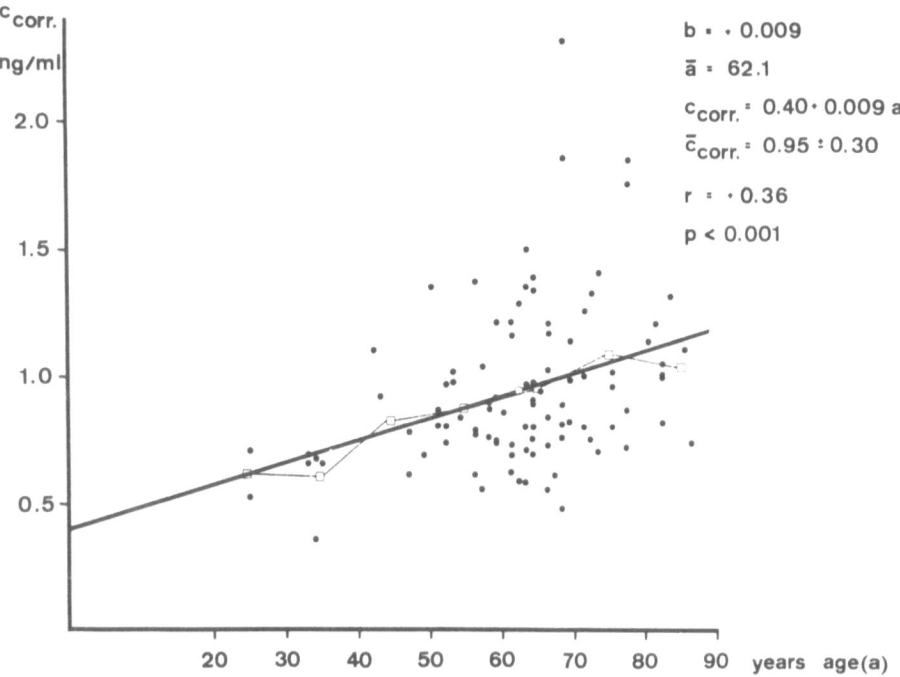

Fig. 35.3. Correlation between age and corrected digoxin serum concentration (c) per 0.25 mg digoxin daily and per 69.28 kg body weight according to regression equation of Fig. 35.2. N = 96. Normal serum creatinine, digoxin maintenance dose 0.25 or 0.375 mg, no interfering drugs

fall from decade to decade, reaching roughly half the value at 20-29 years in the 80-89 years age bracket (Siersbaek-Nielsen, 1971). Similar age dependence was found earlier for inuline clearance and PAH clearance (Dost, 1968). The age dependence of the digoxin serum level troughout all age brackets almost quantitatively reflects the age dependence of digoxin renal clearance.

If the digoxin serum level is not only corrected for the daily maintenance dose, but also for body weight and for age (n = 66, age 40-69 years), the mean concentration remains almost unchanged (0.96 ng/ml), and the standard deviation falls from 0.35 to 0.31. A considerable variation remains due to factors such as technical errors, forgetfulness of patients, variable absorption, obesity, and variable physical capacity. Obesity gives higher digoxin blood levels for a given body weight (Ewy et al., 1971) and so does lack of physical training.

Digoxin blood level determinations provide certainly more than an alibi against the reproach of malpractice. I found them particularly useful in detecting the interference of other drugs with the digoxin blood level. For that purpose, digoxin serum concentrations corrected for maintenance dose, body weight, and age were compared. Striking increases of digoxin serum levels were found for two dose groups of spironolactone (25-50 and 75-100 mg daily) and for amiodarone (Fig. 35.4). Seven patients having digoxin serum level determinations before and after adding spironolactone showed a significant mean concentration increase by 62%. This finding is not surprising in view of other investigations (Steiness, 1974). In both Drugs the rise of digoxin serum level may be technical at least in part. Amiodarone is a potent antianginal and antiarrhythmic drug. It contains iodine and has some electrophysiologic and metabolic effects in common with hypothyroidism (Burger et al., 1976; Singh and Vanghan Williams, 1970). In hypothyroidism, the distribution volume of digoxin seems to be reduced, producing higher blood levels (Doherty and Perkins, 1966). The same may apply to amiodarone.

Of four patients receiving quinidine, all had unexpectedly high digoxin serum levels, two were toxic. In one case, after having stopped quinidine without changing the digoxin dose, the digoxin serum level dropped from 3.5 to 2.1 ng/ml, and the multiform ventricular bigeminal rhythm disappeared (Table 35.1). Digitalis toxicity may sometimes subside by stopping an additional drug instead of digoxin.

For other drugs, no evidence of consistent effects on digoxin serum levels could be furnished. But there is little doubt that some drugs may affect the reel digoxin serum level. Overt digitalis toxicity was rare in this series. In 6 out of 173

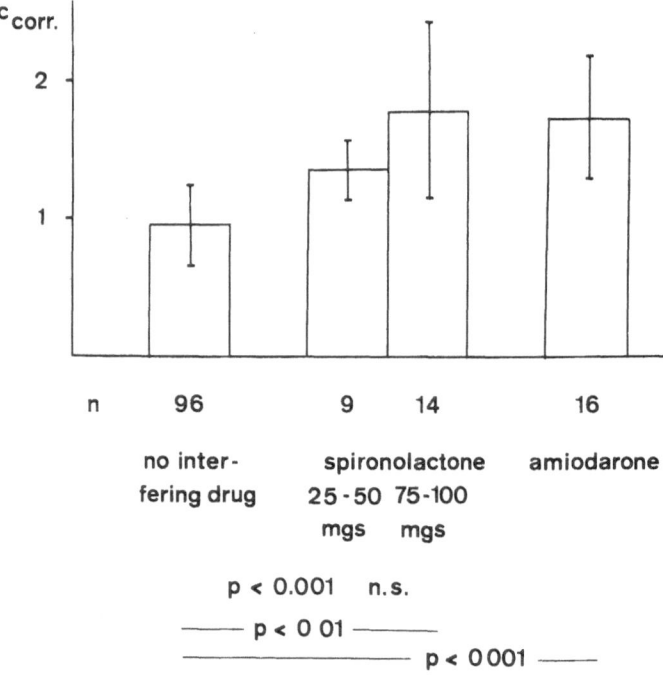

Fig. 35.4. Raised digoxin serum concentration (corrected for dose, body weight, and age) on digoxin maintenance treatment combined with spironolactone (two dose ranges) or amiodarone (100-200 mg daily). Means and SD

Table 35.1. Digoxin serum level (ng/ml) and quinidine

	Digoxin dose mg	Quinidine dose g	Digoxin serum level (ng/ml)	
			Digoxin alone	Digoxin plus quinidine
a	0.375	0.75	2.1	3.5 T^b
b	0.25	0.75	1.2;0.95	1.65 T
c	0.125	0.75	—	1.0
d	0.375	1.0^a	0.65	3.0

[a]plus verapamil. [b]toxic.

patients, overdigitalization was taken for granted, in two it was suspected. Similarly low percentages were described when digoxin dosage was adjusted to body weight, creatinine serum concentration, and old age (Aronson and Grahame-Smith, 1976).

Of the eight toxic or suspected toxic patients, three had digoxin alone, five had additional drugs. Six out of eight had digoxin serum levels above 2 ng/ml, but 17 other patients with raised serum levels had no toxic symptoms (Table 35.2). Overlapping of toxic and nontoxic digoxin serum levels is no argument against their validity.

A single digoxin serum determination does not give the full answer to the problems of digitalis need and digitalis tolerance in a given patient. The results have to be interpreted carefully, otherwise they do more harm than good. Blood level measurements of digoxin are not necessary in each patient treated with digoxin or digoxin derivatives, when the appropriate dose is calculated. For patients with normal serum creatinine concentration, the above correlations furnish a simplified formula to predict the digoxin serum concentration (c, ng/ml)

Table 35.2. Digitalis toxicity

	probable	6
	suspected	2
	Total toxicity	8
Total of patients on digoxin	173	
Digoxin serum level ⩽ 2 ng/ml	149	2
> 2 ng/ml	24	6
> 3 ng/ml	4	3

related to the maintenance dose (d = number of 0.25-mg tablets digoxin daily), body weight (w, kg), and age (a, years):

$$c = d \; \frac{0.6 \, (45 + a)}{w}$$

When an optimal therapeutic digoxin serum level of 1.4 ng/ml is wanted, the approximate calculation of the daily number of digoxin tablets becomes very simple

$$d_{th} \sim \frac{w}{0.4 \, (50 + a)}$$

Males and females did not show a significant difference of corrected digoxin serum level. Therefore, correction for sex seems not to be necessary. In raised serum creatinine up to 2 mg per 100 ml, I follow the recommendation to halve the calculated digoxin dose (Larbig and Haasis, 1975). In more severe renal function disturbance, a further reduction to one-third may be sensible. Digoxin blood level determinations are helpful in suspicion of toxicity or underdigitalization, and furthermore in situations where digoxin serum concentration is difficult to predict, particulary is heavily disabled patients, in obesity, in patients below 40 years, and when one of the interfering drugs mentioned is involved.

Having said so much of a classic heart glycoside, the question arises, are we happy with digoxin, are others happy with digitoxin, or do we need new glycosides? Before we look to the future, I would like to briefly discuss the heart glycosides which appeared on the market during the last 20 years. A new glycoside is usually introduced by one of two claims: Either it has less inhibiting effects on av-transmission and less side-effects, or it is absorbed more easily than digoxin. The first claim applies to nondigitalis glycosides. I mention peruvoside, which has considerably interested clinical pharmacologists (Kramer et al., 1969; Lahrtz and van Zwieten, 1968) but has proven to be a relatively weak compound. Proscillaridin, when tested on the isolated heart muscle, is more potent than digitoxin and digoxin. In man, it produces effects on ejection time and preejection period similar to those of classic digitalis glycosides (Heierli, 1971). But the concentrations determined in the blood are extremely low (Belz and Brech, 1974; Belz et al., 1974). Unpublished findings suggest that the majority of proscillaridin is rapidly transformed into active metabolites not yet identified. In such a situation, the evaluation of the absorption rate is difficult. There is no guideline for individual dosage other than clinical observations. I am not convinced that proscillaridin has less inhibitory effects on av-transmission and less side-effects than the digitalis glycosides.

The other group of newer heart glycosides concerns digoxin derivatives with the attempt to improve absorption and maintain the relatively short half-life of digoxin. I will not deal with ephemeral compounds but shall concentrate on the two most interesting substances, β-acetyl-digoxin and β-methyl-digoxin. β-Acetyl-digoxin, developed by Haberland (Haberland, 1965) and manufactured by Beyersdorf with the trade name Novodigal, is more completely absorbed than a digoxin tablet with optimal bioavailability. To reach the same serum concentration, the oral maintenance dose is reduced to four-fifths of the digoxin dose. One tablet of Novodigal contains 0.2 mg β-acetyl-digoxin equivalent to 0.25 mg digoxin. If the substance is offered by other firms or in combination with other drugs, one has to make sure that bioavailability coincides with that of the original Novodigal. β-Acetyl-digoxin is a labile ester of digoxin split within the gut wall. After oral ingestion, minimal amounts of the original compound are detected outside of the intestinal tract. The further fate of β-acetyl-digoxin is the fate of digoxin (Rietbrock and Abshagen, 1973; Ruiz-Torres, 1972; Wirth et al., 1972). All the information collected on the pharmacokinetics of digoxin, drug interferences included, are also applicable to β-acetyl-digoxin. For practical purposes, β-acetyl-digoxin may be regarded as digoxin with chemically improved bioavailability.

In β-acetyl-digoxin, there is still a difference between the serum concentrations after intravenous injection and after oral intake of the same amount. This difference is not present in β-methyl-digoxin, an almost completely absorbed digoxin ether manufactured by Boehringer Mannheim with the trade name Lanitop. Methyl-digoxin is remarkably stable. Part of it is excreted unchanged, part is transformed to digoxin in the liver. The half-lives of the two substances seem to be similar, but their pharmacokinetics are different. Methyl-digoxin has reduced renal clearance and perhaps increased biliary excretion when compared to digoxin (Kramer and Scheler, 1972; Rietbrock and Abshagen, 1973; Rietbrock et al., 1972; Risler et al., 1976; Wirth et al., 1972).

Methyl-digoxin is a truly new heart glycoside with a more complex fate than that of digoxin. Many points related to clinical pharmacology are still controversial. I should mention the degree the variation, and the temporal sequence of demethylation (Rietbrock et al., 1972; Wirth et al., 1972), the distribution volume, which is smaller than that of digoxin according to some investigators (Rietbrock and Abshagen, 1973), equal according to others (Kramer and Scheler, 1972; Larbig and Haasis, 1975). These problems are not only of theoretic interest. If the distribution volume is indeed smaller than that of digoxin, this will partially explain the lower dosage of methyl-digoxin needed to reach the same serum level. For maintenance treatment, the dose ratio of digoxin, β-acetyl-digoxin and β-methyl-digoxin is 5:4:3 (Greeff et al., 1975; Larbig and Haasis, 1975). When changing from one of these three glycosides to another, tablet contents of 0.15 mg methyl-digoxin instead of 0.1 mg would be desirable. Furthermore, the early and high peak concentration of methyl-digoxin is perhaps an advantage when one wants to have a rapid digitalis effect in a nondigitalized patient, e.g., in paroxystic tachycardia. In such a situation, Lanitop tablets may replace an intravenous digoxin injection. In maintenance treatment, the significance of high peaks is controversial.

According to comparisons of old and new Lanoxin, better absorption also means more regular absorption (Shaw et al., 1974). In this respect, methyl-digoxin seems to be optimal. But we do not know if the smaller variation of absorption (Larbig, 1975) is compensated by a more variable elimination of the drug. I do not necessarily believe that methyl-digoxin needs less blood level determinations than digitoxin or digoxin. It is too early to settle if methyl-digoxin is suited to replace the classic glycosides for the patient's benefit, or if we are better off with digitoxin and digoxin, the latter perhaps in a galenically or chemically improved form.

So much for the present position of digoxin derivatives. The question "is there a need for further new heart glycosides" is ambiguous. The pharmaceutic industry has its legitimate needs. For patients and physicians, however, I would not find it desirable to encounter a new glycoside with entirely new characteristics on the market every few years before the predecessors have been exhaustively evaluated. We have to remember that all the potent heart glycosides known are drugs with a very narrow therapeutic range. That is why there is a need for more investigations rather than for new glycosides.

These critical remarks do not mean that I am entirely happy with the positive inotropic substances currently available. The heart glycosides show the unique combination of positive inotropism and inhibition of atrioventricular impulse transmission. They will perhaps remain the ideal drugs for treating tachycardic atrial fibrillation. They are not ideal for other sorts of heart failure. Physicians, and particularly cardiologists, are still waiting for one or more positive inotropic substances with a broad therapeutic range and a reasonably long half-life, not influencing or rather enhancing impulse transmission, and lacking dangerous arrhythmias. Such compounds may be manufactured some day by the pharmaceutic industry, but — to paraphrase a title used by Dr. Lukas (Lukas, 1972) in an editorial some years ago — the answer probably will not be given by toads and flowers.

References

Aronson, J.K., Grahame-Smith, D.G.: Digoxin therapy: textbooks, theory and praxis. Br. J. Clin. Pharmacol. 3, 639-648 (1976)

Belz, G.G., Brech, W.J.: Plasmaspiegel und Kumulationsverhalten von Proscillaridin bei Niereninsuffizienz. Klin. Wochenschr. 52, 640-644 (1974)

Belz, G.G., Stauch, M., Rudofsky, G.: Plasma levels after a single oral dose of proscillaridin. Eur. J. Clin. Pharmacol. 7, 95-97 (1974)

Beveridge, T., Kalberer, F., Nüesch, E., Schmidt, R.: Bioavailability studies with digoxin-Sandoz and Lanoxin. Eur. J. Clin. Pharmacol. 8, 371-376 (1975)

Burger, A., Dinichert, D., Nicod, P., Jenny, M., Lemarchand-Béraud, T., Vallotton, M.B.: Effect of amiodarone on serum triiodothyronine, reverse triiodothyronine, thyroxin, and thyrotropin. J. Clin. Invest. 58, 255-259 (1976)

Chavaz, A., Balant, L., Fabre, J.: Digoxinémie et digitalisation. Schweiz. Med. Wochenschr. 104, 65-74 (1974)

Chavaz, A., Balant, L., Simonin, P., Fabre, J.: Influence de l'âge sur la digoxinémie et la digitalisation. Schweiz. Med. Wochenschr. 104, 1823-1825 (1974)

Doherty, J.E.: Serum digitalis level — practical value. In: Chung, E.K. (ed.): Controversy in Cardiology. New York-Heidelberg-Berlin: Springer-Verlag 1976, p. 77

Doherty, J.E., Perkins, W.H.: Digoxin metabolism in hypo- and hyperthyroidism. Studies with tritiated digoxin in thyroid disease. Ann. Intern. Med. 64, 489-507 (1966)

Dost, F.H.: Grundlagen der Pharmakokinetik, 2nd. ed. Stuttgart: Thieme 1968, p. 324

Ewy, G.A., Kapadia, G.G., Yao, L., Lullin, M., Marcus, F.L.: Digoxin metabolism in the elderly. Circulation 39, 449-453 (1969)

Ewy, G.A., Groves, B.M., Ball, M.F., Nimino, L., Jackson, B., Marcus, F.L.: Digoxin metabolism in obesity. Circulation 44, 810-814 (1971)

Greeff, K., Strobach, H., Verspohl, E.: Ergebnisse radioimmunologischer Bestimmungen von Digoxin, Digitoxin und g-Strophanthin am Menschen. In: Jahrmärker, H., (ed.): Digitalistherapie. Berlin-Heidelberg-New York: Springer-Verlag 1975, p. 52

Haberland, G.: Darstellung und Eigenschaften von Glykosidestern. Arzneim. Forsch. 15, 481-483 (1965)

Heierli, Ch., Schweizer, W., Burkart, F.: Der Einfluß von Herzglykosiden auf die Systolendauer. Ein Vergleich zwischen Proscillaridin und Strophanthin. Schweiz. Med. Wochenschr. 101, 638-642 (1971)

Kaufmann, G.: Digitalisbedingte Arrhythmien und Diphenylhydantoin. Bern-Stuttgart-Wien: Huber 1972, p.p. 146, 179

Kaufmann, G., Neumann, P.: Der Digoxinspiegel — Abhängigkeit von Körpergewicht und Alter. Schweiz. Med. Wochenschr. 107, 1695-1699 (1977)

Kramer, P., Scheler, F.: Renale Eliminationskinetik verschiedener Herzglykoside. Dtsch. Med. Wochenschr. 97, 1485-1490 (1972)

Kramer, P., Willms, B., Horenkamp, J., Scheler, F.: Blutspiegelkinetik und renale Clearence von ^{3}H-Peruvosid. Klin. Wochenschr. 47, 1157-1166 (1969)

Lahrtz, Hg., van Zwieten, P.A.: The influence of kidney or liver disorders on the serum concentration and urinary excretion of ^{3}H-peruvoside, a tritium-labelled cardiac glycoside. Europ. J. Pharmacol. 3, 147-152 (1968)

Larbig, D., Haasis, R.: Radioimmunologische Bestimmungen der Konzentration von Digoxin und Digoxin-Derivaten. In: Jahrmärker, H. (ed.): Digitalistherapie. Berlin-Heidelberg-New York: Springer-Verlag 1975, p. 62

Larbig, D.: Herzinsuffizienz: Digitalistherapie. Therapiewoche 25, 48-61 (1975)

Lukas, D.S.: Of toads and flowers. Circulation 46, 1-4 (1972)

Rietbrock, N., Abshagen, U.: Stoffwechsel und Pharmakokinetik der Lanataglykoside beim Menschen. Dtsch. Med. Wochenschr. 98, 117-122 (1973)

Rietbrock, N., Rennekamp, Ch., Rennekamp, H., v. Bergmann, K., Abshagen, U.: Demethylation and cleavage of glycosidic bonds of 4'''-methyldigoxin in man. Naunyn Schmiedebergs Arch. Pharmacol. 272, 450-453 (1972)

Risler, T., Grabensee, B., Jesdinsky, H.J., Grosse-Brockoff, F.: Unterschiedliche renale Elimination von Digoxin und β-Methyl-Digoxin. Verh. Dtsch. Ges. Kreislaufforsch. 42, 370-372 (1976)

Ruiz-Torres, A., Burmeister, H.: Stoffwechsel und Kinetik von β-Acetyldigoxin. Klin. Wochenschr. 50, 191-195 (1972)

Schaumann, W., Wegerle, R.: β-Methyl-Digoxin. I. Cardiotoxizität bei enteraler und parenteraler Gabe. Arzneim. Forsch. 21, 225-231 (1971)

Shaw, T.R.D., Howard, M.R., Hamer, J.: Recent changes in biological availability of digoxin. Effect of an alteration in "Lanoxin" tablets. Br. Heart J. 36,
85-89 (1974)

Siersbaek-Nielsen, K., Mølholm Hansen, J., Kampmann, J., Kristensen, M.:
Rapid evaluation of creatinine clearance. Lancet (1971) i, 1133-1134

Singh, B.N., Vaughan Williams, E.M.: The effect of amiodarone, a new antianginal drug, on cardiac muscle. Br. J. Pharmacol. 39, 657-667 (1970)

Steiness, E.: Renal tubular secretion of digoxin. Circulation 50, 103-107 (1974)

Wirth, K., Bodem, G., Dengler, H.J.: Resorption, Ausscheidung und Stoff-
wechsel von Digoxin und digoxinverwandten Verbindungen. In: Schröder,
R., Greeff, K., (eds.): Aktuelle Digitalisprobleme. München-Berlin-Wien:
Urban & Schwarzenberger 1972, p. 51

Discussion

Schaumann: I think the day-to-day variation in the glycoside concentrations in
patients under maintenance treatment is a problem which has not been adequately investigated yet. In patients treated with β-methyl-digoxin, we found
about the same variation during intravenous and oral administration, showing
that a variation in absorption is of minor importance. All plasma samples from
one patient were assayed in series; the variation was definitely above the variability of the method. To my mind there are two possible explanations. One is
that there are factors in the serum interfering with the assay which vary from
day to day. The other one, which I favor, is that there are short-term variations
in distribution volume. We are just doing a study on the rate of elimination.
The serum concentrations after withdrawal are measured in the morning and
in the afternoon. In some patients, the serum levels in the afternoon were lower
than would be predict from the time course of the concentrations in the morning. This can only be explained by variations in the volume of distribution
during the day.

Kaufmann: That's an interesting finding. Some of our volunteers were wine
drinkers from time to time. I wonder if this may have influenced the results.

Schaumann: I think I mentioned in my presentation yesterday that the total
clearance which actually determines the mean serum concentration is about
the same for digoxin as for methyl-digoxin. We found only 15% difference on
intravenous administration, which seems to be negligible. So even a variation
in the amount which is demethylated is without practical importance.

Kaufmann: Don't you think that the renal clearance of digoxin and methyl-
digoxin is different?

Schaumann: The renal clearance of methyl-digoxin is about two-thirds that
of digoxin. On the other hand, there is hardly a difference in the total clearance,
and Rietbrock and colleagues have found a larger proportion after intravenously

injected radioactive β-methyl-digoxin in the feces. So, abiously, the lower renal clearance of methyl-digoxin is due to higher extrarenal elimination.

Concluding remarks

Dengler, Bonn: The concluding remarks will be as short as possible. I'd like to tank the speakers, and I'd like to thank the participants in the discussion. I'd like to thank the audience and finally the Boehringer Company, the sponsor of our meeting. I think even if we were sometimes short of time we had a lively discussion, and I hope that everybody had the apportunity to express what he wanted. Again, thank you for coming, for being here, and hopefully au revoir.

Smith, Boston (for the participants): We thank the sponsors, Boehringer Mannheim, for their warm hospitality. In particular, on behalf of all of us, we thank Prof. Dengler and Dr. Bodem for their superb job of organizing the meeting and for the way in which they have provided an atmosphere conducive to a very lively and informative exchange of ideas.

Subject Index

Abklingquote 211 f.
absorption
 — rate 211 ff.
 —, intestinal 319
accumulation 113
acetyl-digoxin 26, 126, 212, 254,
 320, 419
 —, biliary excretion in man 284
 ff., 292
acetylstrophantidin tolerance 275,
 391
acidosis 308
aludrox 319
amiloride 413
amiodarone 412
anhydrodigoxigenin 57
anorexia 109, 329
antacids 233
antiarrhythmics 232, 367 ff.
antibodies
 — antidigoxin 3, 374
 — — cross reactivity 3, 6
 — with high affinity for digitoxin
 384
apolarity
 — of cardiac glycosides 93
arginine hydrochloride 349
arrhythmias 347
 —, digitalis-induced 134, 339,
 358, 369
automaticity 369
atrial fibrillation 121
av-block 315, 316

bioavailability 46, 171, 181, 187 ff.,

199, 206 ff., 211 ff., 273, 321
 — of digoxin in the diseased patient
 181 ff.
β-blocking agents 350, 358

calcium antagonists 413
canreonate-K 392
cardiac glycosides (see digoxin, digitoxin, ouabain)
 — transplantation 135
cardiotoxicity (see digoxin, digitoxin)
catecholamines 232
charcoal 290
cholestyramine 191, 233, 284, 367
codeine 169
color vision 109
compartment model 109, 110, 121,
 218, 224, 274
cortisol 26
creatinine clearance 270, 310
cross reactivity 62, 63

decay rate 211 ff.
delirium 109
demethylation 290
dextran-coated charcoal method 5
diarrhea 329
digitalis (see digoxin, digitoxin, ouabain)
digitoxigenin 37, 61, 62, 69
 — bisdigitoxoside 69
 — glucuronide 61 f.
 — monodigitoxoside 62, 69
 — monodigitoxoside glucuronide 61 f.

— monodigitoxoside-4-glucuronide 63
— sulfate 61
digitoxin 3, 26, 36, 52, 61, 121, 254, 284, 298, 315, 317 ff.
— - bisdigitoxoside 61
— clearance 403
— determination in the serum 1
— excretion
— —, fecal 36 ff., 66
— —, renal 48, 66, 388
— - glucuronide 61
— - 16'-glucuronide 62
— half-life 64, 72, 78, 292 ff.
— intoxication 332 ff., 363 ff., 367, 384 ff.
— metabolites 36 ff., 46, 64 ff., 74 ff., 296
— —, dihydroderivatives 74 ff., 296
— —, enterohepatic circulation in the dog 85 ff.
— —, epiderivatives 296
— —, β-hydroxylation 64
— —, ketoderivatives 296
— — under rifampicin treatment 401 ff.
— pharmacokinetics 36 ff., 64, 292, 317, 384, 401
— — in renal disease 74 ff., 292 ff., 304 ff., 317 ff.
— protein binding 404, 417
— radioimmunoassay 64
— steady state data 301
digitoxosides of digitoxigenin 46
— of digoxigenin 42, 46
digoxigenin 26, 36, 38, 61
— acid 58
—, acid-hydrolyzable derivatives 36, 41
—, acid-labile derivatives 45
— - bisdigitoxoside 61, 296
— conjugates, enzymatic hydrolysis 38
— - glucuronide 61
— - 3-glucuronide 63
— - monodigitoxoside 61, 296
digoxin 1, 2, 22, 26, 31, 36, 52, 61,

62, 63, 123, 126, 242 ff., 292, 315, 317 ff., 374
— absorption 163, 167, 200
— — rate 186
— biotransformation 40
— brain concentrations 98, 113, 128, 133
— chronotropic effects 274
— clearance 97, 100, 161 ff., 265 ff., 270
— CSF levels 121
— determination in the serum 1 ff.
— disposition 284
— — in jejunoileal bypass 167 ff.
— enterohepatic cycling 284
— enzyme immunoassay 7, 22
— excretion, biliary 284
— —, fecal 36 ff.
— —, renal 28 ff., 36 ff., 161 ff.
— — —, in dogs 110 ff.
— - glucuronide 61
— - 16'-glucuronide 62
— half-life 36 ff., 116, 162, 288, 321
— inotropy 141, 274, 390
— intoxication 109, 123 f., 130, 273, 304 ff., 326 ff., 346 ff., 358 ff., 367 ff., 374 ff.
— — score 358
— metabolites 30 ff., 46, 52 ff.
— —, chloroform-soluble 31, 52 ff.
— —, water-soluble 52 ff.
— microsomal-bound 147
— - monodigitoxoside 26
— myocardial concentrations 126 ff., 135 ff., 266
— pharmacokinetics 64, 159, 199 ff., 211 ff., 242, 274, 326
— plasma concentrations 135 ff., 227, 245, 254, 273, 304, 358
— predistribution phase 335
— preparations
— —, dissolution rate 200
— steady state data 40, 67, 159, 282
— - 1-^{14}C-tetraacetate 37
— tissue distribution 98, 109 ff., 126 ff., 135 ff.

— tolerance in uremic patients
304 ff.
— vasoconstrictor effect 121
— volume of distribution 84, 162,
219, 265 ff., 324
dihydrodigitoxin 74 ff.
— volume of distribution 84
dihydrodigoxin 3, 4, 20, 32, 35, 83
20-22-dihydrodigoxin 63
discomfort, abdominal 329
diuretics 233, 313
dizziness 109
dosage
— clinical parameters 211
— regimens 310
dose (of digoxin/digitoxin)
— effect relationships 254
— fraction absorbed 163
— response curves 259
— single and multiple 113
double isotope dilution derivative
assay 11, 36
D-xylose excretion test 170

ECG parameters 222, 254
— PQ interval 256
— ST-depression 261
— T flattening 256
— — inversion 261
echocardiography 221
efficacy, maximum 256
effectiveness 326
enzymic isotope displacement assay 7
3-epidigitoxigenin 37, 38, 69
epidigitoxigenin glucuronide 61
— sulfate 62
— 3-sulfate 63
3-epidigoxigenin 36, 41
—, acid-hydrolyzable derivatives 42
ethambutol 401
extrasystoly 109, 134

Fab fragments 385, 391
first pass effect of cardiac glycosides
36

gas chromatography 12, 75

gastrectomy 191
glucagon 350

heart failure 71, 181, 317
hemodialysis 314, 317 ff., 367
— intermittent maintenance 317
hemofiltration 367
hepatitis 71, 290
high pressure liquid chromatography
12
horseradish peroxidase 22
hypercalcemia 232
hyperglycemia 349
hyperkalemia 136 ff., 158, 232, 307,
349
hypermagnesemia 307
hypocalcemia 307
hypokalemia 232
hypothermia 350
hypothyroidism 416
hypoxemia 134
hypoxia 349

IgG, specific 387
isodigoxigenin 58
isoniazid 401 ff.

kaopectate 191, 233

lidocaine 349, 369
liver
— blood flow 288
— cirrhosis 46, 287
LVET 255

maintenance therapy 64
malabsorption 167
mass spectrum 58, 75
membrane-ATPase 8, 10, 28, 135 ff.,
247, 368, 374
mental confusion 109
metabolites (see digoxin, digitoxin)
— chloroform-extractable 28
— conjugated 68
— hydrophilic 28
— hydroxylated 67
— nonpolar 34

425

– polar 28, 34, 68
– water-soluble 31, 52, 60, 85

methyldigoxin 28, 191, 292, 419
β-methyl-digoxin 26, 93 ff., 110, 126
  212, 287
  – absorption 93 ff.
  – cerebral content 98
  – clearance 97
  – elimination 100
  – renal excretion in man 110 ff.
  – renal and fecal excretion in dogs
  110 ff.
  – spironolactone treatment 392 ff.
  – tissue distribution 98 ff.
monodigitoxoside of digitoxigenin
  50, 65
motility, gastrointestinal 202
muscle
  – , left ventricular papillary 127
  –, right ventricular papillary 128
  – skeletal 127

nausea 275, 329
neomycin 191, 233
nomogram 270, 319

ouabain 5, 62, 110, 123, 350, 374

pharmacokinetics (see digoxin)
phenobarbital 233, 401
phenylbutazone 233, 401
phenytoin 233, 288, 368, 401
polyethylene glycol 190
potassium
  – in glycoside-dependent arrhythmias 368
prednison 26
progesterone 26
pronethalol 370
propranolol 370
proscillaridin 374
protein-binding 288, 297
  – – of digitoxin 404

QS$_2$ 255
QTc 255
quinidine 370, 412

radioimmunoassay 3, 24, 30, 64, 73,
  126, 171, 211, 228, 284, 319, 412
[86]Rb uptake of human erythrocytes
  9, 60, 83, 228, 245, 254,
reentry phenomena 369
renal failure 75 ff., 131, 181, 232,
  265, 282, 292, 298, 304, 308, 310,
  317
reserpine 349, 413
Resorptionsquote 211 ff.
rifampicin 401 ff.
safety in digitalis therapy 307, 326
Scatchard analysis 385
scotoma, central 109
shock, hemorrhagic 349
sodium depletion 349
solid-phase tube technique 22
spinal fluid 123
spironolactone 26, 392 ff., 412
strophantin 292

thyroid hormone 17

  – status 159 ff., 232
thyrostatic agents 159
time intervals, systolic 254, 305
tissues, "slowly equilibrating" 118
triamterene 413

verapamil 369
vision, blurring of 109
Vollwirkdosis 211
volume of distribution 161, 164, 223
  f., 265 (see digoxin)
  – of dihydrodigitoxin 84
vomiting 109, 275, 329

weariness 109

International Boehringer Mannheim Symposia
Ventricular Function at Rest and During Exercise
Ventrikelfunktion in Ruhe und während Belastung
Editors: H. Roskamm, C. Hahn
1976. 59 figures, 8 tables. XVIII, 183 pages
(77 pages in German).
ISBN 3-540-07707-3

International Boehringer Mannheim Symposia
Myocardial Failure
Editors: G. Riecker, A. Weber, J. Goodwin
Co-Editors: H. D. Bolte, B. Lüderitz,
B. E. Strauer, E. Erdmann
1977. 172 figures, 52 tables. XII, 374 pages
ISBN 3-540-08225-5
Distribution rights for Japan:
Nankodo Co. Ltd., Tokyo

Coronary Heart Disease
Clinical, Angiographic, and Pathologic Profiles
By Z. Vlodaver, K. Amplatz, H. B. Burchell, J. E. Edwards
1976. 1252 figures including 271 LogEtronic scanned radiographs. XV, 584 pages
ISBN 3-540-90165-5
Distribution rights for Japan:
Igaku Shoin Ltd., Tokyo

W. A. McAlpine
Heart and Coronary Arteries
An Anatomical Atlas for Clinical Diagnosis, Radiological Investigation, and Surgical Treatment
1975. 1098 figures, mostly in color.
XVI, 224 pages
ISBN 3-540-06985-2
Distribution rights for Japan:
Igaku Shoin Ltd., Tokyo

H. Selye
Experimental Cardiovascular Diseases
Two parts, not sold separately
1970. 73 figures, some in color.
XVIII, VIII, 1155 pages
ISBN 3-540-05010-8

Controversy in Cardiology
The Practical Clinical Approach
Editor: E. K. Chung
1976. 99 figures, 18 tables. X, 299 pages
ISBN 3-540-07304-3
Distribution rights for Japan:
Igaku Shoin Ltd., Tokyo

Atherosclerosis IV
Proceedings of the Fourth International Symposium, held in Tokyo, August 24–28, 1976
Editors: G. Schettler, Y. Goto, Y. Hata, G. Klose
1977. 308 figures, 185 tables. XLVI, 797 pages
ISBN 3-540-08421-5

Brain and Heart Infarct
Proceedings of the Third Cologne Symposium, June 16–19, 1976
Editors: K. J. Zülch, W. Kaufmann, K.-A. Hossmann, V. Hossmann
With contributions by numerous experts
1977. 155 figures, 14 tables. XVIII, 349 pages
ISBN 3-540-08270-0

Heart and Circulation
Editors: J. Schmier, O. Eichler
1975. 154 figures, 43 tables. XI, 600 pages
(Handbuch der experimentellen Pharmakologie, Band 16: Erzeugung von Krankheitszuständen durch das Experiment, Teil 3)
ISBN 3-540-07127-X

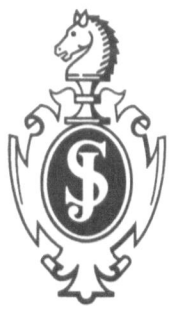

Springer-Verlag
Berlin
Heidelberg
New York

M. Bessis
Corpuscles
Atlas of Red Blood Cell Shapes
1974. 121 figures, 147 pages
ISBN 3-540-06375-7
Distribution rights for Japan:
Maruzen Co. Ltd., Tokyo

M. Bessis
Blood Smears Reinterpreted
Translated from the French by G. Brecher
1977. 342 figures, some in color. XV, 270 pages
ISBN 3-540-07206-3

M. Bessis
Living Blood Cells and Their Ultrastructure
Translated by Robert I. Weed
1973. 521 figures, 2 color-plates.
XXI, 767 pages
ISBN 3-540-05981-4
Distribution rights for Japan:
Maruzen Co. Ltd., Tokyo

Red Cell Shape
Proceedings of a Symposium held June
20 and 21, 1972 at the Institute of Cell Patho-
logy, Hôpital de Bicêtre
Physiology, Pathology, Ultrastructure
Edited by M. Bessis, R. I. Weed, P. F. Leblond
1973. 147 figures. VIII, 180 pages
ISBN 3-540-06257-2
Distribution rights for Japan:
Maruzen Co. Ltd., Tokyo

Unclassifiable Leukemias
Proceedings of a Symposium, held October
11–13, 1974, at the Institute of Cell Pathology,
Hôpital de Bicêtre, Paris, France
Editors: M. Bessis, G. Brecher
1975. 81 figures, 1 color-plate, 38 tables.
VI, 270 pages
ISBN 3-540-07242-X

H. Begemann, J. Rastetter
Atlas of Clinical Haematology
Initiated by L. Heilmeyer, H. Begemann
Translated from the second completely revised
German edition by H. J. Hirsch with an appen-
dix on tropical diseases by W. Mohr
1972. 191 figures in color and 17 in black
and white. XV, 324 pages
ISBN 3-540-05949-0
Distribution rights for Japan:
Maruzen Co. Ltd., Tokyo

Anabolic-Androgenic Steroids
Editor: C. D. Kochakian
1976. 38 figures. XXII, 725 pages
(Handbuch der experimentellen Pharma-
kologie, Bd. 43)
ISBN 3-540-07710-3

Antihypertensive Agents
Editor: F. Gross
With contributions by numerous experts
1977. 120 figures. XV, 779 pages
(Handbuch der experimentellen Pharma-
kologie, Bd. 39)
ISBN 3-540-07594-1

Cardiac Pacing
Diagnostic and Therapeutic Tools
Editor: B. Lüderitz
With an Introduction by G. Riecker
1976. 75 figures, 29 tables. VII, 245 pages
ISBN 3-540-07711-1

Hypertension – 1972
Symposium organized by the Clinical
Research Institute of Montreal under the
auspices of the University of Montreal Medical
School
Editors: J. Genest, E. Koiw
1972. 304 figures. XVI, 617 pages
ISBN 3-540-05755-2

Hypolipidemic Agents
Editor: D. Kritchevsky
1975. 81 figures, 32 tables. XVI, 488 pages
(Handbuch der experimentellen Pharma-
kologie, Bd. 41)
ISBN 3-540-07361-2

**Immunological Diagnosis of Leukemias
and Lymphomas**
International Symposium of the Institut für
Hämatologie, GSF, October 28–30, 1976,
Neuherberg/München
Editors: S. Thierfelder, H. Rodt, E. Thiel
1977. 98 figures, 2 in color, 101 tables.
X, 387 pages
ISBN 3-540-08216-6

Springer-Verlag
Berlin Heidelberg New York